Herluf Skovsgaard, DDS

DANCING HANDS

Herluf Skovsgaard, DDS

DANCING HANDS

Deductions and prescriptions of working methods, skills, assistance, teamwork, precision vision, working postures, equipment and organization in dental practice

QUINTESSENCE PUBLISHING

London, Berlin, Chicago, Tokyo, Barcelona, Beijing, Bucharest, Istanbul, Milan, Moscow, New Delhi, Paris, Prague, Riyadh, São Paulo, Seoul, Singapore, Warsaw and Zagreb

A CIP record for this book is available from the British Library.
ISBN: 978-1-85097-263-1

QUINTESSENCE PUBLISHING

Quintessence Publishing Co. Ltd,
Grafton Road, New Malden, Surrey KT3 3AB,
United Kingdom
www.quintpub.co.uk

Editing: Quintessence Publishing Co. Ltd, London, UK
Layout and Production: Quintessenz Verlags-GmbH, Berlin, Germany
Index: Indexing Specialists (UK) Ltd
Printed and bound in Germany

PREFACE

A new paradigm for dentists' and assistants' clinical competence
And a wake up call for the priority of manual skills

For more than 40 years, during courses I have observed dentists as well as assistants working very differently, and with very varied uses of time and energy. The majority of dentists have been working with methods that are unnecessarily tiring, with repeated disturbances to their concentration, and problems with visual and instrumental access to their focus of work. Unfortunately dentists very often work in bad working postures resulting in musculoskeletal discomfort, stress, and pain, which in the long-term may endanger their health.

This unhappy situation is a result of the working methods used, but most dentists are not aware of the fact that their practical work can be performed differently, and with a different outcome.

A dentist's manual abilities are a central part of essential working skills, and the assistant's professional competence too.

Very often dentists, independent of country, say that they scarcely or have never received training in manual skills. This aspect of a dentist's working life is however too difficult and much too important to leave to "self experience."

Dancing Hands presents a new paradigm: All dentists and assistants should learn and train to perform basic manual skills

This book presents a **prescription** for what all dentists and assistants can learn, and in straight words, **should** learn.

Dancing Hands describes and shows the basic function of "practical management and manual skills," which are all rather easy to learn by repeated training. Furthermore, also presented here are the principles of the dental equipment designed to support best working methods.

Experience has shown time and time again that even small deviations from the prescriptions given in this book may have negative consequences, such as bad work postures, difficult visual and instrumental access to focus of work, disturbance of concentration, loss of time, and unnecessary fatigue.

Quality and performance depend on well-trained hands interacting with equipment that supports good manual skills.

Like the musician who practices manual skills to be note perfect, the dentist must fine tune manual dentistry skills.

Like the ballet dancer who trains for perfection of movement, the dentist must train the hands for perfection of performance.

Like the footballer who exercises for perfect interaction with team members, so must dentists and assistants.

I have written this book for all my colleagues and assistants in all countries, in order to help you make your working life to be as fulfilling and enjoyable as possible.

Good luck and kind greetings,
Herluf Skovsgaard

For reservation of conferences, courses or live internet-based courses, email: dancinghands@mail.dk

ACKNOWLEDGEMENTS

Warm thanks to Alexander Ammann and Johannes Wolters, of Quintessence Publishing for inspiration and guidance. Many thanks also to Anya Hastwell at Quintessence London for intelligent language editing, patient attention and guidance of all the procedures of making this book. And thank you for the kind communication on so many emails.

I am very thankful to my wife Margit for her motivation, inspiration, incentive and patience while I have spent hundreds of hours by the computer, after a long and busy working week in practice.

I want to thank my inspiring assistants Avigalia and Gentiane for engaged participation in perfecting assistance and teamwork – to Avigailia for being the ideal assistant on hundreds of photos in this book – and to you both for creating a friendly, warm ambience in the practice, working with relaxed high efficiency.

And thank you to our patients, who you will see in *Dancing Hands*: our daughter-in-law Stephanie and our son, Daniel, who demonstrated what not to do; and to two of our six grandchildren Alexander and Isabella, as well as our patients, Amy and Tina.

And many thanks to the tens of thousands of dentists and assistants who have participated in courses and lectures, and confirmed the importance of the methods and principles communicated in *Dancing Hands*. They have demonstrated in practice that they can be learned in a limited time, ready to be used in practice. And most of all, they have demonstrated the value of training manual skills.

ABOUT THE AUTHOR

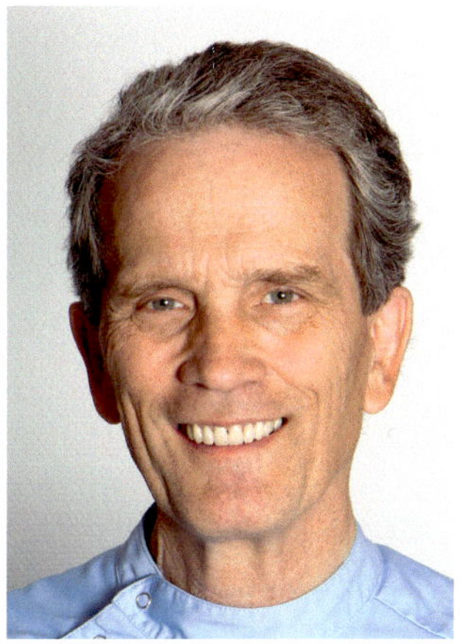

Herluf Skovsgaard, DDS, graduated from the Royal Dental College in Aarhus, Denmark in 1968. From 1970, he was running his own full-time dental practice in Assentoft, Randers, and still does today when not teaching or lecturing for courses (some 25 to 30 days a year). With around 1,000 lectures under his belt, and 40–50,000 dentists and dental assistants attending his courses, Herluf Skovsgaard is the most well-known, reputed and experienced specialist in dental ergonomics and ergonomics-related subjects in Europe.

The courses and lectures have been tailor-made for large groups of many hundreds of dentists, as well as demonstration courses for smaller groups of 50 to 100 dentists. About 500 of his courses have been intensive hands-on practical training courses for 2 or 4 teams, as well as phantom head preparation courses for 2 to 4 dentists.

As well as conducting many lectures in universities, the author has taught courses held in England, Germany, Holland, Belgium, France, Poland, Czech Republic, Austria, Switzerland, Italy, Spain, Portugal, Turkey, Denmark, Norway, Sweden, Finland, Russia, Estonia, Latvia, Korea, Japan, USA, and Dominican Republic. He speaks English, French, German, Danish, and some Italian and Spanish.

Herluf Skovsgaard teaches demonstration courses, as well as hands-on training courses in:

- Work postures, working methods, teamwork, four-handed dentistry, assistance, solo dentistry. Visual and instrumental access to all surfaces of teeth.
- Preparation techniques and methods, use of rotating instruments.
- Practice organization, organization of instruments and materials.
- Workstation design, equipment design, practice design.
- Training programs for dentists and assistants. Training programs for students.
- Service management and marketing for the dental practice.

Besides conducting lectures and courses, Herluf Skovsgaard has personally and as a consultant,

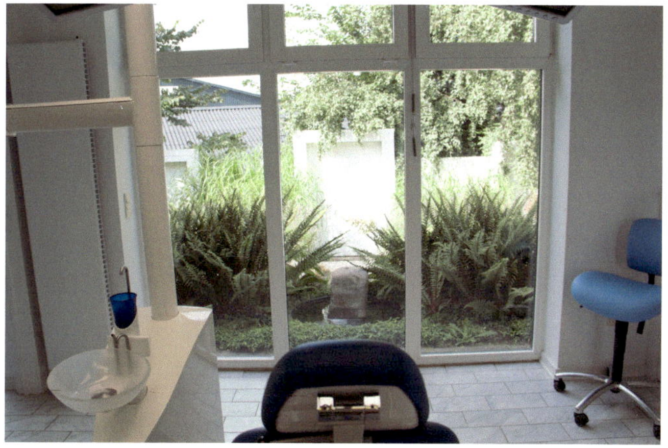

continuously invented, developed and constructed patient chairs, six generations of dental units (delivery systems) and five generations of workstations, all of the highest technical, functional and ergonomically-sound quality.

Herluf Skovsgaard, DDS
Dentist and Lecturer,
Storegade 59, Assentoft, DK 8960 Randers SO,
DENMARK.

For information and reservation of courses (including live web courses), email: dancinghands@mail.dk

CONTENTS

DANCING HANDS

WHAT MANY DENTISTS DO NOT KNOW, IS THAT THEY DO NOT KNOW

If you do not know what you do not know, or are not conscious to what you do not know, then you do not have the reason or the incentive to seek new knowledge or to learn new skills.

If you do know that there is something you don't know, then you may choose to achieve new knowledge or learn new skills.

WHY READ *DANCING HANDS*

- To stay healthy and prevent discomfort, musculosceletal problems, or occupational disease.
- To enjoy being less tired and have more energy.
- To work efficiently and be relaxed at the same time.
- To learn, know, train and perform skills for quality dentistry.
- To develop your teamwork to the highest standard.
- To learn about the specifications of equipment, and be able to profit by a complete workspace based on interactive design.
- To save about 25% of your time (or more).
- To enjoy your profession, whether dentist or assistant.
- To care for and create a positive experience for the patient.

TRAINING SKILLS

Musicians train and learn new manual skills to play a new piece of music. Dancers train new skills to learn a new dance. Dentists and assistants may also train their manual skills.

Many think it will be very difficult to change manual working methods. New skills can, however, be learned easily and quickly. You repeat the movements of the skill until you have learned it.

Experience from hands-on courses has shown that the basics of the working methods presented in *Dancing Hands* can be learned in about 2 days.

INTRODUCTION

Dedication to hands and brain

The title of this book, *Dancing Hands*, is a metaphor for comparing a dentist's hands with a dancing couple or a musician's hands performing precise, well-trained complex sequences of movements, elegant, relaxed and with perfect cooperation to others – without having to think about it.

The structure of *Dancing Hands* reflects the structure of our work in the treatment room and has an interlacing structure like a mesh, where everything interacts and influences each other.

Dancing Hands is dedicated to the eyes, hands and the brain of the dental practitioner, chairside assistant and hygienist, and to their teamwork in the dental treatment room.

The ambition is to transfer to the reader 40 to 50 years of knowledge, experience and practical routine related to training dentists and assistants. Many dentists are using the knowledge, skills and methods of *Dancing Hands*, either by developing the methods themselves by a drive for perfection, or as tens of thousands of assistants and dentists have done, as a result of being on courses and hands on trainings.

But – many dentists don't know or are not aware of the knowledge, skills and methods presented in *Dancing Hands*.

The author presents *Dancing Hands* in the belief and knowledge that almost all dentists can profit from this book, independent of type of practice, of experience, and age and whether the reader is a general practitioner, a specialist, a teacher at a university, or a student, assistant or hygienist.

Everything described in *Dancing Hands* has been tested by thousands of teams and can be relatively easily learned, and used in daily practice.

Habits are blinding eyes, hands and reason

Our daily work is performed in sequences of habits. Many of these habits are achieved during clinical work as a student or at the very beginning as a dentist. It seems to be rare that these habits are established as a result of deliberate training programs. The reason most often referred to is that the university did not offer education about these subjects.

The same habits or unhappy rituals may be repeated every day for a lifetime. We pass through our daily routines, and do what we are used to doing, following our habits without thinking about it, and without being conscious about it. We don't know what we are doing, and therefore believe that nothing can be different.

Habits can make us blind to the fact that our manual work may be performed differently and can create different outcomes. Knowledge and practical training to achieve new skills is presented in *Dancing Hands*.

This book is based on reason and the consequences of reason. The ambition is not to describe how and with what dentists are working, but to describe what there is REASON TO DO and making reasoned deductions and conclusions on this basis.

Dancing Hands is therefore not descriptive, but reaches a prescription as the logical result of deductions from basic principles and axioms.

The equipment and physical surroundings

Dentists and assistants interact with their physical surroundings, including the patient chair, operator's stools, dental unit, and the workstation. Therefore, all these physical elements have to be constructed to support teamwork, good working postures, and be of the best quality.

Today, there are fine patient chairs and dental units on market, that support ergonomical working methods – and many that do not. It is almost impossible to find an ergonomic workstation where a dentist can work and store instruments in cabinetry behind the patient. Therefore, the author has created a standard for today's workstation for *Dancing Hands*.

Dancing Hands leaves details in composite technique, endodontics, prosthodontics, surgery, etc, to the specialist in these topics.

However, some microergonomic features in the use of rotating instruments are presented.

10 STEPS – FROM READING TO DOING

The mental process from reading to finally doing is long, and energy is needed to follow the path described below.

You can:

1. READ in order to
2. UNDERSTAND

You can

3. SEE the photos and illustrations in order to
4. IMAGINE and remember them.

To take new work methods into practice, you have to

5. VISUALIZE the situations and
6. MAKE A MENTAL ANIMATION FOR THE MOVEMENT (a feed-forward plan). Making a mental plan for the sequence of movements you are going to perform is an important part of learning
7. DO/PERFORM THE MOVEMENTS
8. REPEAT THE MOVEMENTS so many times that you learn to use the movements without attention and conscience
9. MOVEMENTS ARE AUTOMATIZED
10. STOP THINKING AND ENJOY your fast, precise, coordinated, elegant dancing hands!

ABOUT THE VOCABULARY

Dancing Hands is expected to be read by dentists of different nationalities, although it is written in English. Here are some basic descriptive words that are used:

- Treatment room is the word used for the surgery, or operatory (for all kinds of treatments including surgical procedures).
- Dental unit is used for what is sometimes called a delivery system, but includes also the cuspidor system (spitton and cup filler) and the suction holder.
- Unit instrument is used as generic description for all the dynamic instruments of the dental unit (also known as "hand pieces"). Examples of unit instruments are: the 3-in-1 syringe, micromotors, turbine, ultrasonic scaler, air scaler, polymerization lamp, intraoral camera. When dealing with the micromotor-mounted instruments they are called "contra-angles" (if they are so), or straight hand pieces, etc.
- High-speed contra-angles are positioned on micromotor-mounted 1:5 multiplication contra-

angles with two red rings, which use the same size diamonds and burs as turbines. The speed can be regulated up to 200,000 rotations per minute.

- The workstation must be distinguished from a simple line of drawer modules used by the assistant and dentist. The workstation is an important and integrated part of the whole work system of dentist and assistant. The workstation has specific and well-defined functions, measures and storing facilities.
- The word ergonomics is almost never used. The reason is that the word had been misused especially for marketing purposes.
- Instead the expression interactive design is used, indicating a different perspective, which also requires user training.
- The term four-handed dentistry is generally not used. When assistant and dentist are working in a team, what is interesting is the purpose and the outcomes of these activities. Therefore, the best standards of assistance are described, which makes it possible to describe an actual teamwork as creating an outcome, eg, say 60% of the best standard of assistance.
- In Dancing Hands, the dentist is generally referred to as being male, and the assistant, female. This is by no means a generalization of how things are (there are many female dentists and male assistants).

THE 12 BASIC PRINCIPLES

The 12 basic principles (or axioms) are the starting position for deductions. *Dancing Hands* is based on deductions from basic principles, with the 12 most important being listed here. These axioms will result in reasoned conclusions, leading to the methods and prescriptions presented in *Dancing Hands*.

Working DUO: dentist and assistant

1. The dentist and assistant should work in good working positions, feeling physically well and relaxed.
2. During the working day, the dentist and assistant should have short periods (eg, 1 minute) of intensive physical exercise for selected muscle groups.
3. The dentist should be able to have visual access to all the exterior surfaces of every tooth, as well as all interior surfaces in any cavity at any place, in a good working posture.
4. The dentist should be able to have instrumental access to all exterior surfaces of every tooth, as well as all interior surfaces in any cavity at any place, in a good working posture.
5. The dentist should perform precision dentistry, and when there is indication for it, minimally invasive dentistry.
6. The dentist should be able to keep undisturbed concentration on the object of work – as long as necessary and comfortable.
7. The assistant should be able to provide maximum assistance with a workplace that has everything, including unit instruments, within reach.
8. The assistant should be able to prepare instruments and materials for any treatment in a minimal time.
9. The dentist's and the assistant's hands should be highly trained and work coordinately, guided by protocols.
10. DUO–SOLO working: If the assistant is not able to assist the dentist for shorter or longer periods, there should be a well organized workstation and working methods to optimize the dentist working a part of the time DUO working and part-time SOLO, while allowing a fast switch between DUO and SOLO.
11. SOLO working: A dentist working SOLO should be able to prepare for any treatment in minimal time.
12. Patients should feel comfortable and experience a concentrated dentist and assistant working with elegant, relaxed efficiency.
    - Working completely SOLO – see Chapter 6.
    - Hygienist working SOLO – has the same demands as a dentist working SOLO.

COMMENTS TO THE 12 BASIC PRINCIPLES

You may test the relevance of these 12 axioms by testing the negation (the opposite and negative version):

- It is better to – work in fine working positions – than not to do so.
- It is better to – be able to see all surfaces of the teeth – than not to do so.
- It is better that – the patient experiences a concentrated dentist – than not to do so.

Presented in this way, almost everyone will agree with these basic principles or axioms. So is it a problem to work and perform dentistry that conforms to the aforementioned axioms?

The short answer is YES!

Remembering about 500 hands-on courses with (in most cases) 3 to 4 teams of one dentist and one assistant per course and furthermore visiting many more dental practices, I will describe examples of problems of complying with the basic principles.

1. It is rather rare – with exceptions of course – to see dentists working in good working postures for all procedures. Many are twisting their spine, bending their neck, placing their head inclined, lifting up the elbow and arm, and sitting with a rounded back with a strong lumbar kyphosis.
2. Concentrated working in a sitting position should be balanced by active exercises maintaining a considerable force of muscles in order to maintain a good working posture. This is essential for all work as a dentist and as an assistant.
3. The problems really are big *if* principle 3 is combined with principle 1. Many dentists need to learn the solutions, by using different clock positions according to the direction of vision, and learn to use a mirror efficiently in the maxillary, as well as the mandibular jaw (on distal molar cavities).
4. For achieving instrumental access and performing precision dentistry, several aspects will interact. These include: a precise instrument grip in different pen grip modifications, perfect finger support, and well-trained hand and finger biomechanics.
5. Preplanned movements using feed-forward working methods. This is one example of a combination of principle 1 and principle 3, micro/mini-invasive techniques, and special diamonds and burs.
6. In order for the dentist to achieve undisturbed concentration, the unit instruments and hand instruments should be grasped without looking away from the patient's mouth AND working with an assistant who can grasp and transfer unit instruments, hand instruments and materials to the dentist's hand according to the work protocol.
7. Workplaces providing this are rare. Most arrangements with modules for the assistant are basically only a line of drawer modules, like in a kitchen. (A new workstation with high functionality is presented here in *Dancing Hands*, Chapter 8.)
8. A lot of different materials must be collected and made ready in order to perform treatments like endodontics or crown and bridge procedures, as well as surgical procedures. Assistants can often take considerable time to find everything needed for these procedures. Short and effective solutions will be presented.
9. Some teams of dentists and assistants have perfect protocols guiding their teamwork, and many do not.
10. If the assistant (in either shorter or longer periods) leaves the dentist to take care of other tasks, then the working methods, dental unit and workstation have to fulfill very specific demands. The dentist will then switch between working DUO and working SOLO.
11. Working alone, SOLO work (never with assistant) needs a specially designed treatment room and an organization that is rarely found. The organization of materials and instruments for working SOLO is extremely important.
12. The concentrated and relaxed dentist, who does not have to look away from the patient time and time again, is seen as being calm and professional by the patient. So too is teamwork between dentist and assistant, especially if performed with a certain elegance, producing a pleasant ambience.

SELECTION OF METHODS

Based on the step-by-step reasoning from the 12 principles

The methods and techniques demonstrated in *Dancing Hands* have been carefully selected and tested by thousands of dentists and assistants.

In *Dancing Hands*, the concept of so-called "schools of thought" is deliberately avoided. The author knows of course a lot of different "schools" or "shared habits," which are closed for critical examination and respond by claiming that criticism is just an other opinion. Therefore, it is important to open up or leave the different concepts of "schools," in order to open for reasoned conclusions.

The introduction and application of more knowledge about working methods, more training of manual skills, together with the introduction of the dental unit, patient chair, stool, suction system and workstation – that have been developed to be integrated in the complete working system – will often completely change the environment and conditions.

The activities in the treatment room are complex, and interact with and influence each other. But to understand what is best practice, the concepts of established schools have to be broken and to be replaced by sound common everyday reasoning. This may be an eye opener as an observer to see what we are doing, and make conclusions from the observations. That is why in the subtitle of *Dancing Hands*, there is the word "deductions," the result of the deduction is then a "prescription."

Can't everything be done differently?

Everyday activity in practice in some countries shows that working methods can be very different. But that will compromise the previously-listed 12 principles.

- Insight is needed to realize, eg, that an instrument grip or hand support can cause very bad working postures.
- That insufficient assistance can also cause very bad working postures.
- That an insufficient position of the dental unit can hinder important parts of assistance.
- Insufficient workstation or dental unit can make it very difficult to optimize assistance.

In *Dancing Hands*, you can follow the lines of reason-based deductions. The author asks you to not call this a "school," but a rebirth of reasoned conclusions from the "bottom line." If you follow these deductions, whether they are done by the author, or occasionally by colleges, the results are almost the same. There may be smaller variations but the final solutions are surprisingly close to each other.

The methods and techniques in *Dancing Hands* can all be learned in a limited time. Methods that need more intensive training are not presented. The author is very aware of the historically based traditions in some countries for placing unit instruments at the right side of the patient, where the assistant cannot reach them and where the dentist has to look away from the patient to take them. This underlines the necessity to look away from old traditions and start from the bottom line, guided by unbiased reason.

A matter of opinion or a question of knowledge and skills?

Often it is argued, especially from the sales staff of dental equipment, that working methods and choice of dental equipment is a matter of opinion.

In *Dancing Hands*, the reader will find logical step-by-step reasoned conclusions, showing that having sufficient knowledge and the training of required skills leads to the solutions presented.

The deductions will be made with diplomatic attention to the fact that the solutions presented may be quite different to the traditional work habits and equipment in some countries. In the section "Straight talking" on page 267, you will find a short, straight and direct resume.

Dancing Hands can be used under different conditions in different countries. The organization of dentistry, public support and payment, regulations and restrictions for dentistry, and conditions, quality standards, legal systems, private insurance costs, etc, for dentistry and patients' own costs vary widely between countries.

There may be remarkable changes just by passing a country border. The spectrum of treatments, as well their organization in dental practices, may be very different from country to country or between regions, and from dental practice to dental practice.

In some countries, general practice may be based on patients who need large and complex treatments – and can pay for it. These practices treat rather few patients during several long appointments. Other dental practices may offer emergency care for patients with limited economical capacities.

In some countries, dentistry may be based on regular recalls with integrated prevention programs and – if necessary – early treatment for the most based on minimal invasive fillings. A practice may have many recall patients per day, because the dental care needed per patient is minimal.

In some countries, childcare is free, and is covered by tax payments. Preventive and early interceptive care reaches almost all children from 2 to 3 years of age. In other countries, this is not the case and parents have to pay in full for childcare (if they can afford it).

In some countries, the value of recall-based preventive and interceptive dentistry is not well known by patients. In many countries, amalgam fillings are allowed and in others, the use of mercury is forbidden.

In some countries, the practice of having dental hygienists is not allowed, and in others it is. Some countries have deregulated the limitations for auxiliaries, where the hygienists may make fillings and the assistants may – under the supervision and responsibility of the dentist – perform scaling, root planing and polishing of teeth, and even fillings. The habits of working with an assistant are different however:

- In some countries, it is normal that the dentist works SOLO, without an assistant.
- Some work DUO–SOLO, sometimes with a chairside assistant and sometimes alone.
- Some always work DUO, with permanent assistance.
- Some always work DUO, supplied with a part-time second assistant (roving assistant).

Group practices are common in some countries where two or several dentist share a practice. Some of the dentists may be specialized in surgery, endodontics, periodontic treatment, orthodontic treatment, and so on.

In some countries, all patients (with rare exceptions) have been treated in a horizontal position for the past 30 to 40 years. In other countries, it is not believed to be possible. In northern European countries, a majority of female dentists graduate. It is probable that female influences and priorities may induce future changes in dental practice and organizations in some countries.

Chapter 1

THE PROBLEMS

MOST FREQUENT PROBLEMS

- How not to sit
- How not to work
- Discomfort and pain
- Occupational diseases and fatigue.

THE POSTURE

It is astonishing how often dentists' working postures are "quite far from being good." If the dentist is young and is in good physical health, he or she may work with a bad posture without any noticeable or major physical symptoms. But 10 to 20 years later, these symptoms may become manifest or even become chronic. So if a working method implicates health risks, it is beneficial to use principles to prevent them.

When performing precision work, the dentist has to sit still. This is achieved by maintaining a static muscular tension. If the posture is inclined, twisted or bent, the muscles become extraordinarily tense in order to maintain the awkward position. This very often causes discomfort and pain in the muscles of the lower back, shoulders, neck and arms, as well as headache.

Over the course of time, these muscular tensions can become chronic and even disabling for working as a dentist. When the dentist or the dental assistant is working, very often they have to lean forward in order to look into the mouth of the patient. For many dentists, this is done by rounding the lumbar back in a kyphosis, resulting in a strong compression of the front part of the intervertebral discs, creating painful overload, deformation or the ultimate collapse of intervertebral discs. The resulting pain from discus hernia (prolapsed disc) with compression of nerves and/or osseous contact between spiculae on the corpus vertebrae (vertebral body) can disable and prevent the dentist from working.

The same unfortunate condition may result if the dentist lowers the head (in order to reduce eye to object distance), creating an excessive bending of the neck with compression of the anterior part of intervertebral discs.

Arthrosis or arthritis

If a dentist works with arms and elbows elevated, then acquired deformation in the articulation of the shoulder and/or the elbow is a risk. This can lead to "tennis elbow," or "frozen shoulder."

Destabilization of the hip joint

This can be a risk if thighs are "expanded" by sitting on a wide saddle chair, thus overstretching tendons, ligaments and the capsule of articulation.

Soft tissues

Pain and discomfort caused by pressure from the median part of saddle stools can be an infection risk for women, and cause reduced blood circulation for men.

Vision difficulties

Difficulty in seeing and working on certain surfaces, especially in maxillary molars, premolars, and distal cavities in the mandibular jaw, may force the dentist into awkward working postures. This can cause problems when working with a mirror and spray, with the dentist working almost without visibility.

Work difficulties

Difficulties when working can include:

- The aspiration and retraction of soft tissues is insufficient and disturbing.
- Working with movements with visual feedback is difficult to automatize.
- Working with the sensorimotor feedback system, which is tiring and time consuming.

The changing direction of vision

The dentist can lose concentration when working on a patient's mouth, while having to look away to pick "something" up and put it back, several to many hundreds of times per hour.

Working alone with an assistant

If a dental unit is in a position that the assistant cannot reach, then the dentist is working more or less alone, even with an assistant present. The dentist will be reaching for hand instruments, unit instruments and materials, having to change rotating instruments him or herself. Storage modules arranged in a "kitchen-like" sequence rarely support the assistant.

Dentist is asking for "everything"

If there is no protocol for cooperative teamwork, then the assistant cannot predict the dentist's stages of work. The dentist then has to ask for everything.

Waiting for "everything"

If the assistant leaves the patient to prepare planned or unplanned treatments, then "jogging assistant syndrome" is the result. The assistant moves around, rather than assists the patient.

Stress

Physical and mental stress causes fatigue and loss of energy. Here are a number of examples of bad work postures to follow in Figs 1–1 to 1–17; often they are much worse.

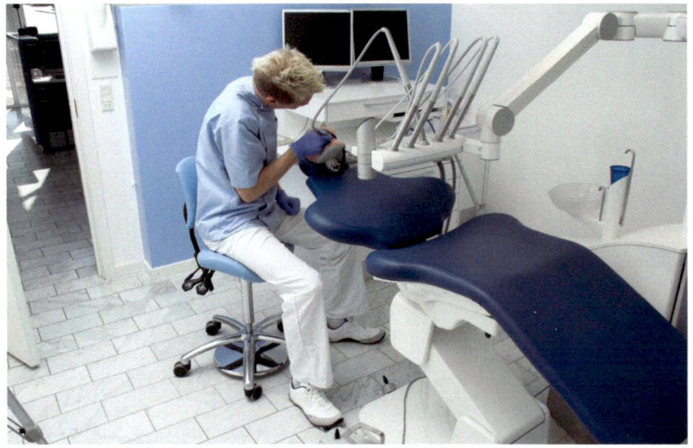

Fig 1–1 Twisted spine. The foot controller is on the right side of the patient's chair base.

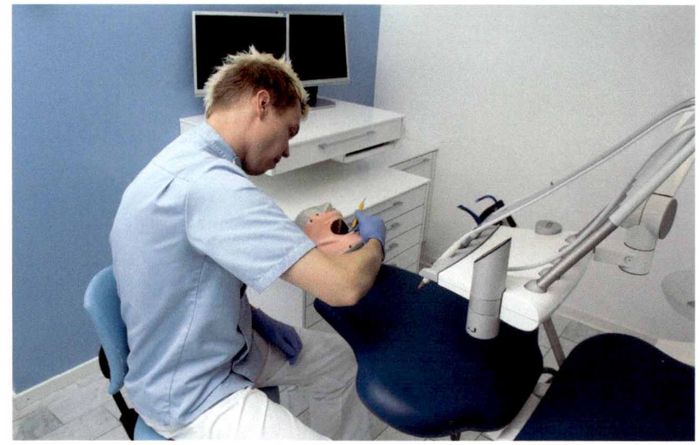

Fig 1–2 Insufficient side-bending of working part of the hand scaler forces the dentist to use the scaler lingually in the mandibular front teeth, with the hand in a 7 o'clock position and the head in an 11 o'clock position.

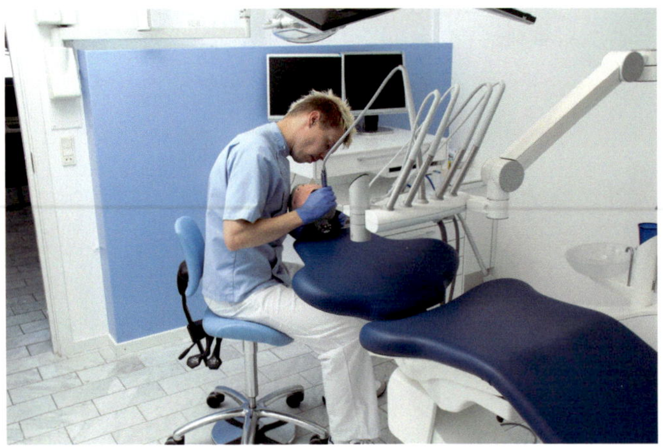

Fig 1–3 The dentist positioned at 10 o'clock, with head positioned at 1 o'clock.

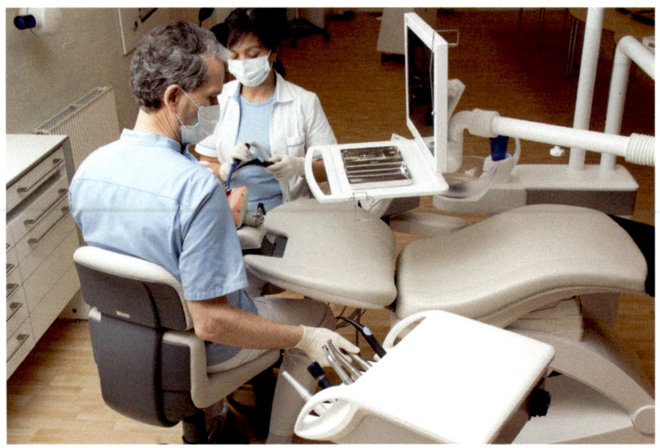

Fig 1–4 The dentist takes an instrument from the unit at the right side of patient. He has to look away from the patient to do it.

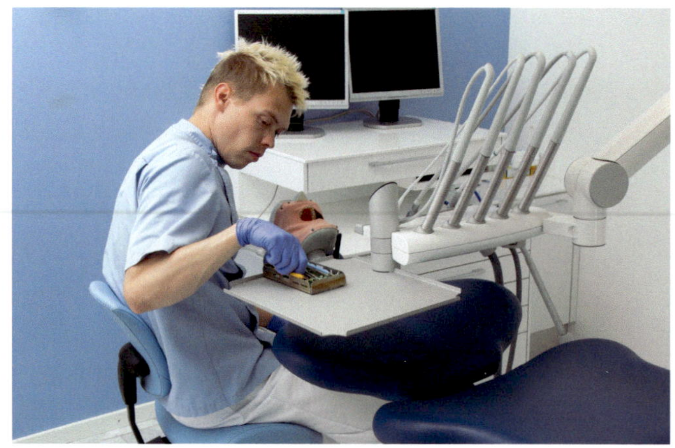

Fig 1–5 The dentist sits in a 9 o'clock position in order to look at surfaces at the patient's right side. He is twisting himself to take the hand instrument and is looking away from the patient.

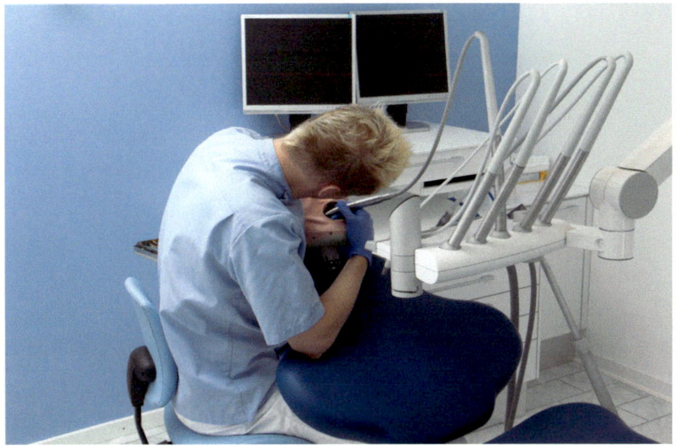

Fig 1–6 The dentist is positioned at 9 o'clock – looking at tooth 17 (occlusal). The patient's chair is not horizontal.

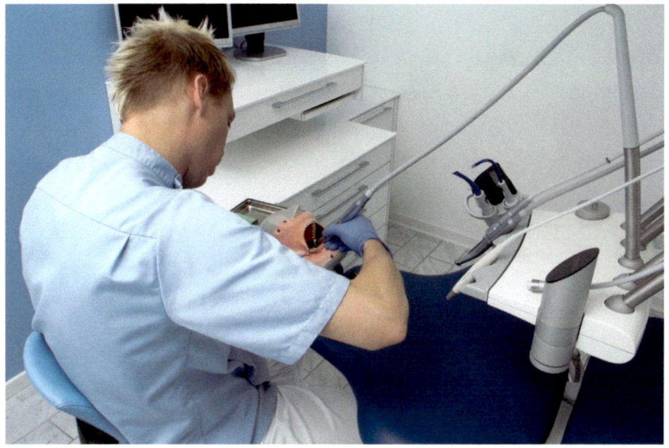

Fig 1–7 The dentist is positioned at 10 o'clock – working at tooth 44 (vestibular) with pen grip and right elbow high. The head is inclined left to align with the tooth axis.

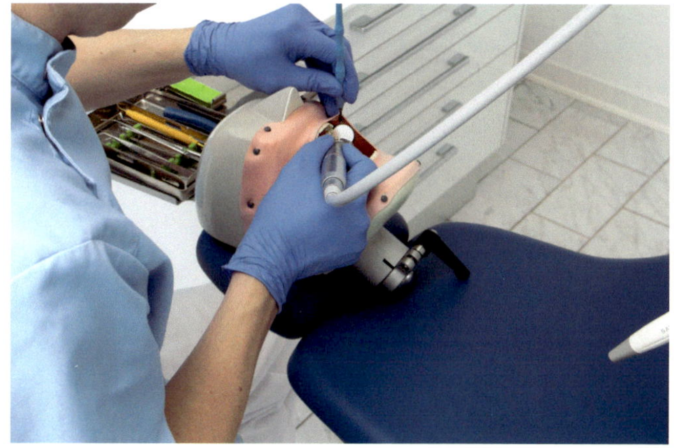

Fig 1–8 The dentist is positioned at tooth 11 – looking at tooth 26 (occlusal) in the mirror. He retracts the soft tissue himself; note that the left arm is elevated. If present, the assistant is not able to help, so the dentist works solo.

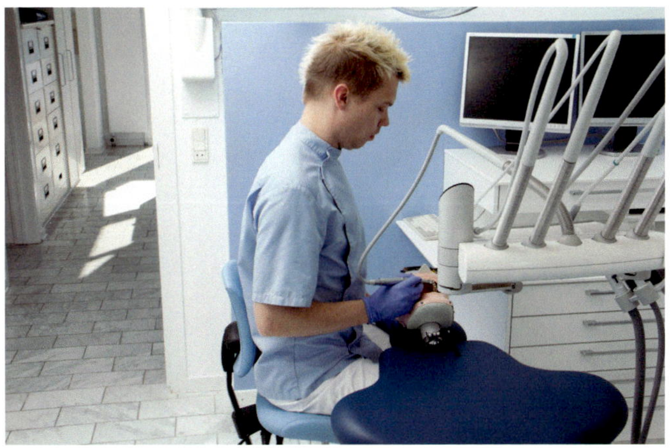

Fig 1–9 Dentist positioned at tooth 11, with horizontal lower arms, and a 60 cm eye to tooth distance.

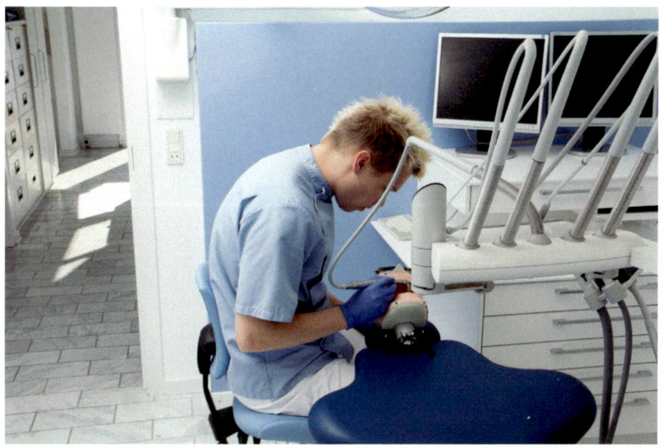

Fig 1–10 Dentist with a horizontal lower arm, bending down to 32 cm eye to object distance and rounding the back. This posture is a health risk as it causes heavy compression of the forward part of the intervertebral discs in the lumbar region.

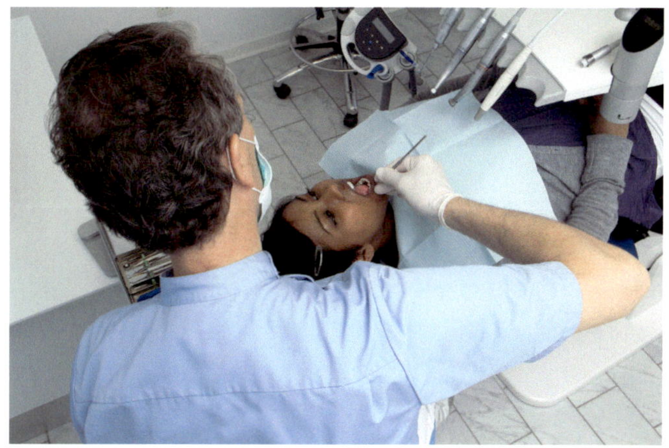

Fig 1–11 The pen grip here leads to a bad posture with an elevated right arm.

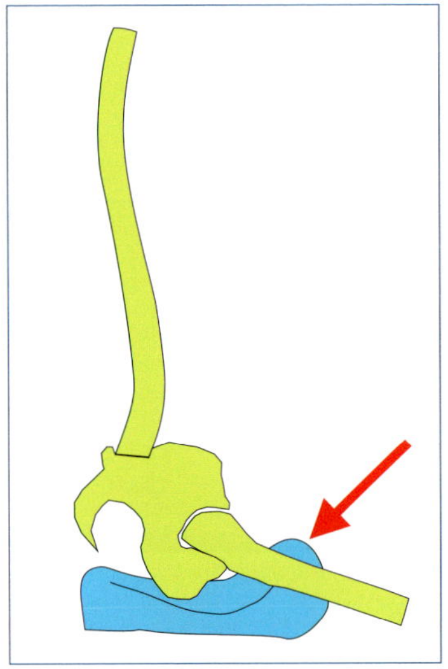

Fig 1–12 Dentist at saddle stool. The middle part of seat causes inconvenient compression of soft tissues.

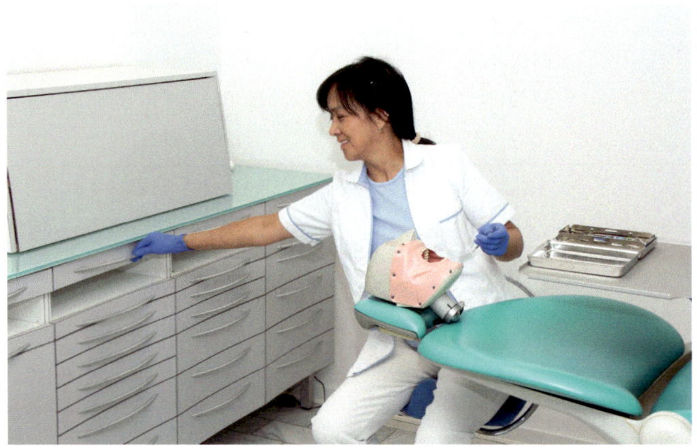

Fig 1–13 The patient's chair is positioned 80 cm from workstation front. The assistant cannot reach the workplate without leaving the patient.

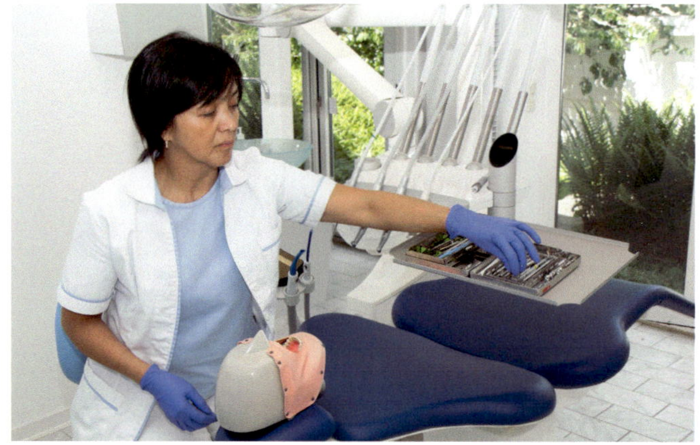

Fig 1–14 The assistant tries to pick up hand instruments from the unit in a very inconvenient position, blocking the dentist's access to the unit instruments.

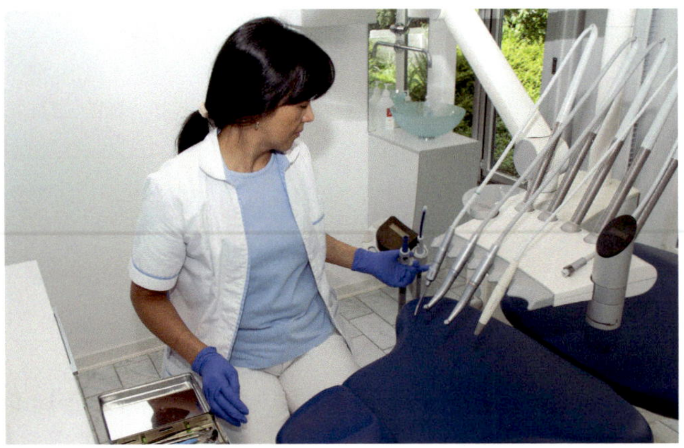

Fig 1–15 Assistant takes a suction tube from the left side behind her back, 30 cm or more away from unit instruments, in an inconvenient suction holder position. The suction holder could be placed correctly by the unit, and close to the unit instruments.

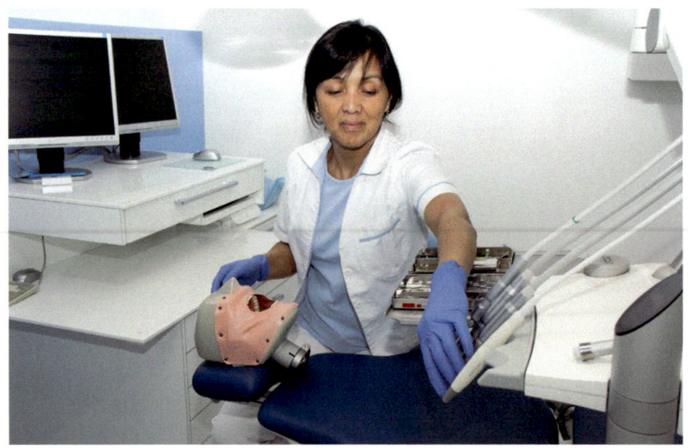

Fig 1–16 The unit instruments are placed on the right side of the patient's chair to leave space for the hand instrument table on the assistant's side of the unit. The assistant cannot (or only with difficulty) reach the unit instruments to prepare them and transfer them to the dentist.

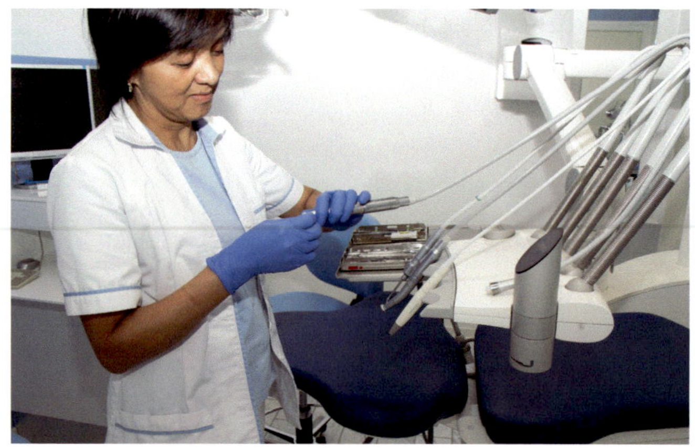

Fig 1–17 Here the unit instruments are placed on the right side of patient. There is the same problem whether the instruments are suspended or hanging; the assistant has to walk to the right side of the patient to change burs and diamonds (jogging assistant!).

WHY ARE MANY DENTISTS TIRED AFTER A WORKDAY?

- The short answer is that their work is tiring.
- It is tiring to work in bad postures.
- It is tiring to work by a patient chair where you cannot sit properly while leaning forward in order to look into the mouth of the patient.
- It is tiring to work sitting on a stool, where you cannot sit in a balanced position.
- As work postures (for the most) are a result of instrument shape, instrument grip, hand support, and movement of hands, working is tiring if these factors are not improved.
- It is tiring to work if your muscles in the shoulders and back are weak.
- It is tiring to work by a dental unit where it is difficult to grasp the instruments.
- It is tiring to have problems seeing the external or internal surface of the tooth from where you are working.
- It is tiring to try to work in a mirror if you cannot see what you need to see in it.
- It is tiring to try to retract soft tissues while working at same time.

It is tiring to have to look away from precision work in the patient's mouth. to take a unit instrument, hand instrument or a material, say 100 times for prep, excavation, filling and polishing a composite filling. This is around a 200 times back and forth change of direction of vision, convergence of eyes, accommodation to another distance and adaptation to different levels of light. If you try to simulate this just 10 times, most dentists feel irritated and suffer eye tiredness.

That is just the part of the problem that the eyes play in changing the direction of vision. Every time you look at something, you will have to perceive it, and that is brainwork in say 0.6 seconds, and double that if you need to take a micro decision concerning the visual input.

- These processes are tiring, but the work itself is not.
- The micro-stress of being interrupted in the flow of work is tiring.
- It is tiring to wait for materials or instruments or unit instruments because it stops workflow.
- It is tiring to ask for everything.
- It is tiring to have to think during the work instead of concentrating about the movements of your hands.
- It is very tiring to do most of the work by yourself, solo, even if an assistant is present by the chair.
- It is tiring to work with an instrument that is not the best for the specific task.
- It is tiring to work if the assistant cannot assist well, because the workplace does not support it.

Are these problems often present?

Yes, very often.

May all problems be presented by one dentist?

Yes, often.

Are the dentists themselves aware of these problems?

In many cases, they are not. *Dancing Hands* provide the solutions.

So to answer the question, "Does a dentist need to be tired after a workday?"

In most cases – NO.

YES, BUT –

Every dentist has to do it his/her own way. Things can be done differently.

This may be a good point, but what if there unwanted and negative side effects such as bad work postures?

It is difficult to sit and to work in perfect body positions!

That is right, because body positions are often secondary – caused by many other elements in the work system. These elements include:

- the necessary direction of vision
- the position of the patient's head
- the position of the dentist
- use – when needed – of a mirror
- mirror dried with air when working with unit instrument with spray
- instrument grip, finger or hand support
- the biomechanics of movements.

So good body positions can, and have to be learned, by learning working methods that support good work posture.

My treatment room does not work for assistance.
Well then redesign can be considered. A good workstation and work methods may save so much time, thus making the repayment period for a new workstation, for example, very short.

Habits are difficult to change.
That's right, it does not come by itself. You have to work for it and train yourself, like a pianist prepares for a concert by constantly repeating movements of the fingers, until the actions become automatic and the music sounds melodious.

I am not interested in working faster.
The different elements of work simplification presented here may reduce the time for a task, by eliminating disturbing and unnecessary activities.

But you decide how to use this time. You can use the time you gain to work in a more relaxed manner, or to work less, for having one or two afternoons free, for longer pauses, having longer holidays, or for improving the practice, or … the choice is yours!

Dental unit on the patient's right side

In some countries, dentists have the habit of working with the dental unit positioned at the right side of the patient's chair, believing that the patient does not like to see the unit instruments in a central position over themselves. Yet they accept that the unit instruments are placed very visibly in front of the waiting patient, while the chair is horizontal.

If the unit is placed here, the dentist in a 9 o'clock position will have difficulty accessing the instruments.

The 9 o'clock position is often used while working, as it gives vision from right the side of the patient AND works the midplane of the body of the dentist, without twisting the head, neck and spine.

If the unit is placed on the right side of the patient, then the assistant has no access to the instruments, and none of the assistant's activities involving the unit are possible. The assistant is "amputated." Providing good assistance is therefore not possible.

Another complication is the habit in some countries of the assistant sitting with her legs to her right side of the dentist's legs, a habit that may have been established many years ago when the assistants (or nurses) were wearing skirts, prohibiting the dentist and assistant from sitting in front of each other. When the assistant is turned away from the unit, she cannot integrate assistance with the unit instruments.

In Europe, except UK and Ireland, the dentist and assistant sit in front of each other and in most cases with legs intercrossed, so certainly one can sit like this. It is done by maybe 75,000 teams in continental Europe.

The practice of having the unit in a central position placed over the patient is dominant in the Nordic countries, the Netherlands, Belgium and France, Spain and Italy, as well as by ergonomically conscious dentists in North America during the past 30 to 40 years.

So why are some dental units sold with the unit instruments placed on the right side of the patient, when the negative consequences for the dentist's unit instrument grip and quality of assistance are so large?

For the author, there seem to be two more reasons. One is that dentists are not aware of how fast old habits can be changed by training. The other is a lack of knowledge of the remarkably better quality of assistance and ease of unit instrument pick up that can be achieved by centrally positioning the unit instruments.

Isn't it best to work directly without mirror?
Yes of course, but NOT to the cost of your health. Many surfaces of teeth can be seen directly, without a mirror.

The patient is asked to move the head in different positions. Back, forward, left or right, which is combined with the dentist's position (eg, 9-, 10-, 11-, or 12 o'clock).

In some cases, the patients accept lying with their head and neck tilted backwards so much that some work tasks, even in molars in the maxillary jaw, can be performed directly. For patients aged 30 years+ or disabled, this is often not possible.

Distal surfaces and narrow distal cavities in molars can never be seen directly, in either the maxillary or the mandibular jaw. So both the dentist's and the assistant's (if there is one) skills for using a mirror have to be highly developed.

Everyone can intuitively find his or her solutions.
Not everyone, but some dentists have an extraordinary intuition for practical work combined with a never-ending search for improvement, and simplification.

The author has often met such extraordinary colleagues. Colleagues who – on their own – have worked and found solutions very close to or identical to those described in this book. All these colleagues are also of different nationalities. Nevertheless, the methods converge to be very similar.

But only few can go all the way alone.
That's why *Dancing Hands* was written.

In short, if you want to sit well, see well and work well – in a team or a mixed duo-solo work method – and want to do it without making compromises, then all the possible individual systems have solutions in *Dancing Hands*. Often it is the lack of functional quality in the "total workplace" in the treatment room that can hinder the above.

The author feels obliged to promote the 12 basic principles (and more besides) in the hope of establishing and describing what has made the GOLDEN STANDARD FOR PRACTICAL ERGONOMICS in dental practice, for the past 40 years, to the present day.

Can the work be performed differently as described in this book? NO! is the short answer. There are very few or no variations possible without compromising visual and instrumental access, team performance, undisturbed concentration, efficiency and FINE WORK POSTURES. However slight differences occur for dentists who prefer to work with a mirror, and also in cases where direct vision is possible.

Chapter 2

THE SOLUTIONS

WORK POSTURE – SIT WELL!

When a dentist performs work in the patient's mouth, a maximal level of concentration is necessary in many phases of work. The body and arms must establish a stable base of fine hand and finger motor work. Therefore the whole dentist's body should be as relaxed as possible in a position without twisting and bending, and with the joints in as close as possible to a natural, relaxed posture.

To maintain a fine and healthy work posture, you need strong back and shoulder muscles. This means that regular muscular training will be necessary. Poor sitting positions can compromise your health (Fig 2–1).

Leaning forward

In order to look down into the patient's mouth, often the dentist must lean forward. This work demand is different than many other professions. The forward-leaning working position requires special solutions in order to maintain good work postures.

Traditional sitting position with horizontal thighs

When leaning forward, it is very difficult to maintain lumbal curvature (lumbar lordosis) because the angle between the thighs and body now is less than 90 degrees. For most people, this induces a roundness in the lumbar region of the back, with a compression of the forward part of the intervertebral discs.

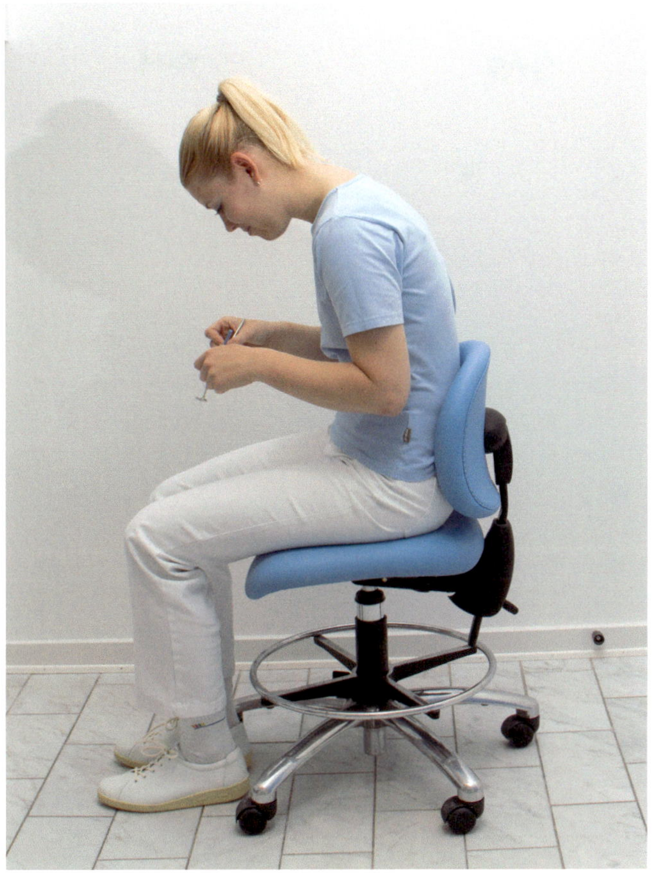

Fig 2–1 Dentists are often working like this!

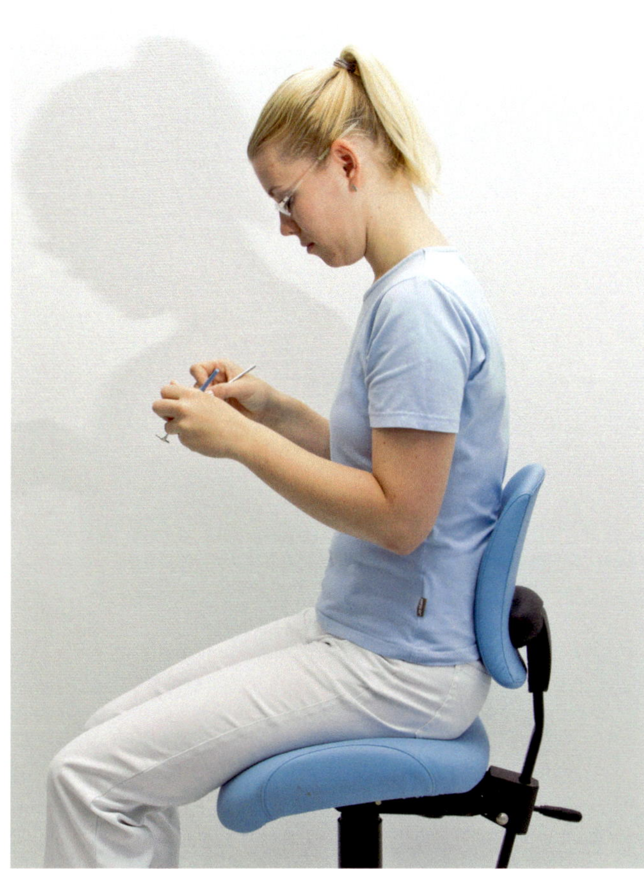

Fig 2–2 A good working posture.

A good work posture

The following all contribute to maintaining a good work posture (Fig 2–2):

- The focus of work should be in the midsaggital plane ("midplane") of your body.
- Don't twist, bend or incline your head or body.
- A balanced sitting position – maintain lumbar lordosis, also when leaning forward.
- Keep an open angle between the thighs and body by having inclined thighs (the seat of the stool has been constructed for this sitting position). These principles have been generally accepted in Northern Europe for 40 to 50 years.
- Incline your eyes downwards as much as is comfortable, in order to keep your head up as much as possible.

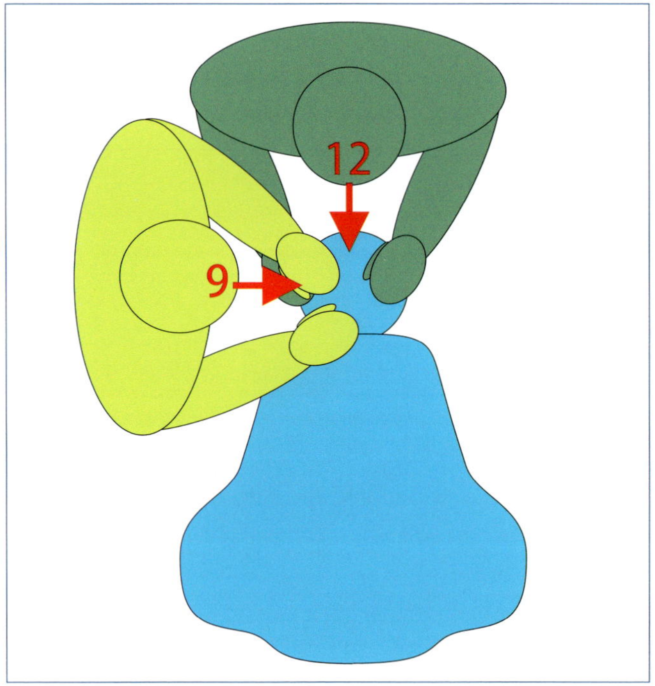

Fig 2–3 The dentist is sitting in a 9, 10, 11, 12 o'clock position, depending on direction of vision.

- Move your focus of work (the patient's mouth) up until you can see with necessary precision without bending down, and with lower arms as inclined as necessary to achieve this.
- Keep your elbows in light contact with your body, and use an instrument grip which supports this.
- Your wrists should not be more than slightly bent.
- Careful and secure hand and/or finger support for both hands.

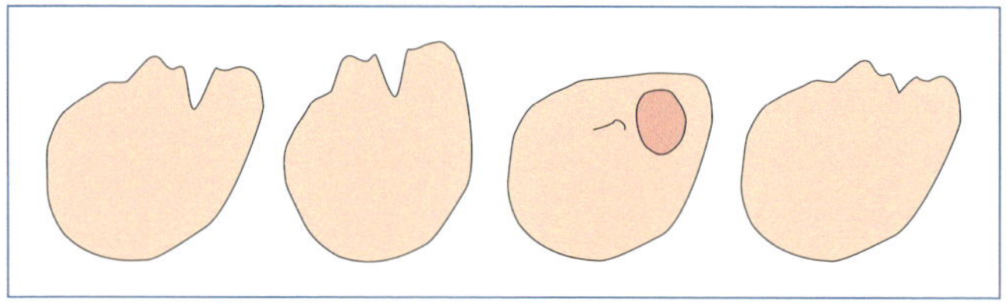

Fig 2–4 The patient is turning the head forward, back, right, or left to facilitate ease and direction of vision.

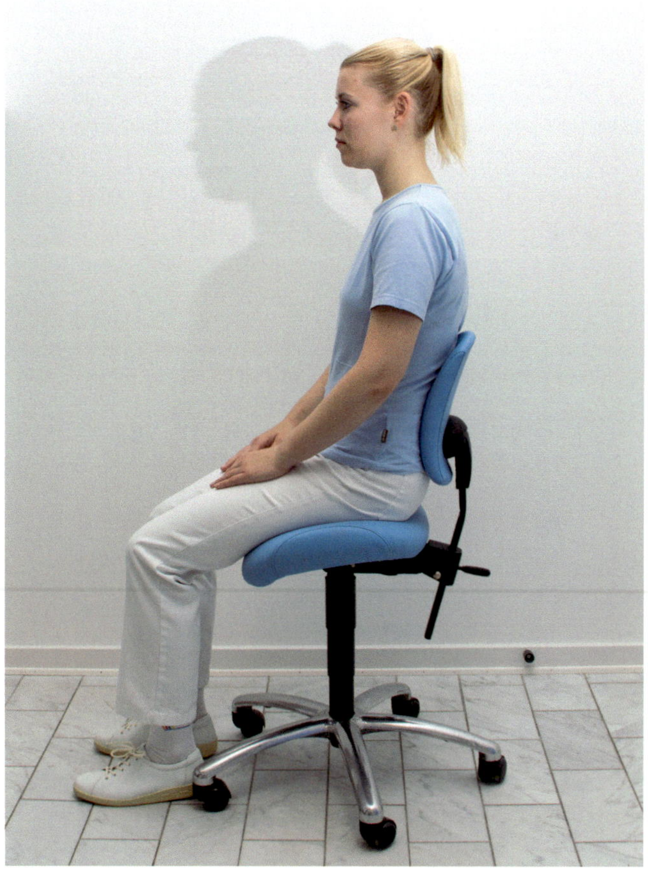

Fig 2–5 A relaxed sitting position using back support, a horizontal seat and inclined thighs. There is an open angle between the thighs and body.

Working in the midplane

When working in the midplane of the body:

- The sitting position will depend on the direction of vision.
- The surfaces of the teeth have different directions, and accordingly we need different directions of vision to see these surfaces. This is achieved by the dentist using different "clock-sitting positions," each decided by the direction of vision (Fig 2–3). This is combined with the patient turning slightly to the side to allow better vision (Fig 2–4).
- When direct vision in a good posture is not possible, a mirror has to be used.

In Chapter 3, you will see systematic and specific solutions to this.

Relaxed sitting posture – triple support

A relaxed sitting posture with triple support and leaned more or less backwards is depicted in Fig 2–5. The thighs are inclined, and the body has two supporting points/areas, which are firstly the ischiatic tuberosity (tuberositae ossi isciatici). With local soft tissues, together these two bones transfer our weight to the surface where we are sitting.

Leaned more or less backwards, the spine (vertebral column or columna vertebralis) is furthermore supported by the back of the seat. The coccyx (os coccygis) may add a slight support.

This not a good working posture as it is difficult or even impossible to look into the patient's mouth from this position.

Leaning forward

In order to look into the patient's mouth it is – in most cases – necessary to lean a little (or more) forward.

Leaning forward on a horizontal seat, with the thighs also horizontal, means that the angle between the thighs and the pelvis/spine will be less than 90 degrees.

For most people, this is not possible. The muscles of the backside resist stretching to this level. The muscles on the backside of the lumbal spine are not stretched yet. The result is that it is the lumbal part of the spine that bends.

It is very important to avoid creating a lumbar kyphosis (backwards rounding), because this causes a severe compression of the forward part of the intervertebral discs of the lumbar region. This compression can trigger degeneration of the intervertebral discs and cause a prolapsed disc (intervertebral discus hernia; Fig 2–6).

Balanced sitting working position

To maintain the health of the intervertebral discs, it is important to maintain the lumbar curvature (forward rounding, lordosis) to obtain an even load on the intervertebral discs without compressing of the forward part. In a standing position, the back is in a dynamic balance supported by the muscles, even when leaned forward.

A **balanced sitting position**, especially when leaning forward a little, implies an **open angle between the upper legs and back (spine) (Fig 2–7)**.

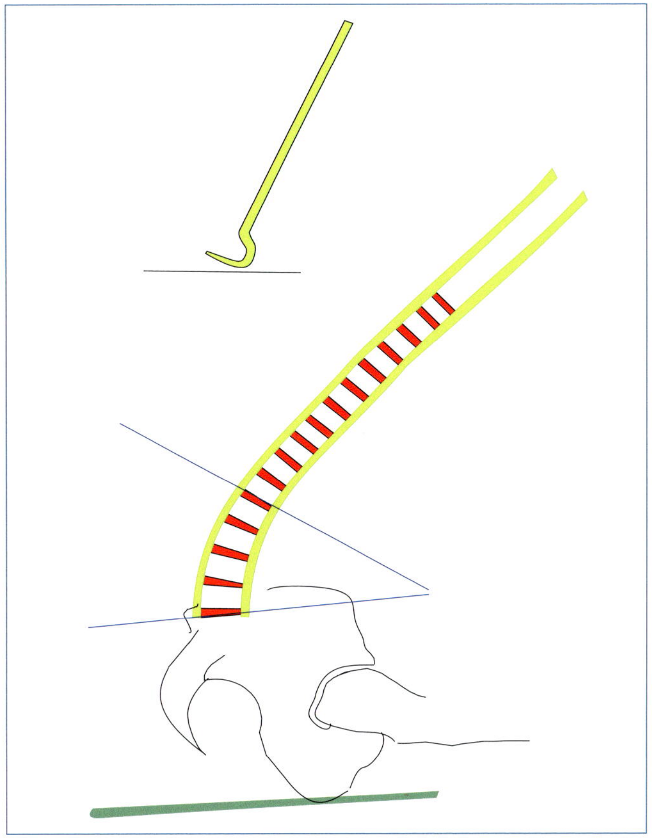

Fig 2–6 Horizontal seat and horizontal thighs. The pelvis is leaned backwards and the thoracic spine leaned forward, with a heavy compression of the forward part of the lumbar intervertebral discs. This posture is a serious health risk.

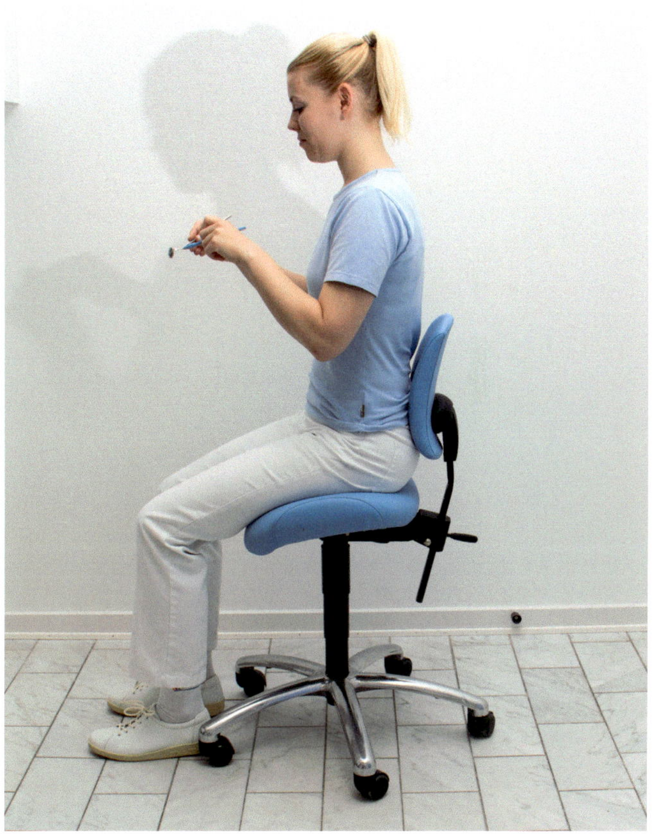

Fig 2–7 A balanced sitting position.

In order to maintain a balanced sitting position, the angle between the thighs and the back has to be about 110 degrees or more. The balanced position when leaning forward a little is maintained by strong back muscles, and is NOT a relaxed sitting position (Fig 2–8). It is recommended to carry out frequent exercises to strengthen the back muscles (see page 22). A balanced sitting position can be obtained by a saddle stool or by so-called balance stools.

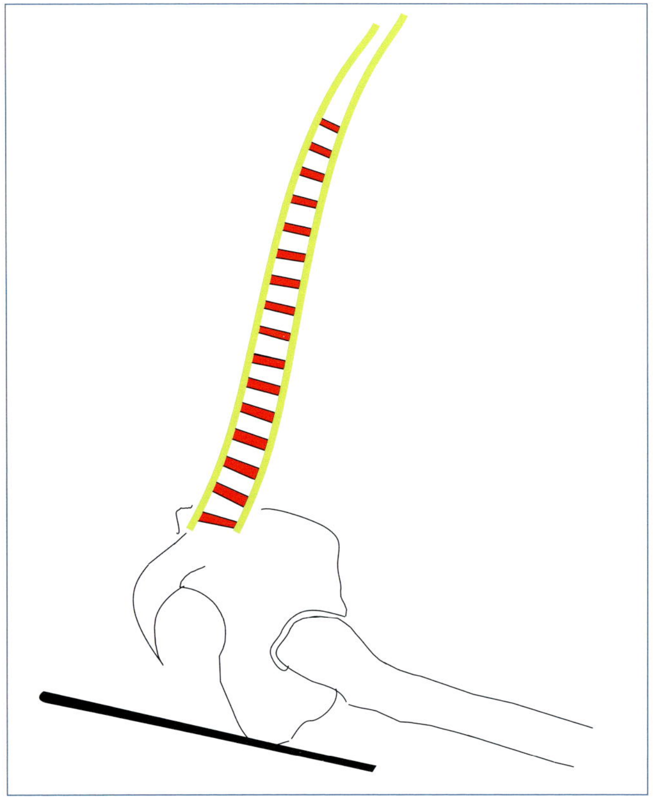

Fig 2–8 The seat is inclined forwards, which may cause the dentist to slide forwards.

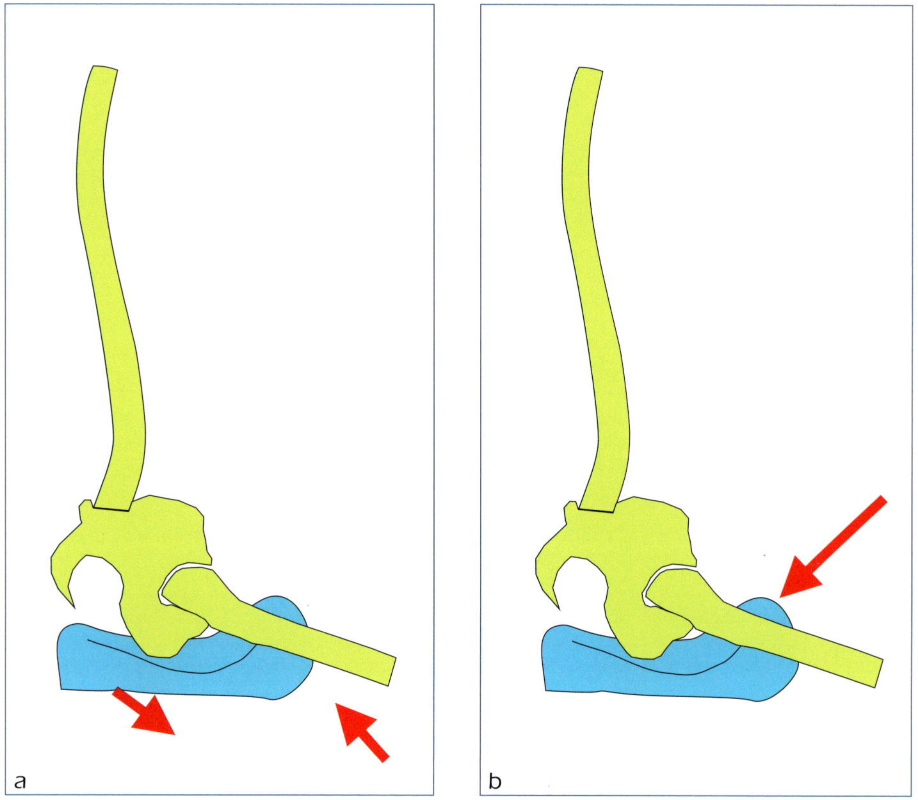

Fig 2–9 In this saddle stool, the support for the isciatic bones is inclined forwards so the dentist here too may slide forwards (a) until stopped by the elevated middle part of the seat (b).

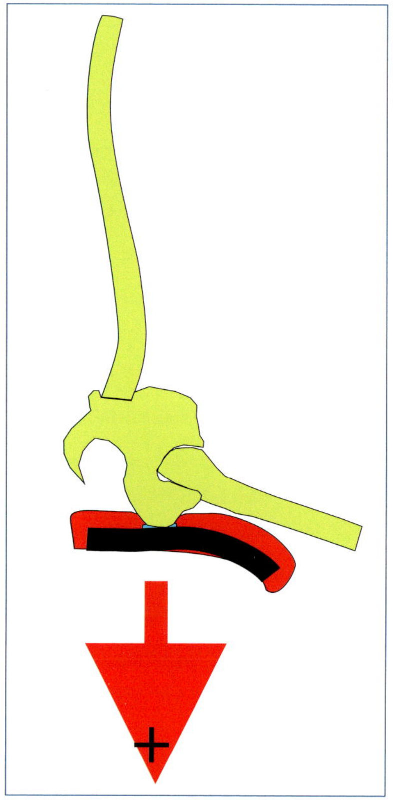

Fig 2–10 Seat of the balance stool, without the risk of sliding forward.

We sit and carry our upper body weight on the tuberositae ischiatica (sitting bone), which supports the sacrum (os sacrum), which in turn supports the spine (columnae vertebralis) and our body. If the sitting bone is supported by a forwards inclined surface, you will of course tend to slide forwards on the seat.

The saddle stool

This tendency to slide forwards can be prevented by elevating the middle–forward part of the seat of a saddle stool (Fig 2–9).

This middle part will stop the sliding by applying a pressure at the soft tissues between the legs. The pressure in this region is particularly uncomfortable (and bad) for men because of the compression. The blood circulation here will be compromised and for women it increases risk of fungal infections.

A wide saddle stool may overstretch the ligaments and articulation capsules, and may destabilize the hip joint (Fig 2–10).

The "balance stool"

Developed by the author, the balance stool is an alternative to the saddle stool (Fig 2–11). The seat is rather short and is rounded at the forward part allowing a comfortable downwards inclination of the thighs with a 110-degree angle to the body.

The support for the ischial tuberosity (the sitting bones) is horizontal so you will not slide forwards on the seat. Therefore, the uncomfortable middle part used with the saddle seat is no longer necessary. You must place yourself on the seat rather deliberately, so the sitting bones are placed right on the horizontal part of the seat. The inclination and height of the seat must be adjusted individually (Fig 2–12).

The seat supports the sitting bones (tuberositae ossei isciatici), carrying your weight at the horizontal part of the seat so you can sit in balance. The seat is curved in front of the supporting area, so you can sit with inclined upper legs and an open angle (about 110 degrees) between the upper legs and back.

Back support

The back should not make contact with the stool's back support when you work leaning forward a little, because this indicates a backward rounded back. The thin back support is used when you relax, leaning backwards in small pauses such as light polymerization, taking an impression, and other waiting periods, as well as conversation with the patient. The thin back support does not limit your mobility.

Height adjustment can be done hands free by a foot-activated disk. A footrest ring for assistants should be fitted for use if the assistant is about 15 cm shorter than the dentist.

Keep your head up

Keep your head up by inclining your eyes as much as comfortable. The direction of vision will depend on your "clock" position and the position of the patient's head.

Occlusal cavities in premolars in the mandibular jaw can be seen on a lying patient in an approximately 45-degree inclined direction of vision. An occlusal cavity in a second mandibular right molar may, however, need an 80-degree inclined direction of vision.

Many dentists have the habit, without knowing it, that their eyes are only inclined slightly downwards. The rest of the inclination is made – for the most part – by the head (Fig 2–13).

Unfortunately, the head can only be inclined around 8 to 10 degrees. An inclination of more than this is done by bending your neck, with a compression of the forward part of the intervertebral discs.

The more you can incline your eyes – within the limits of comfort – the less you will need to bend your neck (Fig 2–14). Some can incline the eyes quite far (more than 45 degrees) without feeling discomfort or tiredness in the eye muscles. For others, the limit for inclination may be 25 degrees.

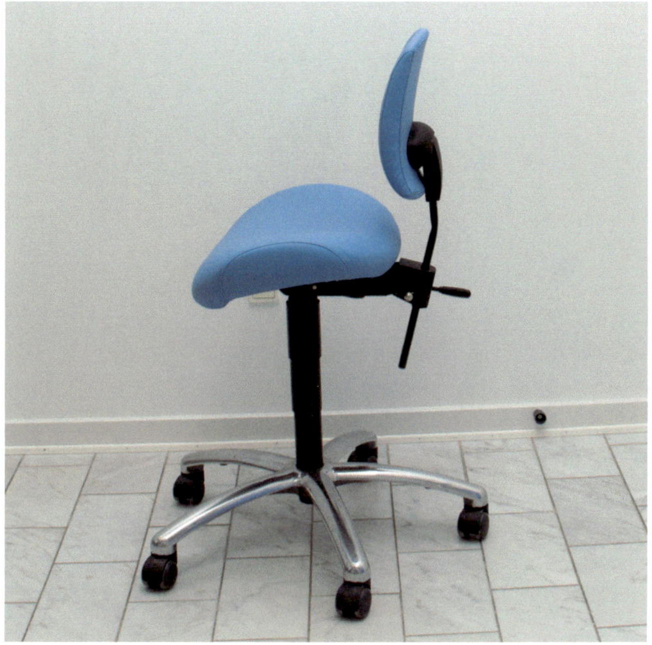

Fig 2–11 A balance stool. One can sit with the upper legs inclined while maintaining the lumbar curvature and the back in balance, and avoid the discomfort of the saddle chair.

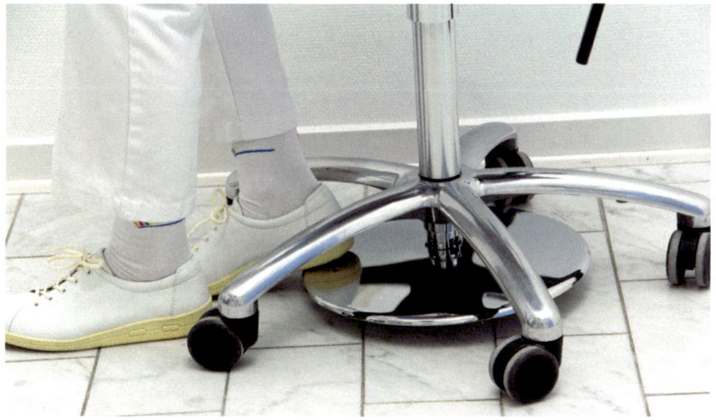

Fig 2–12 The height adjustment can be made by the disk under the stool.

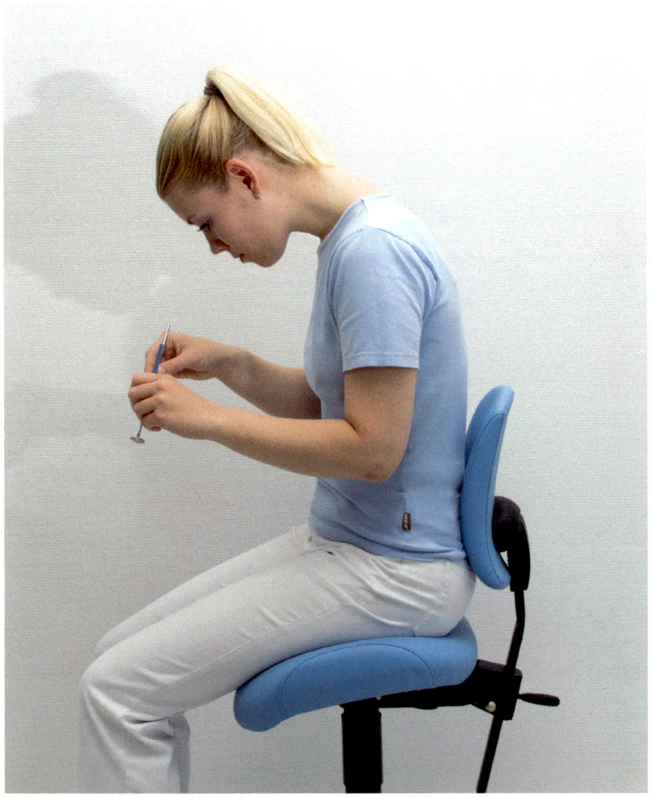

Fig 2–13 Head bent instead of inclined eyes.

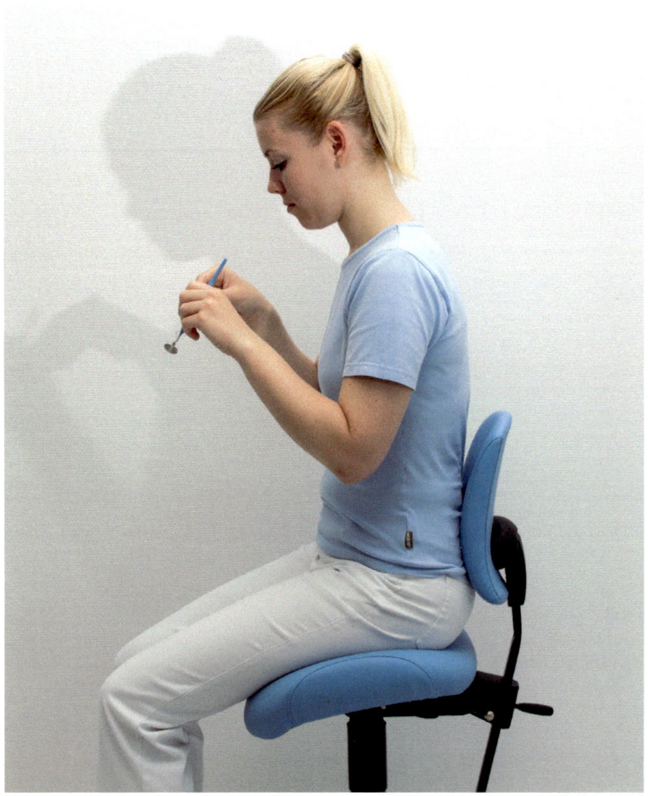

Fig 2–14 Eyes inclined, with the head less bent.

Most dentists can incline their eyes 40 to 45 degrees downwards and maintain comfort in the eye muscles.

But what is the best way to change a habit where the eyes are not sufficiently inclined when working? As habits are normally subconscious, an external feedback is necessary.

One possibility is that the assistant indicates with a little sign (not visible to the patient), that the eyes now need to be more inclined, in order that the dentist can keep the head in a higher position. This may happen so often that the assistant feel a little reluctant to continue to do it. In "hands-on courses," a thin horizontal line has been drawn on glasses to indicate the upper limit for the field of vision.

Working with inclined forearms

It is important to work with forearms inclined upwards (Fig 2–15), in combination with a balanced sitting position. Without loupes, the eye-to-object distance for precision work for most dentists is about 32 cm. For tasks where precision vision is not needed, the distance may be 10 cm more (Fig 2–16).

When the head of the dentist is slightly lowered with downwards-inclined eyes, his or her eyes will be lowered about 10 cm. Their hands will be about 6 to 10 cm higher than the patient's teeth. The upright eye-to-elbow distance can vary from about 50 cm by smaller dentists, to more than 60 cm by taller dentists.

The conclusion of this little calculation is that in order to sit upright and with inclined eyes, the hands of a smaller dentist (with an upright 50 cm eye-to-elbow distance) will have to be working with hands about 15 cm higher than the elbows (Fig 2–17).

The taller dentist (with upright 62 cm eye-to-elbow distance) will have to work with hands almost 30 cm above the elbows (confirmed by the 193 cm-tall author of this book!). If the forearms are not inclined upwards, the dentist bends downwards to obtain a distance for precision vision of about 32 cm, creating a health risk for the spine.

Working with a horizontal forearm position is not possible because it is in conflict with a good upright sitting posture and the need for precision

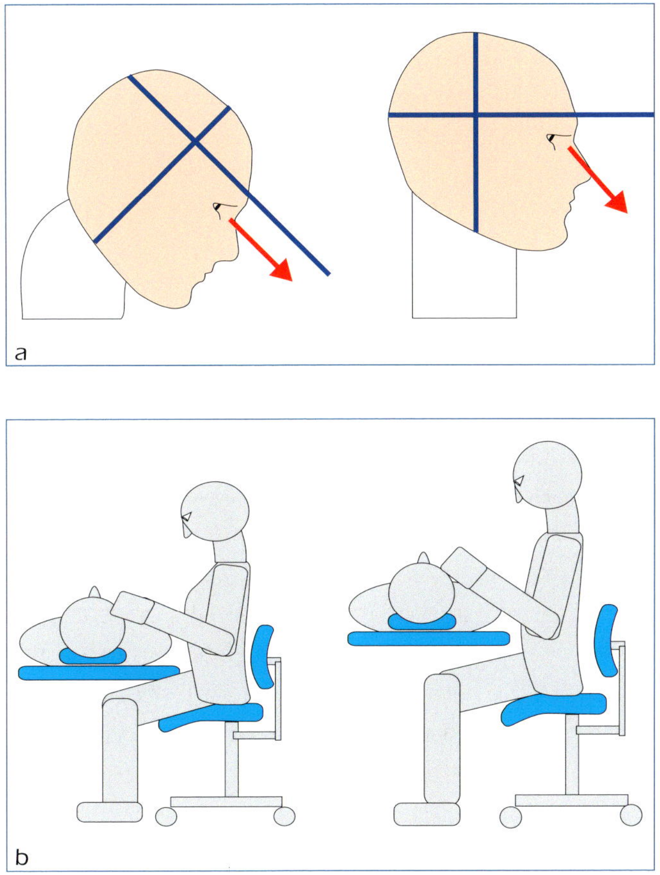

Fig 2–15 (a) Incline the eyes in order to keep the head up. (b) The taller the dentist is, the more the forearms need to be inclined to maintain the same object-to-eye distance.

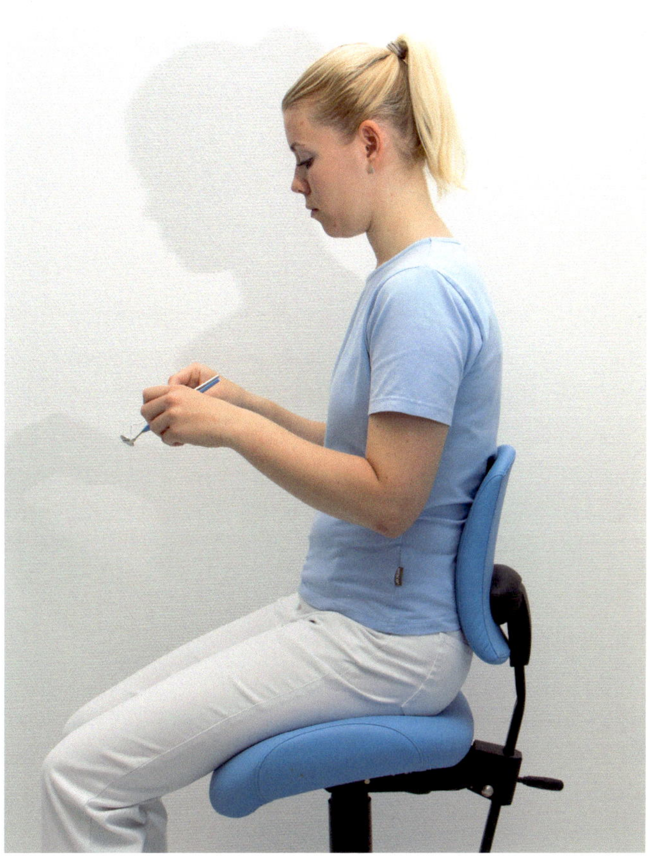

Fig 2–16 Hands and forearm in low position. The eye-to-tooth distance is 45 cm for non-precision vision.

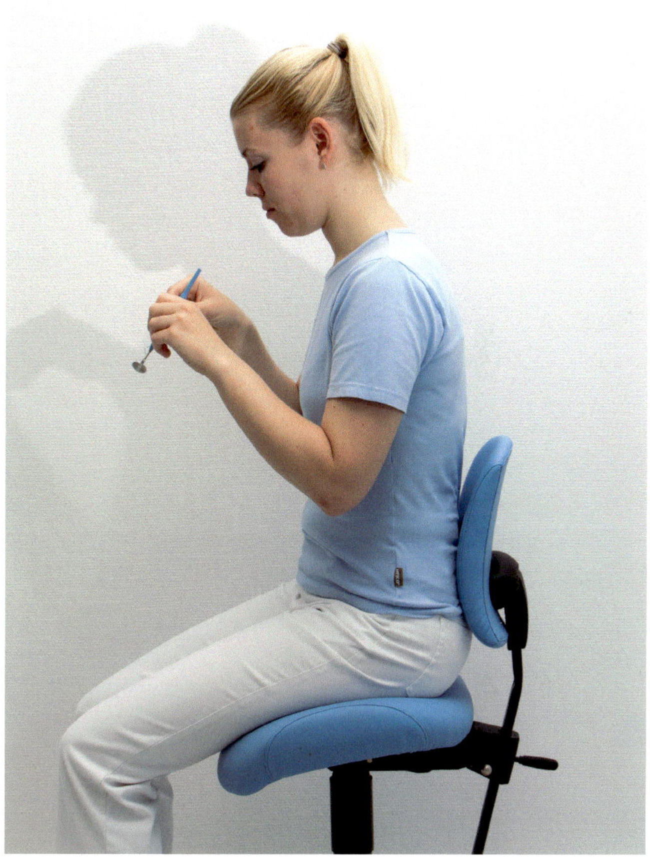

Fig 2–17 Hands and forearm in higher position. The patient chair must be higher. The eye-to-tooth distance is 35 cm for precision vision. This is a good sitting position.

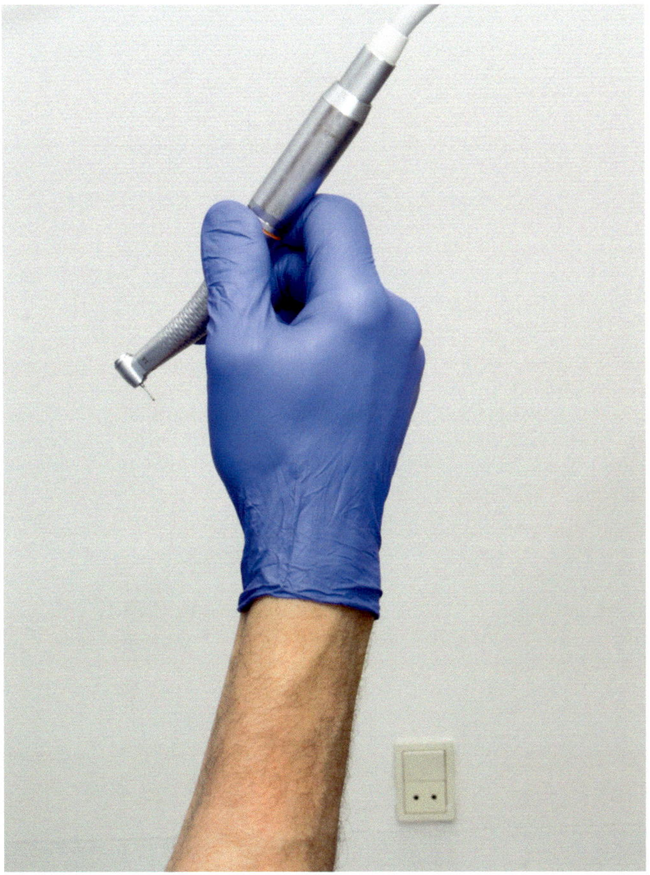

Fig 2–18 The angled grip of the instrument ensures that the shoulders do not need to be elevated.

vision. If loupes are used with an eye-to-object distance of around 40 cm, the forearms will be lowered accordingly.

"What about the shoulders – isn't there a risk that the shoulders will be raised?"
Yes there is, and the solution is here!

You can keep your shoulders down if your instrument grip, especially the grip of contra-angles, is a little more inclined (Fig 2–18; also see Chapter 6).

Furthermore, you should always work with finger/hand support for both for your left and right hands. Then your shoulders do not need to carry the whole weight of the lower arm and hand.

A secure hand/finger support liberates the arms of muscle tensions, in order to try to stabilize the hands. You also relax better with a secure finger/hand support. Keep elbows in contact with your body in order to stabilize your arms, and the wrists should be straight in order to avoid tiring bending, and maintain sensitivity for tension (golgi tendon sensors).

DO 1-MINUTE EXERCISES DURING WORK HOURS

(and more when you are at home)

Take small breaks during work hours – not to relax – but to do selected active physical exercises at high intensity for a minute. This will enable you to concentrate on work.

Our body needs to be physically active. In order to sit still with a good posture and perform precision work, we need well-trained muscles. Consulting physiotherapists recommend selecting three 1-minute exercises for active mini pauses, instead of passive mini pauses. The results are that the blood circulation is increased, and the muscles are strengthened and relaxed afterwards.

Starting training

You will find that your muscles develop rather quickly, but be careful not to accelerate your training too much. Your muscles may develop much faster than muscle attachments, tendons and ligaments. Increase intensity slowly, and the older you are, the more slowly it should be increased. Otherwise you may risk developing symptoms of overload from the muscle attachments, tendons and ligaments. Some guidelines:

- It is recommended to do physical training and fitness training a couple of times per week, and to take a fast walk or other activity half an hour every day.
- Always consult your doctor before you start a new training programme.
- There are no age-related limits. A younger person can profit from training, as well as a person aged 60 years or more.

Upper torso exercises

A good base for precision work is the upper torso muscles that carry your arms and shoulders, and

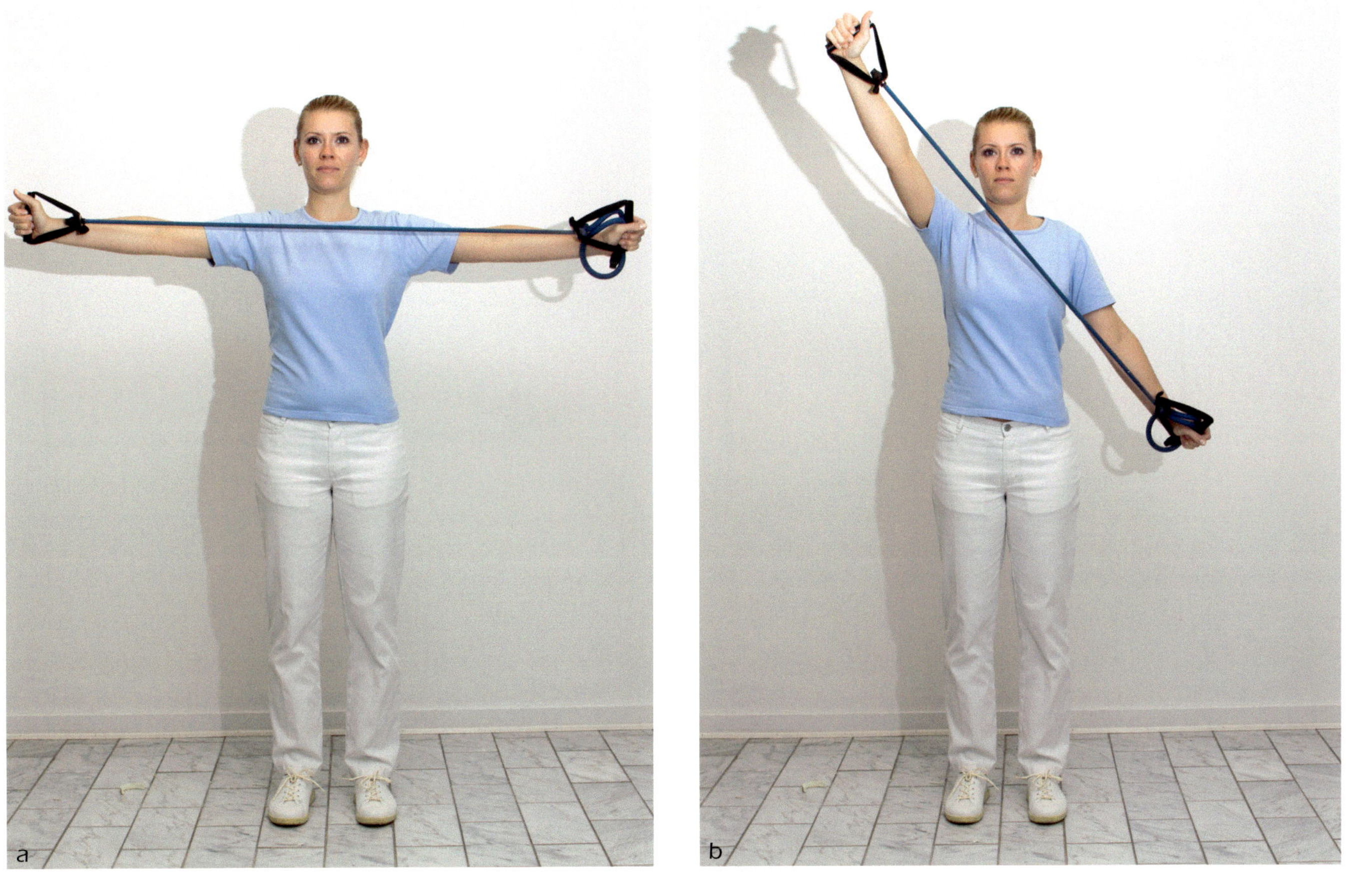

Fig 2–19 (a and b) Upper torso exercises.

provide the tension to keep your arms in a steady position (Fig 2–19a and b).

- Exercise with a resistance elastic exercise band so strong that you will be tired after 1 minute.
- One movement per second, for 1 minute.
- Finish by stretching.

Exercises for legs

"Stepper"

Maintain two steps per second on a mini-stepper machine for 1 minute. Adjust the resistance so your legs will be tired after 1 minute (Fig 2–20).

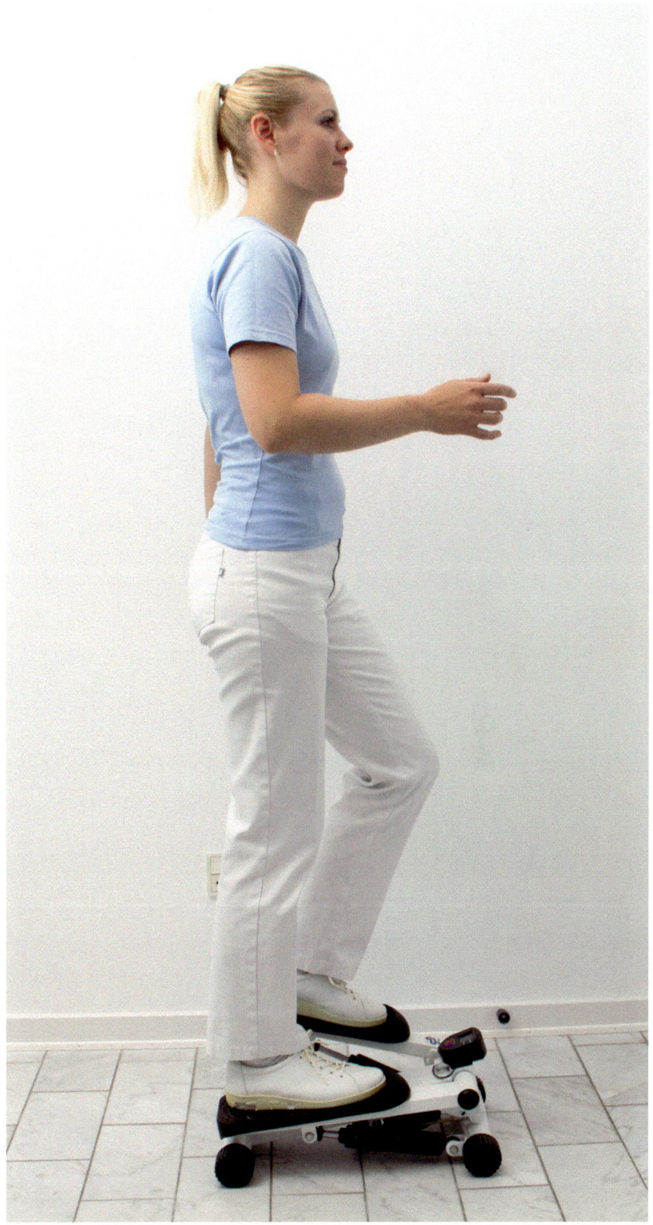

Fig 2–20 Exercises for the legs.

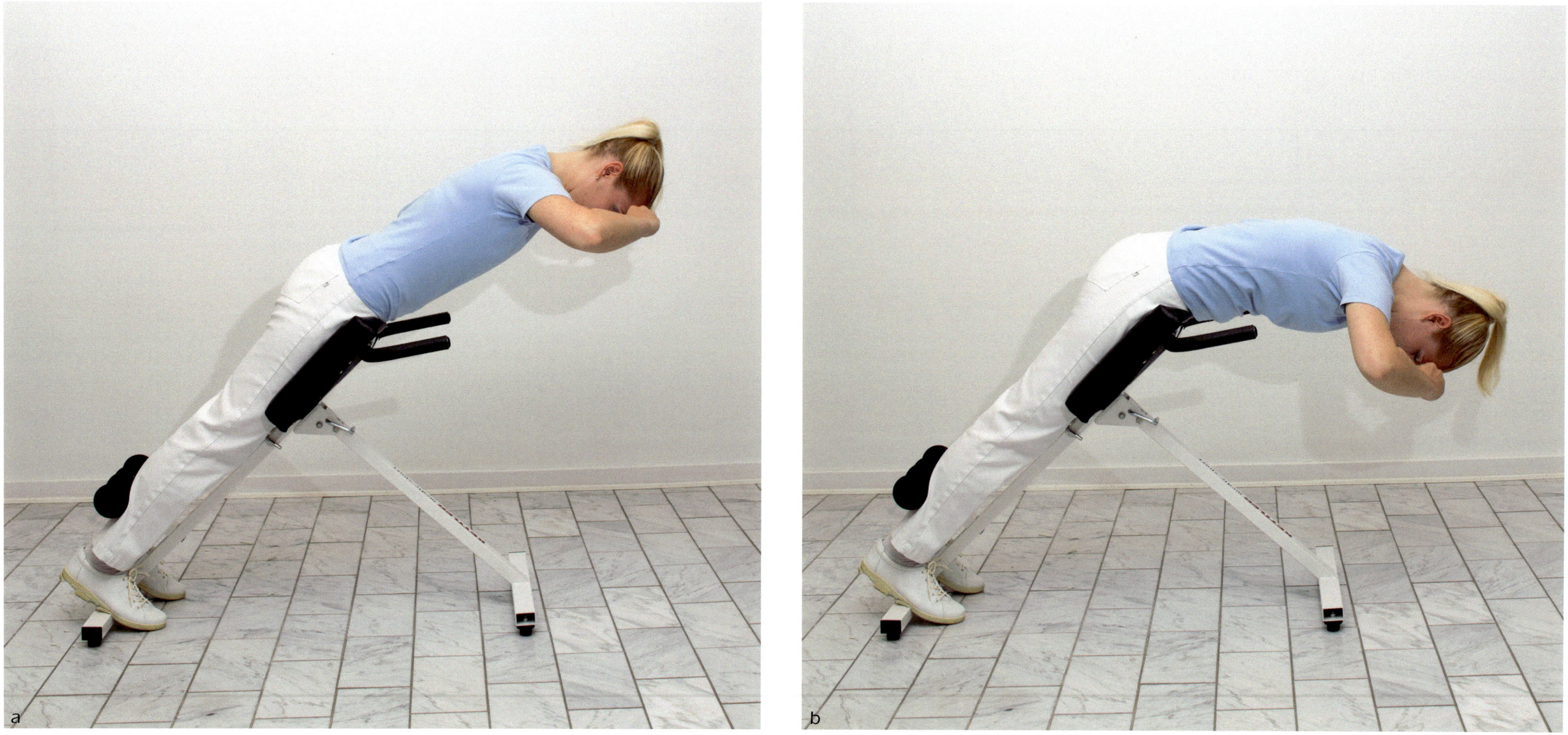

Fig 2–21 (a and b) Exercises for the back.

Exercises for the back muscles and buttocks

Use a back trainer 10 to 15 times a minute, with so much weight in your hands that you will be tired after 1 minute (Fig 2–21a and b).

THE PATIENT CHAIR

A basic principle to apply to the patient chair, is this: "The equipment of the clinic must be adapted to best work methods," and not the reverse.

The objective is that the patient can be examined and treated while lying in a comfortable horizontal position, so both assistant and dentist can look into the patient's mouth while they are sitting in good work postures.

The patient chair should be comfortable for the patient and, for the dentist, allow best possible visual and manual access to the patient's mouth (Fig 2–22).

Comfort for the patient

If leg support is inclined downwards, the seating is easier for the patient. This should particularly help when the patient has to use the cuspidor (spittoon) for mouth rinsing, making it more convenient to lean forward (Fig 2–23). The presence of an armrest or no armrest is not a major point. If armrests are chosen, the right-side one can be dismounted to facilitate access to the chair for disabled persons.

When the back of the patient chair is horizontal, it will tend to stretch the back of the patient's clothes. Reducing the length of the back of the patient chair while moving backwards prevents this discomfort. These principles are reflected in the construction of a patient chair:

- When the backrest is horizontal, and the patient is lying, there should be a convenient support for the arms of the patient.

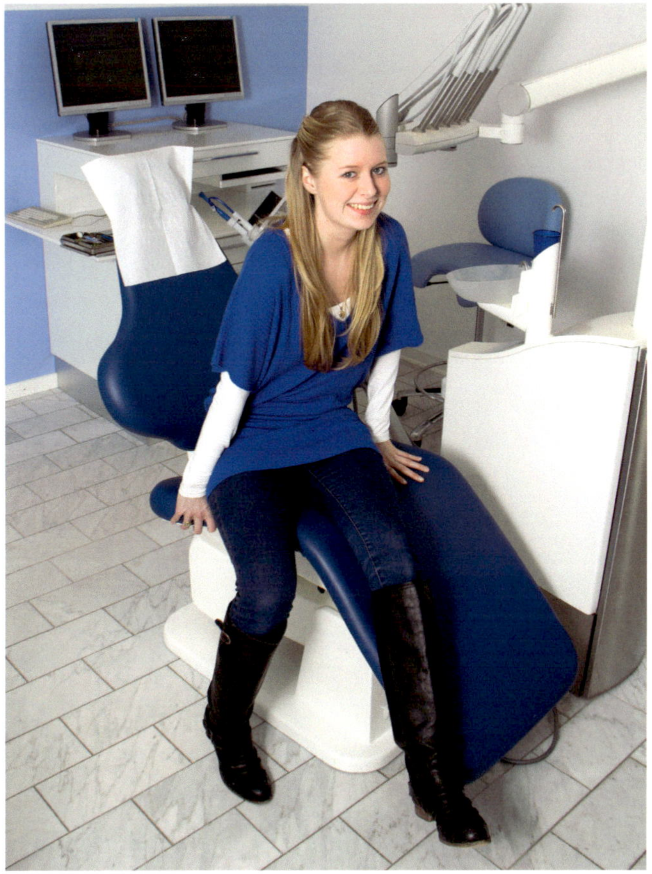

Fig 2–22 Patient seating.

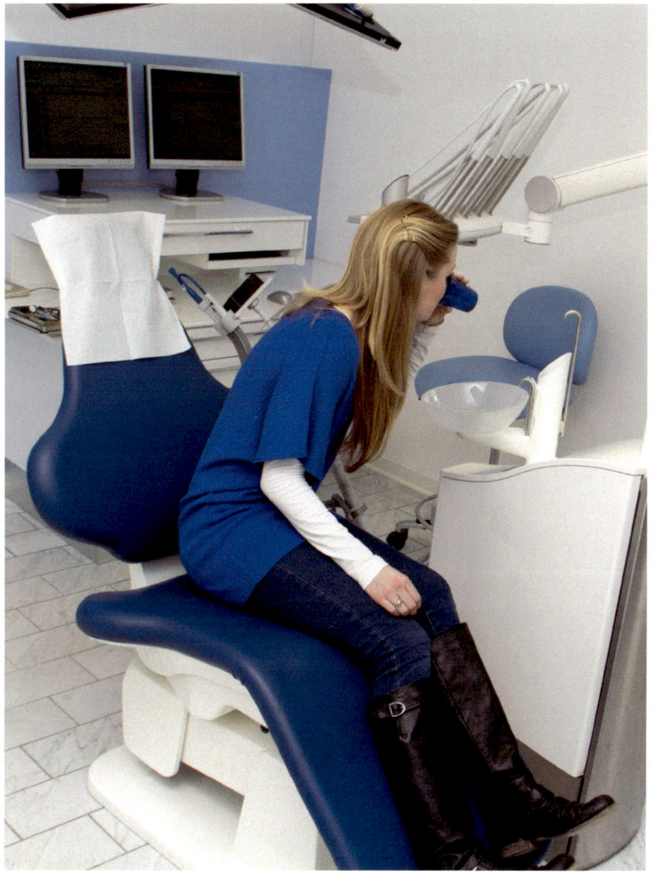

Fig 2–23 Patient rinsing.

- The upholstering should be soft and pleasant to compensate for the different "anatomy of the patient" while lying down.
- On the other side, the back of the patient chair must be thin enough to allow access for the dentist's and assistant's legs.
- The back of the patient chair should be so short that the headrest can be adjusted to the neck and the lower part of the back of the head. A great deal of patient chairs have a backrest that is too long to achieve this if the height of the patient is below average.

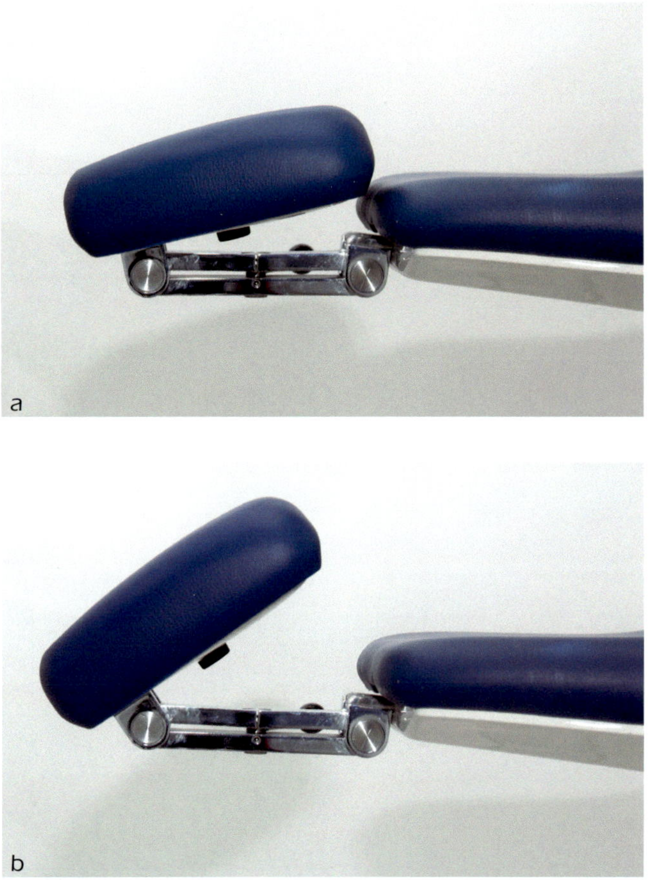

Fig 2–24 (a and b) The headrest position depends on the patient's head size and shape, and the position needed for visual access to the patient's mouth.

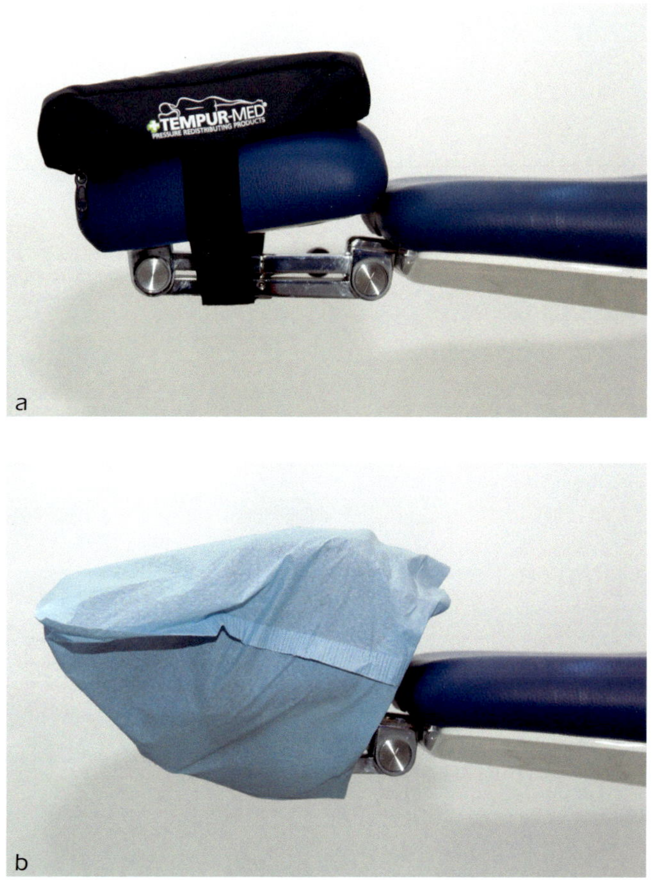

Fig 2–25 (a) Foam pillow on headrest. (b) Paper cover on foam pillow.

- If the headrest has a double articulation it is easy to adjust to patients' needs.
- The headrest often has to be elevated for increased comfort, especially for elderly patients. Sometime the elevation may be up to 15 cm for tall patients with a rounded back and neck (Fig 2–24).
- The headrest should have a comfortable shape, and many headrests are too hard to be comfortable for the patient. Your patients would be pleased if you used a thin (30 mm) supersoft foam "pillow" as a cover on the headrest (Fig 2–25a).
- It is important that the foam pillow is thin, and so flexible that the head compresses the middle of the foam pillow to a thickness of few millimeters.
- The headrest and foam pillow should both be covered with a hygienic paper bag covering, which is changed between patients (Fig 2–25b).

The horizontal position of the patient chair is very important for visual and manual access to the patient's mouth. When working in maxillary molars with distal cavities (with a distal direction of vision into the cavity), the mirror has to be placed BEHIND the tooth, and so much to the back of the mouth, that the head of the patient must – if possible – be turned backwards (Fig 2–26).

It is the same case for working in small distal cavities in molars in the mandibular jaw – the mirror is placed BEHIND the tooth. The horizontal position of the patient enables a good visual access to the mouth for the dentist. Young patients may be able turn their head backwards, but the majority of older patients find it inconvenient or impossible to do (Fig 2–27).

As the assistant does not use a mirror, her visual access to the mouth while maintaining a fine work posture is dependent on the horizontal position of the patient. It is necessary to insist on a patient chair constructed for horizontal positioning. Unfortunately

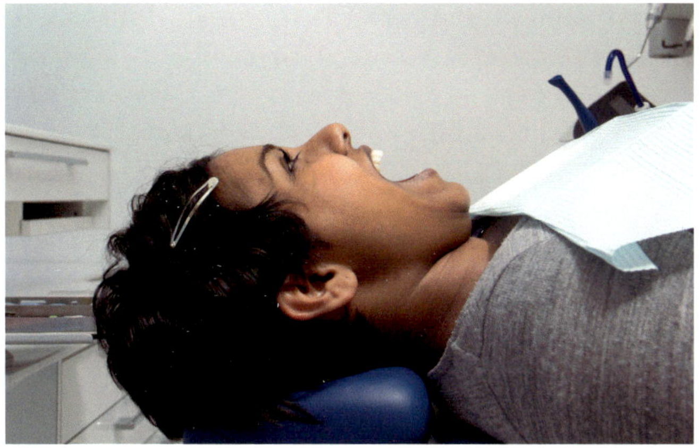

Fig 2–26 The head of the patient is placed horizontally.

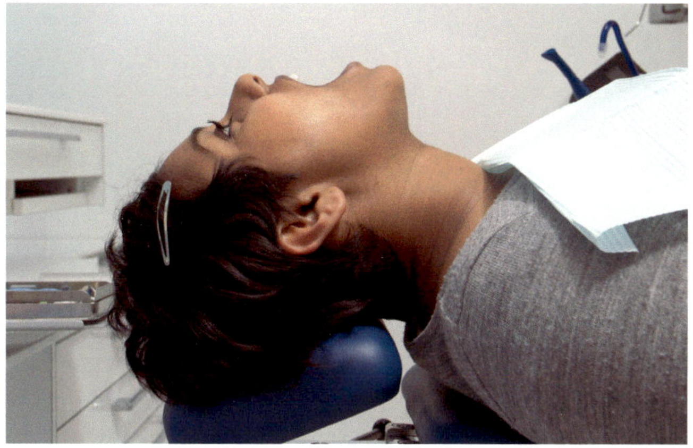

Fig 2–27 A position allowing direct vision to the occlusal and mesial aspects of the maxillary jaw – a possibility for young patients. The head of the patient is inclined backwards.

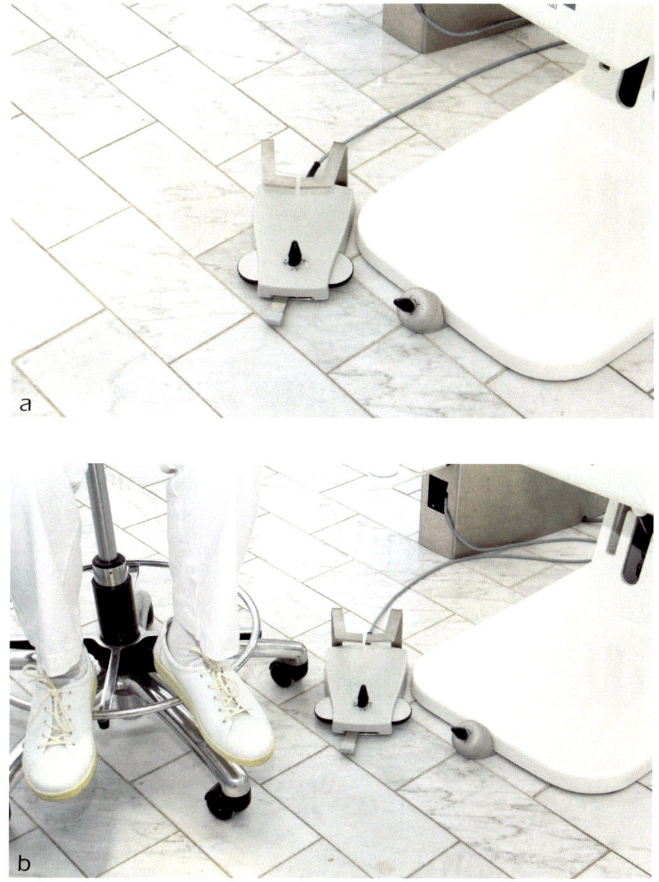

Fig 2–28 (a and b) The base of the patient chair is small.

there are several combinations of dental unit and patient chair, which propose to fulfill these requirements, yet do not do so.

A frequent reason is that when the patient chair is reclined in a horizontal position and in the correct height over the floor, a centrally placed dental unit with instruments cannot be placed over the patient for use. The support of the unit instruments is either too low so they cannot be placed over the patient, or the arm system carrying the unit instruments is so low that it touches the patient.

Important

When the backrest is placed in a horizontal position, it should be at least 80 cm above the floor, and for taller dentists from 157 to 180 cm, it should be 90 cm above the floor.

The patient chair must be moved upwards into a position that the dentist is able to work in, with a distance for precision vision of about 32 cm (sometimes less for younger dentists), and be able to sit well (maintaining lumbar curvature, keeping the head up while working with inclined eyes).

The height of the dentist's and assistant's sitting position will depend on the inclination of the thighs while sitting in a balanced position. The back of the patient chair while in a horizontal position should, for tall dentists, be about 90 cm and for dentists under average height, about 60 cm.

The base of the chair

The patient chair should be small enough (Fig 2–28) that there is sufficient room under the chair for the foot controller at the left side of the midline. This position of the foot controller allows the dentist to work in the different "clock positions" (9, 10, 11 and 12 o'clock) without having to move it any further, because it is placed close to the center of this quarter of a circle-movements.

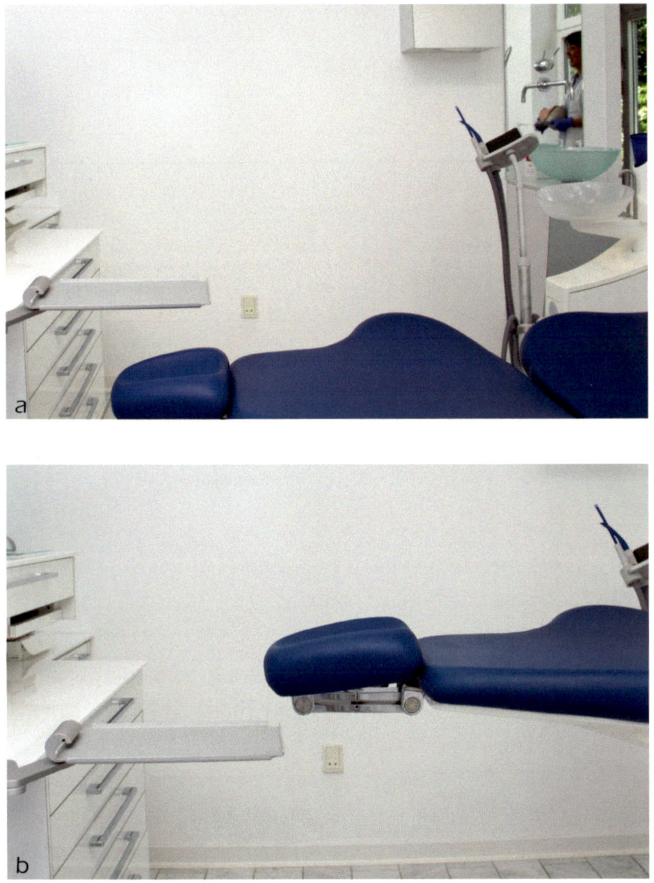

Fig 2–29 (a and b) Measuring horizontal movement when the chair is moved up.

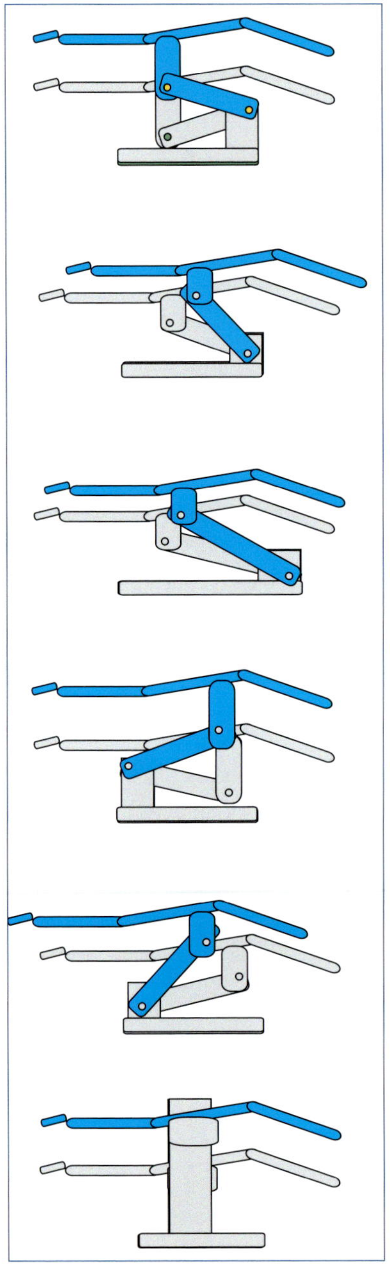

Fig 2–30 The horizontal movement of the chair when moved upwards is dependent on the geometry of the supporting "arm system."

Attention! Many patient chairs move horizontally when they are moved upwards

When close to their top height position, chairs with a floor-base move in the direction of the patient's feet. This is caused by the "parallel arm system" carrying them. The horizontal movement may be up to (and sometimes more) than 15 cm (Figs 2–29 and 2–30).

The higher the patient chair is positioned, the more it moves in the direction of the patient's feet. This influences the measurements for the positioning of the patient chair. The patient chair has to have a precise relation to the workplace, therefore the measurements of the exact position of chair and dental unit must be calculated both with the chair back in a horizontal position, and also in a vertical working position for the dentist who going to use it, depending on his/her sitting position and how tall she/he is.

Children in the patient chair

For small children, the movement of the patient chair back could be a bit frightening. The chair could be adjusted to a horizontal position before the child arrives to the treatment room. She or he could be lifted to the patient chair by her/his parents or by the dentist (Figs 2–31 to 2–34).

All children should lie down with their head on the headrest, otherwise the sitting posture of both dentist and assistant will be very bad. With slightly older children, the movements of the patient chair could be made more fun by calling it the "Apollo Airspace Chair," for example.

If the child starts by sitting in the patient chair, she/he – when the back of the chair is reclined to a horizontal position – can be carefully slid up into the chair by pulling under the elbows, until the child's head is placed on the headrest of the chair.

Funny dental unit instruments

To put a nervous child at ease, the multifunction syringe can be mounted with a little toy animal, eg, a cat, and we can talk with the little cat, which wants to blow a bit of air on a finger first, and maybe a little later on a tooth. The dentist takes on the voice of the toy animal.

If, unfortunately, the examination reveals a caries attack, then other instrument supports may be mounted with a teddy bear or other soft stuffed animal, which now start to talk with each other.

With the animals mounted on the dental unit tubing, the child sees the whole visit as fun.

The treatment of children needs a highly skilled team

If children need treatment, the principles of vision and manual techniques are the same as for adult patients. However the visual and manual access to a small mouth is more difficult than for an adult's. In addition, a fast treatment may often be very important, so the skills of the team should be highly trained for treating children. When using a mirror, a smaller version may be preferred.

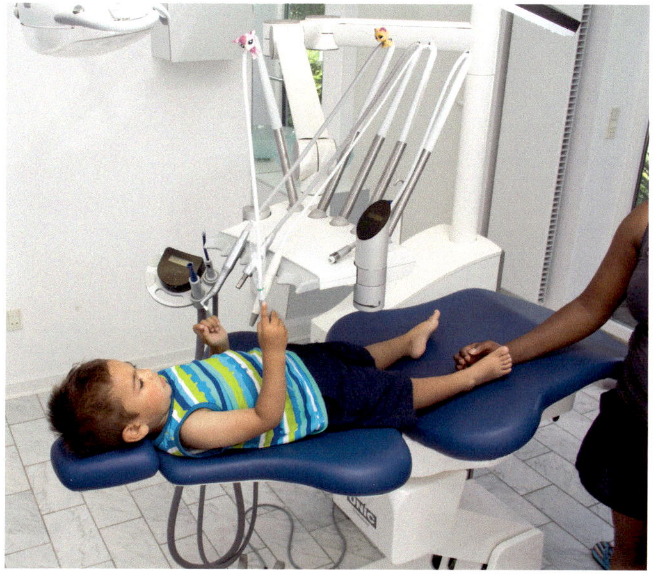

Fig 2–31 Putting a child at ease in the patient chair.

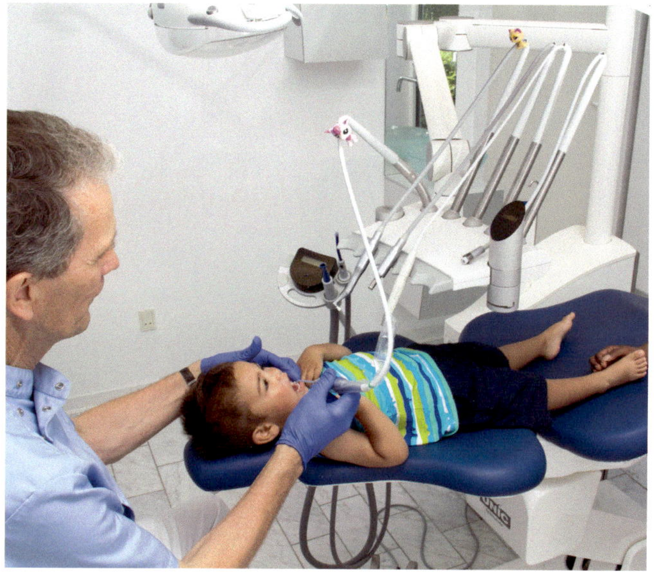

Fig 2–32 The dentist talks reassuringly while preparing the hand instrument.

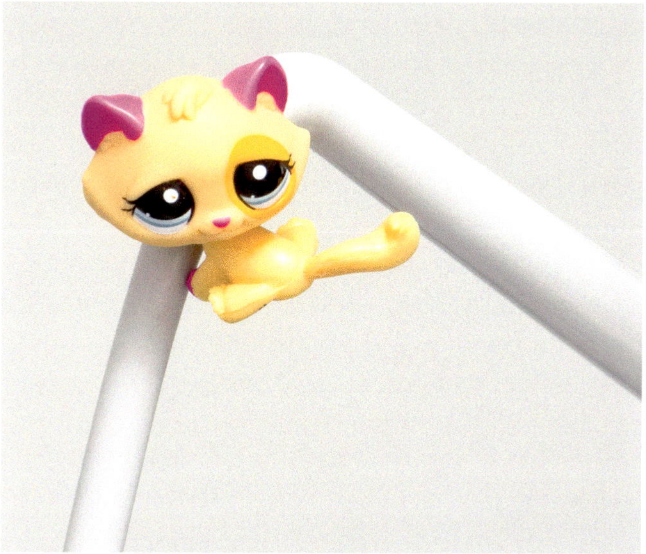

Fig 2–33 A small toy can be mounted on the unit syringe.

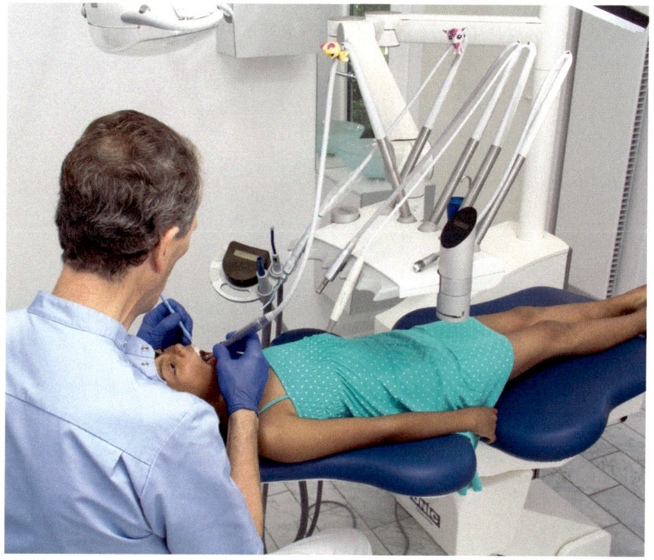

Fig 2–34 The child now relaxed, the dentist works on the teeth.

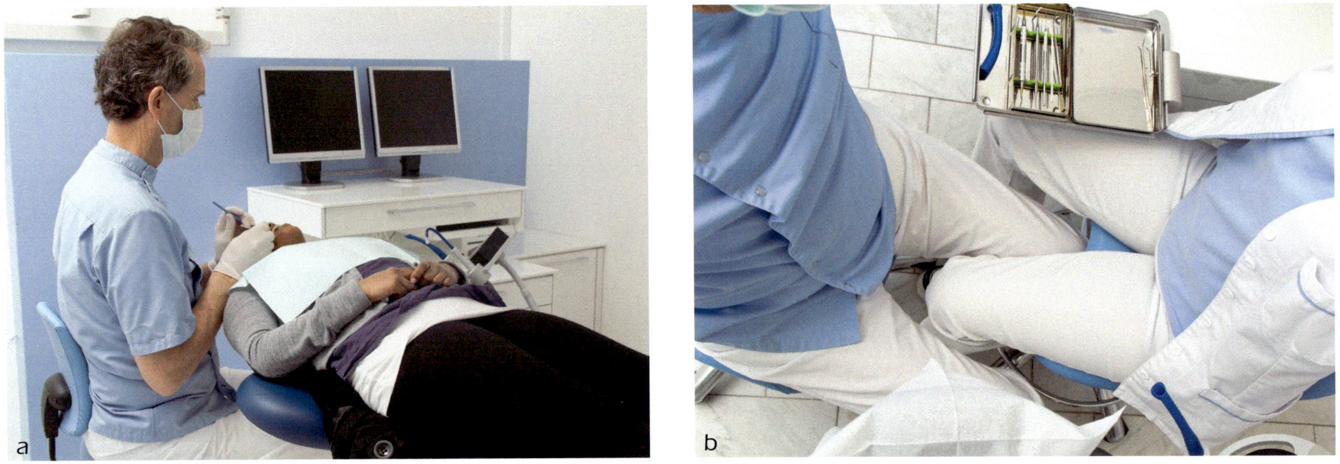

Fig 2–35 (a) Dentist sits at 9 o' clock. (b) Assistant sits at 3 o'clock.

DENTIST AND ASSISTANT SITTING POSITION

While dentist and assistant are working in a team, both have to be able to see the performance of tasks in the patient's mouth.

The need for visual precision is different however. Dentists have to see with a maximum visual acuity of about 0.1 mm for performing precision work, however the visual precision of 2 to 3 mm is sufficient for the assistant to precisely position a suction tip, or for drying a surface with a multifunction syringe.

The dentist needs to be able to work at a 9–10 o'clock position when looking at the right side of teeth (Fig 2–35a).

Meanwhile, the assistant needs to be able to sit in a 3 o'clock position for assisting in the patient's mouth (Fig 2–35b), and furthermore needs to be able to turn about 30 degrees to her right side to be able to prepare materials, mix liner, etc.

The solution to this is intercrossed legs (a technique used for more than 40 years). It is possible to combine both the mobility of dentist and assistant with a balanced sitting position, with the thighs angled forward.

When the dentist is working in a 12 o'clock position in order to look at the left side of the teeth, the patient's head is turned towards the right side (Fig 2–36). This means that the assistant cannot see anything in the left side of the mouth and when she is using a suction tip, she has to be guided by the dentist.

An argument for having a sitting position higher than the dentist is that it improves the vision into the mouth of the patient. But that is not sufficient when the patient's head is turned to the right.

The foot controller is placed for use by the dentist's right foot. The position of the foot controller does not need to be changed when the dentist changes clock position, but may be used by the dentist's left foot in a 12 o'clock position (Fig 2–37).

If the dentist is working in an 11 to 12 o'clock position for a long sitting, then the assistant could sit with both her legs parallel.

If possible, the assistant should sit at the same height as the dentist, but as her legs are partly placed under the back of the patient chair, this limits her vertical position. If the assistant is about 12 cm or more lower than the dentist, then her stool must be fitted with a ring for foot support when she sits at about the same vertical level as the

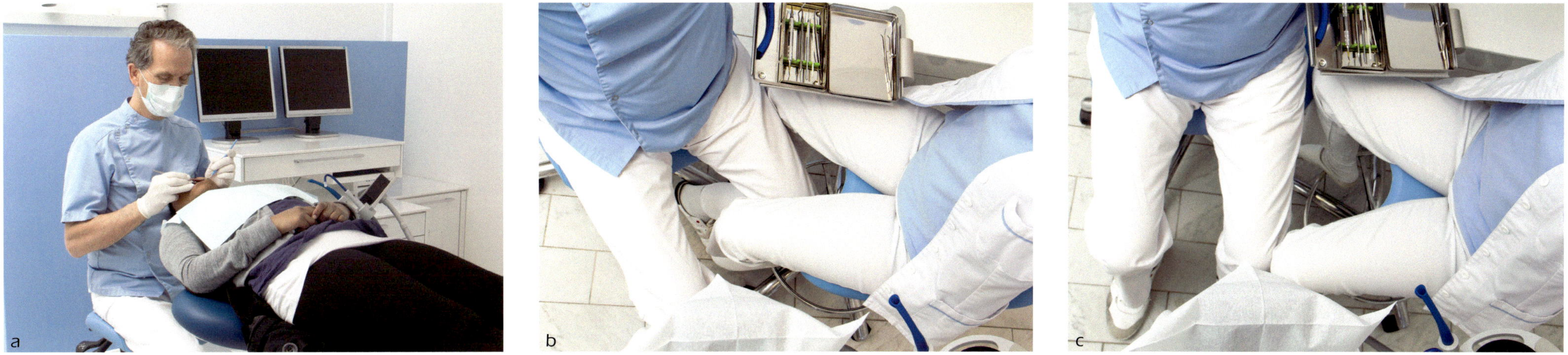

Fig 2–36 (a, b and c) Assistant sits at 3 o'clock, dentist at 12 o' clock.

dentist. When the assistant is preparing materials and instruments, she can turn her stool to the right to face the work module (Fig 2–38).

In photos from early 1960s, one could see a different sitting position, where assistants wearing skirts sat with legs together and beside the dentist. It will be difficult for her to face the patient, and to use unit instruments and a suction holder without twisting to the left. She is sitting higher than the dentist, supposedly to have a better vision, but as described before, the vision is lost in the left side of the mouth in any case when the patient turns their head a little towards the right side to improve vision for the dentist. Sitting higher, she may have trouble finding space for her legs under the back of the patient chair. This habit, although not the most functional, seems to

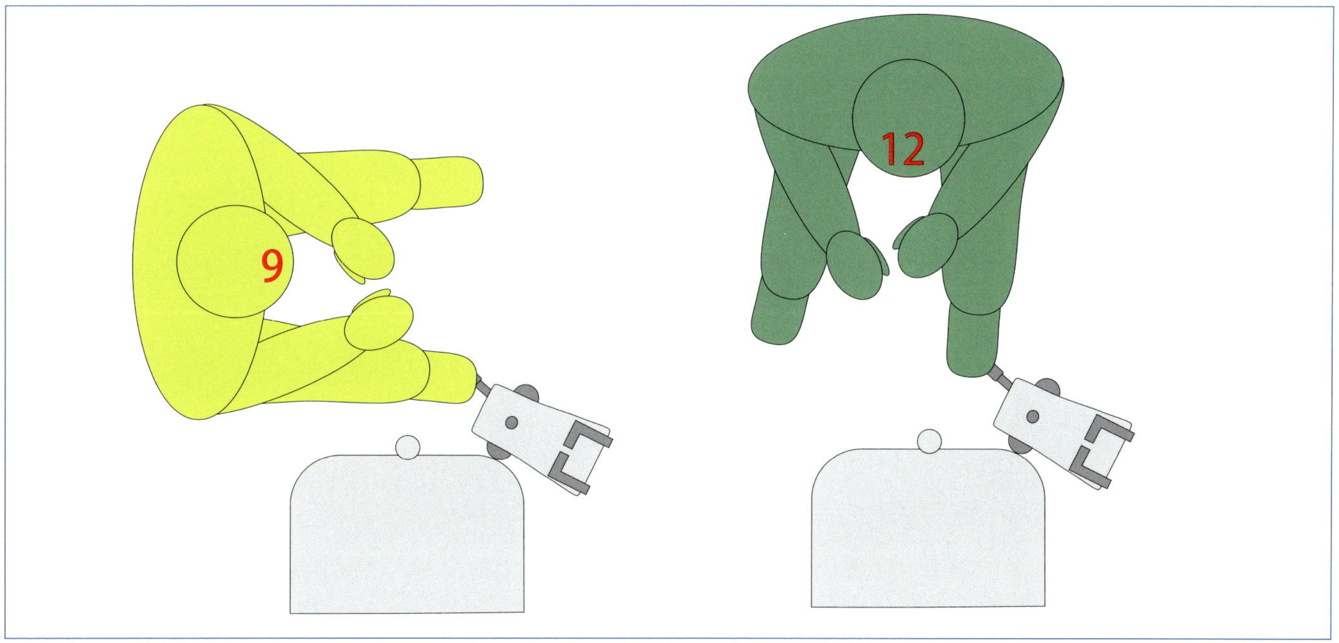

Fig 2–37 The dentist's foot controller.

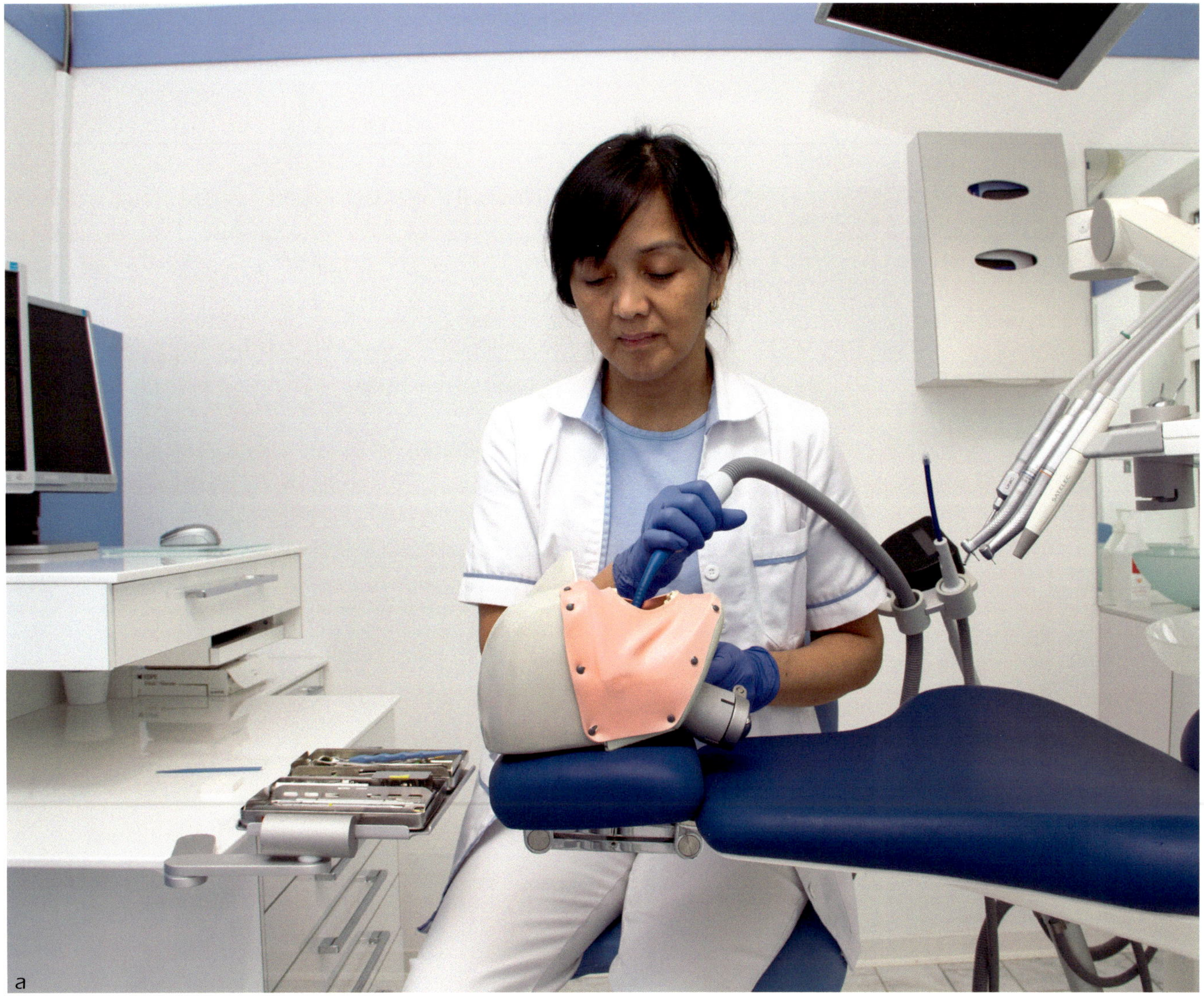

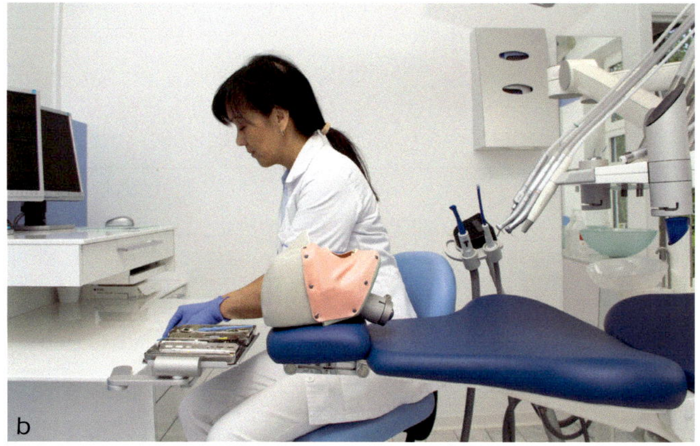

Fig 2–38 (a and b) Assistant turns to the right for mixing materials.

have been accepted in Anglo-Saxon countries without being questioned.

Times have changed since. Skirts are now replaced by a clinical dress with slacks, and a balanced sitting position with thighs inclined forward is the accepted standard (and has been for the past 30 years). Therefore the intercrossed leg position is recommended. It reduces the risk of the assistant twisting her back, and facilitates the use of aspiration tubes placed close to the dental unit, which also aids the simultaneous pick up of the tubes and 3-in-1 syringe, as well as other unit instruments.

HELPING PATIENTS ACCEPT HORIZONTAL POSITIONING

Stepwise adaption

The patient is invited to sit in the patient chair, and in most cases it is easiest to get into the patient chair from the side. After a friendly chat, it is time to look at the teeth.

In order to be able to see into the mouth and sit in good work postures, we now would like our patient to lie down. Moving the back of the chair downwards may sometimes create strong feelings in the patient. The movement of the back of the chair will be felt as a falling motion, without knowing where the movement will stop. This may activate our vestibular reflexes of equilibrium and cause anxiety. If the patients are not prepared for the movement, some remain in a sitting position, even when the back of the patient chair is moving down.

To lie down in front of another person is a position of submission. This too may cause anxiety. Some patients also need a little time for their blood pressure to adjust to being in a horizontal position, and feel a too-fast movement as being physically unpleasant.

How does one take care of the anxious feelings of the patient? You could say something as follows:

Dentist: "Mrs Miller! We would like to make a relaxed examination of your teeth..." *[short pause with eye contact].*

"OK? Therefore Mrs Miller I would like to ask that you are happy for us to move the back of your chair downwards, because then it is very easy to look at your teeth."
[Pause so the patient can process and think about this.]

Dentist: "Is that OK? We will move the back of the chair down in steps so you can adapt to the position, and I will be right beside you."
[Pause for the patient to imagine this.]

If the patient is very anxious, the dentist could slightly touch the right shoulder of the patient while moving the chair back (in most cultures this will be acceptable).

Dentist: "Are you ready Mrs Miller?"
The foot controller is now activated and the back of the patient chair is moving downwards. The dentist is sitting beside the patient ready to interrupt the automatic movement.

About halfway down, the movement is interrupted for a short pause of maybe 15 seconds, so the patient can physically and mentally adapt to the position. The face of Mrs Miller is observed, and if her facial expression becomes tense with signs of anxiety, the movement of the chair back is interrupted in an earlier stage.

When the patient seems to be ready, you can ask if the back of the chair may be moved further in order to improve visibility towards the teeth. The backrest is again moved down, but may be interrupted again, this time perhaps with the headrest 10 cm above the horizontal. The final movement is made later.

The headrest should have a supersoft cover so the patient feels comfortable. Often the headrest for elderly patients is placed much too low – some sleep with two pillows under their head.

It is some dentists' experience that some patients will not accept a horizontal position, while others almost never encounter this, independent of patients, country and culture. The difference lies more with the dentist than by the patient. Using a careful approach, emotional empathy and well-trained contact with the patient, along with a step-by-step motivation and adaption (as in the case of Mrs Miller, left), almost all patients can accept a lying position for dental examination and treatment.

STAYING CONCENTRATED – BLOOD SUGAR MANAGEMENT

The glycemic index of food

Our brain represents about 2% of our bodyweight, receives 15% of cardiac output, 20% of total body oxygen consumption and 10% of blood sugar glucose.

The blood sugar of a healthy person has a level from 4 to 8 mmol/l and can change throughout the day. Variations of the blood sugar level can be different for everyone, independent or dependent of what has been eaten.

Working attention and concentration often has a close relation to blood sugar level. Some persons are sensitive to low levels of blood sugar. The symptoms may include lack of concentration, irritability, fatigue, blurred vision, hunger and the craving for sugar. The symptoms of low blood sugar will disappear 10 to 15 minutes after eating sugar or some other sweet food. But shortly afterwards, the blood sugar level may drop again.

To maintain full concentration throughout the working day, it is important for persons sensitive to low blood sugar to keep a stable blood sugar level. This can be obtained by eating food with a low and slow ability to cause a peak rise in blood sugar, and therefore keep it stable for longer. (This food is described as having a "low glycemic index.") So to maintain good concentration, instead of eating a few large meals, the solution is to eat smaller meals every 2 to 3 hours, consisting of food with a low glycemic index.

Chapter 3

PRECISION VISION

EYES AND PRECISION VISION

As having precision vision is mandatory for precision work, it is important to know some basic functions and aspects of vision that have practical implications for the dentist.

You will as a dentist have to deal with some of the following aspects of vision while at work. When traditionally constructed spectacles or loupes are used, they may lead to serious health risks for a dentist's neck and shoulders. The following chapter provides basic knowledge about how this can be avoided, so you can specify your demands to the optician. Experience shows that you yourself will need to provide these specifications, which are seldom known by opticians. For more information (including illustrations), refer to **www.wikipedia.com**, using the headlines in following pages as search words.

Visual acuity or "sharpness of vision," and its "resolving power" are an indication of the clarity or clearness of your vision. Visual acuity is measured in arc minutes, and defined as the minimal gap between two black lines to be distinguished. Normal visual acuity corresponds to 1 arcminute, and should be measured by test cards. The most used is the so-called Snellen card, with lines of letters in different sizes.

A "normal vision" is described at being 6/6, which means that at a distance of 6 m from a Snellen card, you can see the same as a "normal person." If the vision is for example 6/4, from a distance of 6 m you can see the same as a "normal person" can see at a distance of 4 m. This is considerably better than average vision.

Vision of 6/8 means that from a distance of 6 m, one can see the same as a "normal person" can see at 8 m, which means below average vision.

In the USA, where feet are used as the unit of measurement instead, this will correspond as 20/20, because 6 meters are close to being equal to 20 feet (often described as having "20/20" vision).

A person with so called "normal vision" (6/6) can see a gap of 1.75 mm between two black lines at a distance of 6 m (20 feet). This corresponds to 1 minute of arc, and to a little less than 1/10 mm at an eye-to-object distance of 30 cm.

Convergence of the eye

When looking at an object, both eyes must be directed towards the object. The convergence is connected to the accommodation of the eye. When focusing at an object from a distance, the convergence and accommodation will happen automatically.

Strabismus

Strabismus is a condition where the eyes are not aligned in the same direction. The muscles of the eyes can compensate for strabismus to a certain extent.

However, in the case of a latent strabismus, the muscles become tense in order to direct the eyes towards a visual object, and the eyes may not be able to look inclined downwards as far as 45 degrees. Latent strabismus may also result in making it tiring to focus at short distances.

Loupes may be a solution to augment the working distance (eg, to 40 cm) to reduce the stress caused to the eye muscles to converge.

Pupils

Pupil (iris) constriction has a double purpose. It reduces the intensity of light to the eyes, when the incoming light is extreme. Pupil constriction focuses the incoming light to the middle of the lens where the refraction of light is more precise, and focuses light to the most sensitive part of the retina, the macula.

Accommodation of the lens

The lens is suspended in fibers attached to the ring-shaped ciliary muscles. When the ciliary muscle is relaxed, the fibers are tense and the lens is flatter.

When the ciliary muscle is tense, the fibers are relaxed along with the lens, which contracts into a more convex shape that refracts the light more, allowing the eye to focus on closer objects. If looking to the side, the distance from the object to the right and left eye is different, so accommodation of both eyes is not possible.

Precision vision by both eyes is therefore impeded. For precision vision, the object of vision must be placed in the mid-saggital plane of the dentist's head.

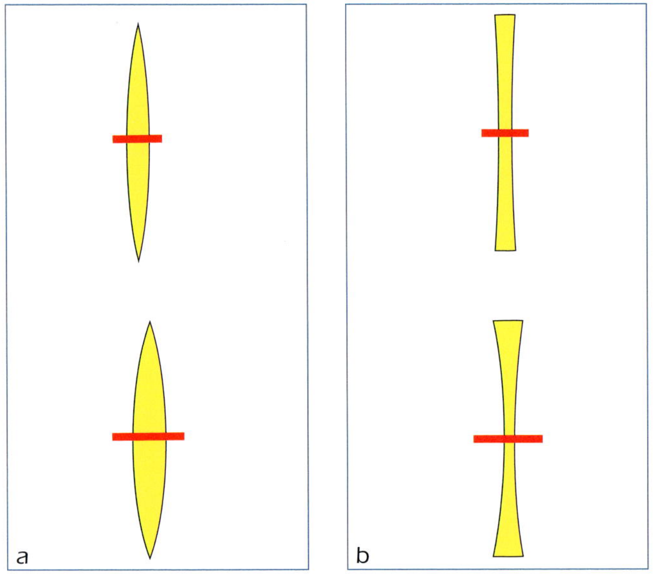

Fig 3–1 (a) Convex lenses. (b) Concave lenses.

Optical correction

If the optical system of the eye does not create a sharp picture on the retina, optical correction with glasses or contact lenses is necessary.

The lenses may be convex (Fig 3–1a) or concave (Fig 3–1b). The curvature is measured in diopters, which is a measure for the lens ability to collimate or dissipate a beam of light.

A lens that collimates a beam of light to a point (burning point) after 1 m has +1 diopter. A lens which spreads (dissipates) parallel light to the point where it meets with the other (burning point) is 1 m behind the lens – 1 diopter (dioptri).

Young children have an accommodation of 15 to 20 diopters, while persons of age 25 have an accommodation of about 10 diopters. For persons aged 50+, the accommodation is reduced to about 1 diopter.

Spherical aberration

Spherical aberration is a distortion of the visual field, which is likened to looking through a prism.

Chromatics aberration

Chromatics aberration is a "rainbow effect" best seen at margins and lines, which is visible while looking through a prism.

These two disturbing "prism effect" aberrations will occur while looking "oblique" through margins of corrective lenses. The stronger the force of the lenses, the stronger effect of the abberations.

Hyperopia (far-sightedness)

With hyperopia, the picture is created behind the retina, which can be corrected with convex lenses. The best vision is gained when looking through the optical mid-axis of the lenses.

Looking at an oblique angle, particularly through the margins, causes disturbing spherical and chromatic aberration. This phenomenon will be intensified the stronger the lens is (measured in diopters).

Myopia (near-sightedness)

For myopia, the picture is created in front of the retina. It can be corrected with concave lenses. The best vision is achieved when looking through the optical mid-axis of the lenses.

As with hyperopia, looking at an oblique angle, especially through the margins, causes disturbing spherical and chromatic aberration. The effect is intensified the stronger the lens is.

Astigmatism

Astigmatism may or may not be combined with hyperopia or myopia. Astigmatism occurs when the front surface of your eye (cornea) or the lens, inside your eye, has a surface that is not even and smooth curved in all directions. The surface may have some areas that are flatter or steeper. Either type of astigmatism can cause blurred vision.

The best solution is by wearing corrective glasses, with a curvature correcting the optics of the eye. The stronger the astigmatismatic correction, the more important it is to look through the mid-axis of the glasses.

Presbyopia

Presbyopia is a loss of focusing range due to aging. The ability to accommodate is gradually diminished because the flexibility of the lens of the eye is reduced.

When the supporting fibers to the lens are relaxed by the contraction of the ciliary muscle, the lens should relax and be more rounded. This effect is reduced when the lens is less flexible. Where young eyes may accommodate for vision, from say 20 cm to infinity, the accommodation to short distances is gradually reduced. The width of accommodation can be measured and calculated by a skilled optometrist.

If the lenses of the glasses are calculated for precision vision from 30 cm as the shortest distance, the width of accommodation will decide the upper limit of precision vision using these spectacles. For example, say it is from 30 to 120 cm. In this case, it will be possible to look into the patient's mouth with precision vision, and also to clearly see people's faces when you are talking to them, with the same glasses.

You will not be able see sharply at longer distances, and you may choose to accept this, as long you are inside the practice working. However, if you do need to see sharply at longer distances, then your glasses should have two forces. This means wearing bifocal lenses, with a weaker upper part and a stronger force at the lower part of the spectacles.

With increasing age, the width of accommodation while wearing your glasses will be even smaller, say from 30 cm to 38 cm. This means you (with the aid of these spectacles) will see sharply from a distance of 30 to 38 cm. In this case, it is very important that the closest distance for sharp vision is 30 to 32 cm and no less (because then the upper limit of sharp vision will be reduced too). The width of accommodation will also have a strong influence on your work posture. A normal distance for reading is about 40 to 60 cm, which means that your spectacles made for distances 30 to 38 cm cannot be used for reading. The distance is too short. You will need spectacles for performing dentistry, and other (weaker) spectacles for reading. Even looking at a computer screen at a distance of 80 cm may even require another pair of glasses with a different strength.

Precision vision is essential for the correct diagnosis and treatment of patients in dental practice. Therefore the dentist's vision should be monitored regularly (ideally at least once a year), to identify any possible need for corrective spectacles.

GLASSES AND WORKING POSTURE

The health risks

The head of the working dentist can only be tilted about 10 degrees forward. Bending the neck makes further inclination. This causes a compression of the forward part of the intervertebral discs, and if done excessively for a long time every day throughout the years, it can lead to arthrosis and/or a partial or total collapse of the discs. A prolapse of the discs, creating compression of the nerves, may also happen. Furthermore, even after a short time muscular discomfort, tensions and further pain can result. To prevent this, the eyes have to be inclined downwards as much as possible (and necessary) within the margins of comfort.

The design of spectacles undergoes the trends of fashion. Sometimes they are very large, sometimes they are small, sometimes there are no spectacle frames and sometimes the frames are prominent. A standard design of spectacles may often interfere working with inclined eyes, and are often in conflict with our needs.

A pictorial description of what dentists should avoid with their glasses is depicted in Figs 3–2 to 3–6.

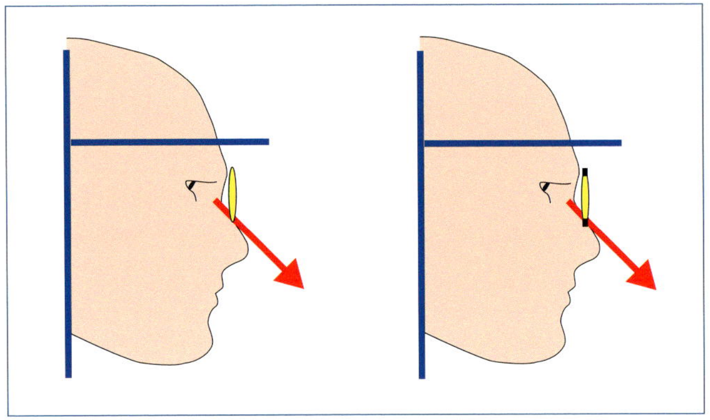

Fig 3–2 The lower margins of the glasses lenses are so high that 45-degree inclined vision is not possible. The frame of the glasses is too thick.

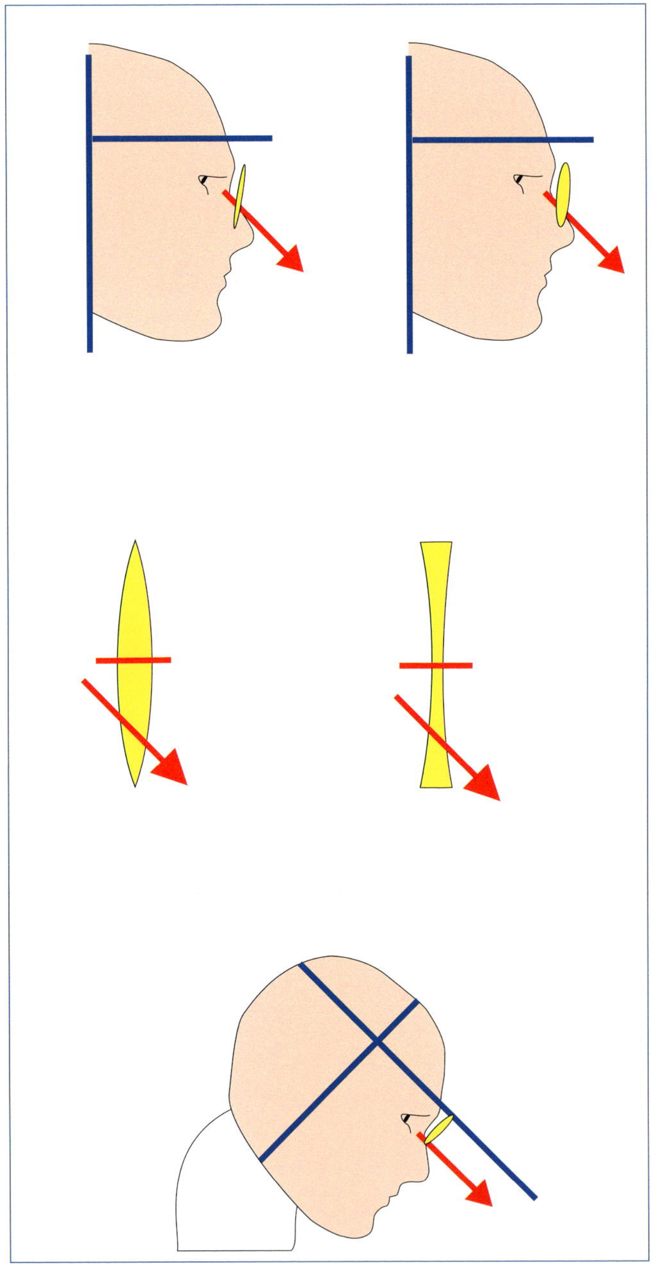

Fig 3–3 The lack of inclination for the spectacle lenses means that the dentist looks obliquely through the lenses. If the strength of the lenses is more than 1 to 1.25 diopters, this will result in visible spherical and chromatic aberration, with a prism effect in the margins of the lenses. If the dentist inclines the neck (and head) in order to look through the lenses in the direction of their geometrical axis, it will create a very bad posture.

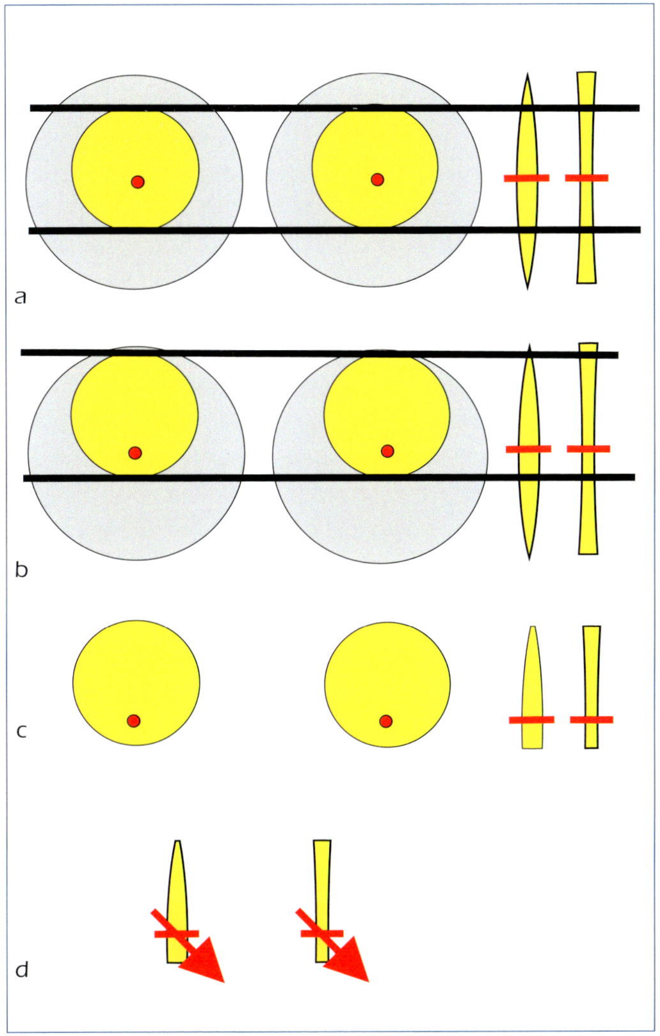

Fig 3–4 The lenses for the glasses (yellow) may be cut from a larger lens (gray) made in a factory. (a) The optical center of the lenses (so-called "pupillary points") is not placed at a low position, according to the inclined direction of vision. (b and c) The lenses are cut so the optical center is 40 to 45 degrees below the horizontal. (d) This means that looking obliquely through the lenses will result in minimal spherical and chromatic aberration.

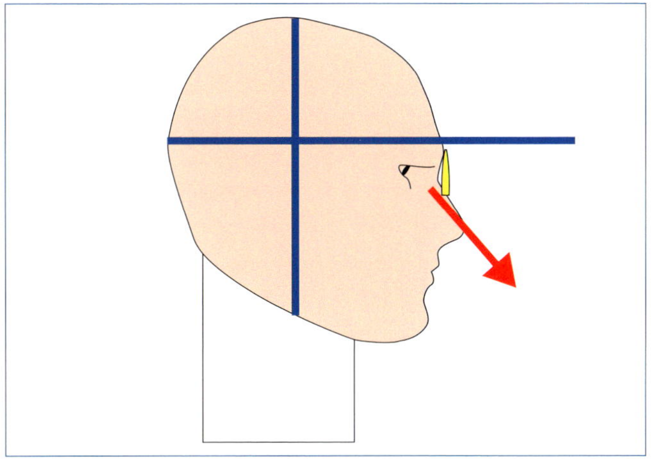

Fig 3–5 Glasses with the lower margin placed high, and with space free under the glasses. The dentist needs to incline the head and bend the neck very much in order to look 45 degrees downwards (and imagine how the posture will be in a situation where vertical direction may be needed).

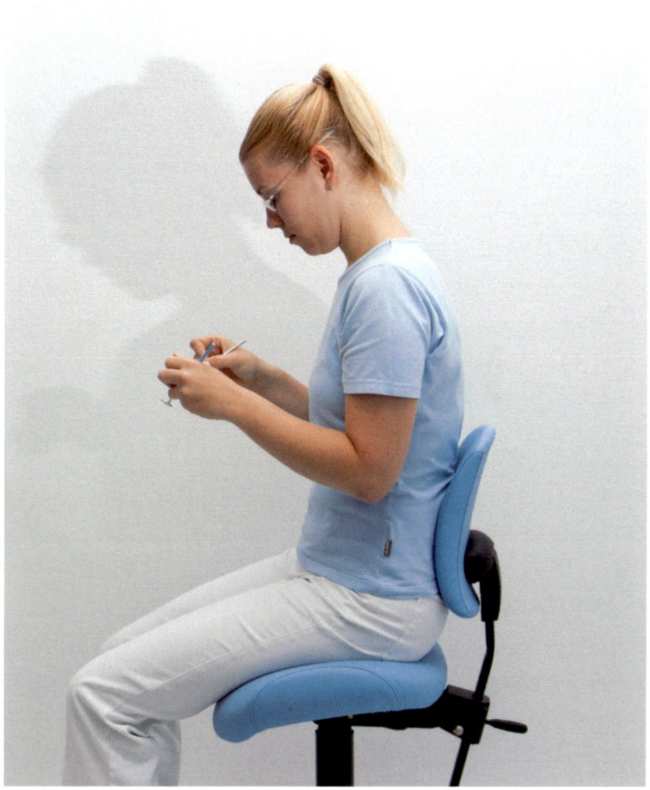

Fig 3–6 The dentist is wearing glasses enabling a 45-degree downwards inclined vision (also see Fig 3-8).

Dentist's responsibility

One would expect that the solutions to these problems are well known to opticians, optometrists or eye doctors. But unfortunately that seems not to be the case. And one has to admit, that some of the "problems" are not easy to solve.

Apparently, we as dentists must take on the responsibility for the design of glasses for use in our profession.

Demands for glasses

There is a demand for glasses to have a 45-degree downward-inclined vision. The lower margins of the glasses must be placed so low that they almost touch the dentist's cheek. The frame of the glasses here must be absent or very thin. As the shape of the cheek is a different size here, the position of the lower part of the spectacles will differ. Therefore, a standard frame often cannot

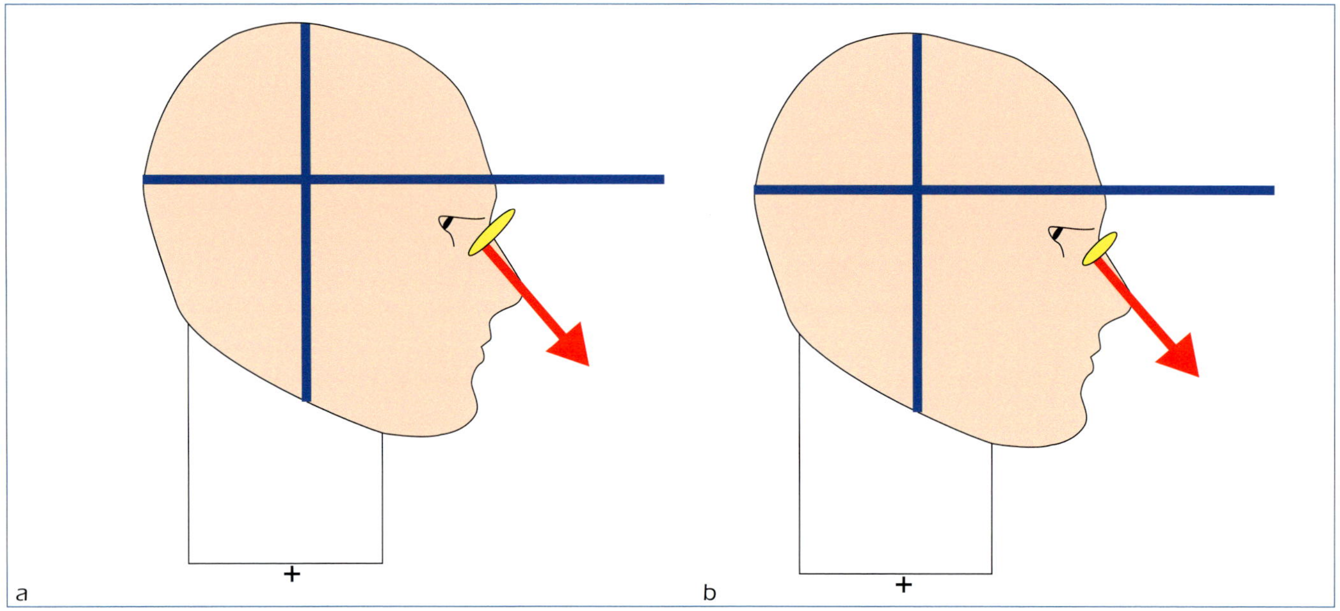

Fig 3–7 (a) The glasses are ideally inclined at the direction of vision. (b) The effect is greater with concave lenses.

be used. Frameless spectacles may be used, where the lower margin of the lenses is cut after individual design.

Ideally, the direction of vision through the lenses of the spectacles should be the same as the geometric axis of the glasses. If that is not the case, the image of the objects seen through the glasses will be distorted (Figs 3–7a and 3–7b).

The reason for this distortion is the "spherical aberrance" caused by the refraction of the rays of light. This effect will be intensified with concave lenses (negative diopters), because the glass here is thick at the margins.

The frame of the glasses must be carefully selected to allow this inclination and take into account that the nose support will have a different width, as compared to standard spectacles.

If the glasses have a threadlike frame of titanium wire for example, the frame can be bent at the base of the ear support to create the best inclination of the glasses. The glasses must be prescribed with the optical center inclined downwards at 35 degrees. The distortion of vision is absent if you are looking through the middle of the lenses in the direction of the lenses' optical axis.

KEEP YOUR HEAD UP WITH INCLINED PRECISION VISION GLASSES

Here is an example of a glasses frame tailor-made for a dentist's precision work:

- Inclination is 45 degrees and the optical center is 35 degrees below horizontal
- The frame is custom-made by hand
- Weight of about 4 g, which is difficult to feel.

The frame of this prototype is handmade by the author, from 1 mm orthodontic wire. The size of the spectacles lenses allows visibility to the "full head" of the patient. If a larger face protector is wanted, it can be used as a supplement. Most patients find **mini-spectacles** smart and professional looking!

The author has made a number of these mini-spectacles for colleagues. Do consider a pair of these precision vision glasses if you need to keep your head up – please visit www.netergonomie.com for further details.

If correction with glasses is needed for general vision above the mini-spectacles, they may be combined with glasses with low margins placed high. The lenses are inclined so the optical axis is almost inclined 35 degrees. Then you will see through the lenses of the spectacles in a direction from 35 degrees ± 10 degrees, which is from 25 to 45 degrees (Figs 3–8 and 3–9).

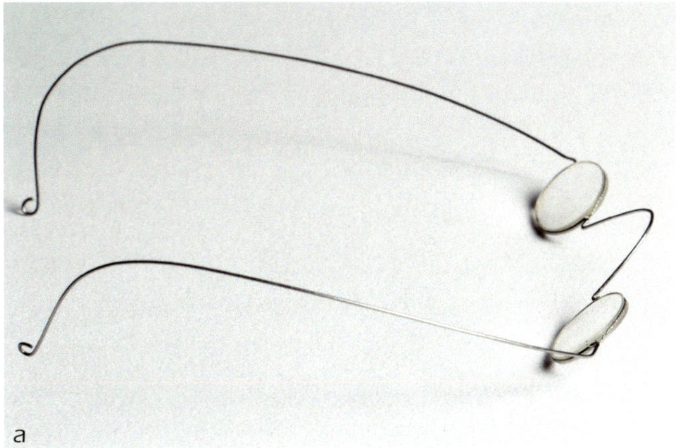

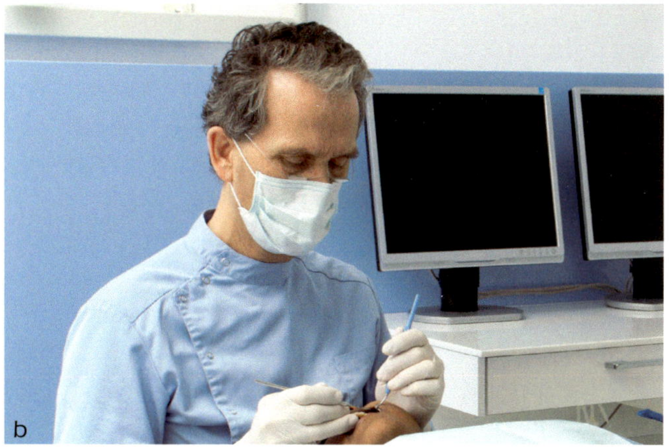

Fig 3–8 (a and b) Inclined precision vision glasses – almost invisible.

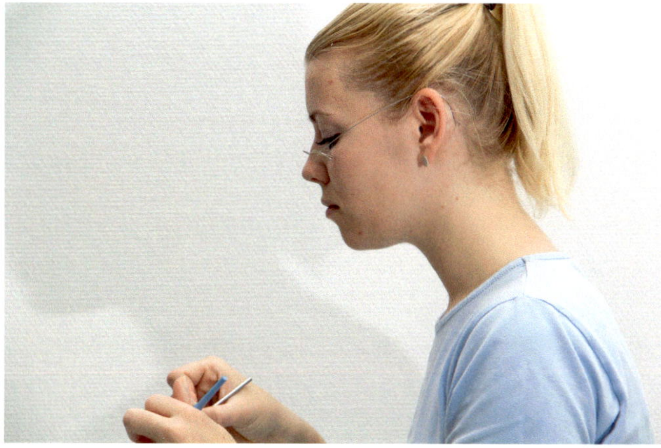

Fig 3–9 The direction of the dentist's head with "dentist's precision glasses."

Acceptable compromises

An acceptable compromise for convex lenses with a maximum of about 1 to 1.25 diopters:

- the frames of metal thread are bent
- the lower margins of the lenses almost touches the cheek
- the optical center is 35 degrees below the horizontal.

If the force of the lenses has a strength of more than 1 to 1.25 iopters, spherical and chromatic aberrance will be more prominent looking obliquely through the spectacles.

In this case, there are three choices:

1. Mini-spectacles may worn be in combination with conventional spectacles with a lower margin, placed high.
2. Loupe systems with a 45-degree inclination, see page 47.
3. Contact lenses can be used for a distance of vision of 35 cm (or your width of accommodation). The contact lenses may be combined with spectacles with a force of the lens, so you can see at longer distances than the working 35 cm distance.

These spectacles have a lower margin so high that they do not disturb your precision vision with your contact lenses when looking downwards. The contact lenses for 35 cm ± precision work may be removed when working hours are finished.

Thus, the dentist has visual correction with two forces: contact lenses for precision work and glasses for more distant vision.

Bifocal glasses

Can two forces be integrated in spectacles, and if so, how should this be done?

If the field for precision vision is large, the direction of the vision can be kept when moving the head of the dentist a little to the sides or up and down, which helps to relax the muscles in the neck and shoulders. Figures 3–10 and 3–11 show lenses with two forces, known as bifocals. The lower field for precision vision is placed almost in contact with the lower margin of the lens, and is so large that the upper limit of it is close to horizontal. The optical center of the field for precision vision is 35 degrees below the horizontal plane of the dentist's head. If the spectacles are tilted forward and the force of the lower part is 1 to 1.5 diopters (maximum), then the spherical and chromatic distortion of visual field is small.

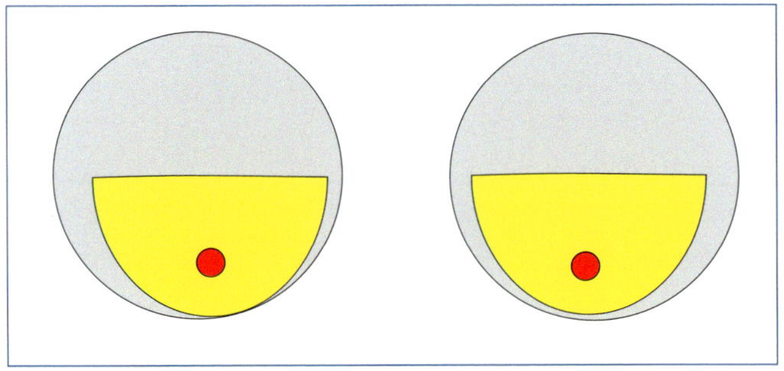

Fig 3–10 Bifocal spectacles; the lower visual field is very large, allowing mobility of the dentist's head (recommended).

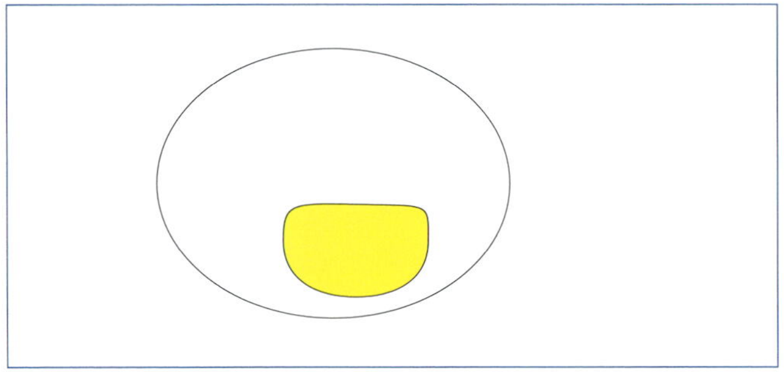

Fig 3–11 A very small field of vision, making movement of the dentist's head while maintaining vision impossible (not recommended).

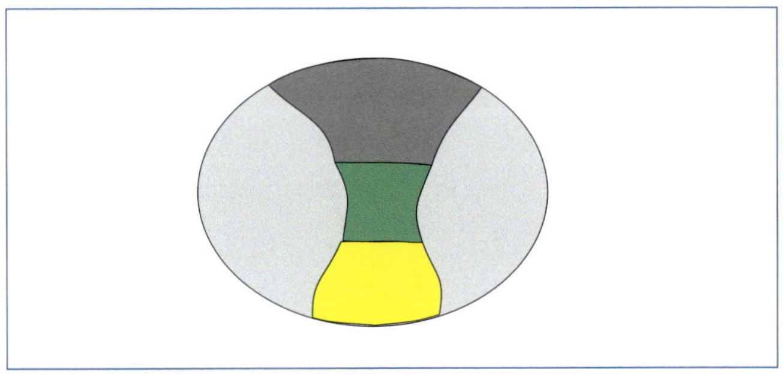

Fig 3–12 The visual field in progressive lenses.

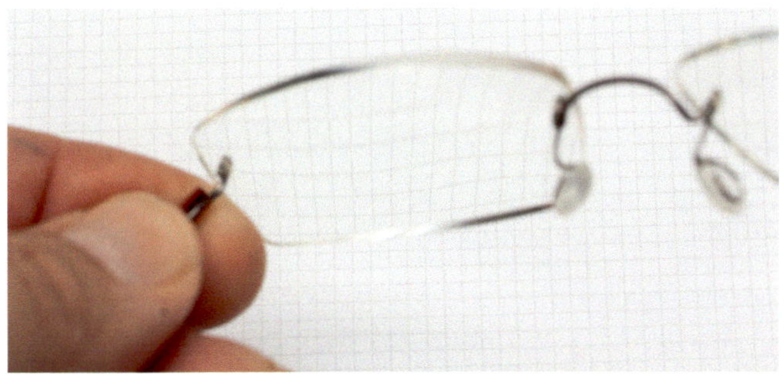

Fig 3–13 Oblique view through progressive lenses – severe distortion.

Some opticians may try to persuade you to try other solutions, so you may need to be quite insistent, or find another optician who can get hold of the special bifocal spectacles from another supplier.

Progressive lenses

If the accommodation of the eye lenses is reduced from presbyopia (see page 36), then different powers of optical corrections are needed depending on the eye-to-object distance.

Are progressive lenses in dentists' spectacles an option?

Looking obliquely through progressive glasses reveals serious distortions of visual field (Figs 3–12 and 3–13). The field of vision has an hourglass shape, and within this margin the force of the glasses is gradually changing. The upper part of the visual field is wide; in the medium part it is narrow, and then it is wider in the lower part. At both sides of the lateral to medium to lower part, is an area with visual distortion.

This causes the following problem for the dentist:

- Looking to side is limited by the rather narrow margins of the visual field. By looking at an object, the possibility to move the head sideways and maintain the direction of vision is limited.
- If the accommodation width of the dentist's eyes is very reduced, the working distance (eye-to-object distance) will depend on the force of the progressive lens in the precise angle of vision.

Looking at a very inclined angle through the progressive lenses, the eye-to-object work distance is shorter than it is when looking at the same object with a less inclined direction of vision, and the eye-to-object distance is longer.

If the dentist has presbyopia (age-related reduced accommodation of the eyes), one may see that progressive lenses cause the dentist to lower his/her head when looking inclined downwards to adapt the shorter eye-to-object distance here – and with less inclined vision, the head is kept higher because the eye-to-object distance is different here.

Lowering the head may especially rapidly produce painful muscular tensions. Instead of progressive lenses, choose bifocal lenses, or in cases where stronger forces are required, glasses with double lenses (Fig 3–14).

Loupe system

If working with the loupe system, the requirements for the direction of vision though the loupe will be the same as described above, with 45 degrees of downwards-inclined vision (see page 36).

Retina

The optical system of the eye forms a picture of what you are looking at on the retina. In the retina, there are light sensitive elements called rods, which are sensitive to light at low intensity, along with three types of cones, sensitive to each of three colors.

At the central part of retina, there is a part called the fovea (fovea centralis), which is a 0.3 mm rod free area densely packed with about 6 to 7 billion cones.

Cones

There are three different types of cones:

- "Red "cones (64%), which are sensitive to red light of 564 nm peak value.
- "Green" cones (32%), which are sensitive to green light 533 nm peak value.
- "Blue" cones (4%), which are sensitive to blue light, 437 nm peak value. As blue is seen with similar intensity as the other colors, the weaker signal for blue seems to be amplified during visual processing in the brain.

The cones provide high-resolution vision as well as color vision, where what we see as colors is created by our brain as a result of the stimulation of a different combination of the three types of cones.

The "red" and "green" cones are concentrated in the fovea, where the blue cones have the highest sensitivity but are mostly outside the fovea, so the visual acuity for "blue" cones is smaller. This means that our most distinct vision is based mostly on the "red" and "green" cones.

The cones' vision adapt to changes in light levels in a few seconds.

Rods

There are about 120 billion rods placed outside the fovea. The rod vision is much more sensitive to weak light, but does not detect color. Their peak sensitivity is green at 498 nm. The rods are dominant in our peripheral vision, which is more light sensitive and responsible for our vision under dim light. Motion is better detected by peripheral vision. The adaptation for optimal night vision may take half an hour.

Color perception

The spectral colors from the rainbow have a one-to-one correlation to light wavelength. Hue is related to the wavelength of the spectral colors. But many mixes of light wavelength may, if combined in right portions, produce the same perception of color, eg, the same hue.

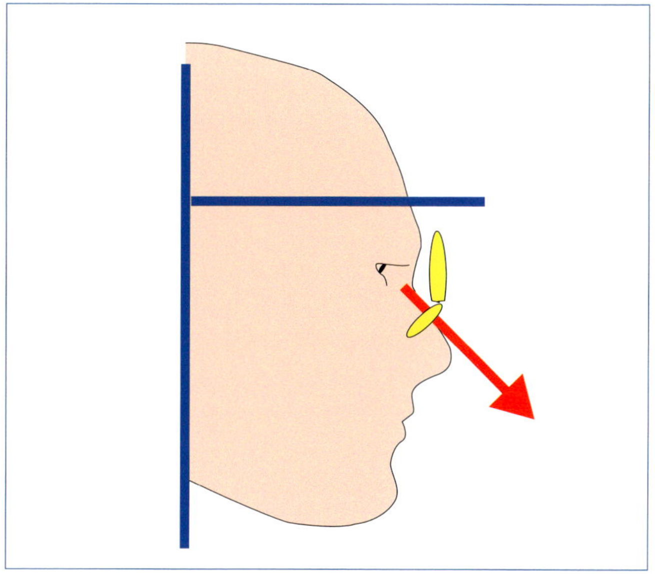

Fig 3–14 Glasses with a lower part for precision vision with optical axis same as direction of vision, and an upper part for general vision. This concept does not (yet) exist.

Several different combinations of two different colors may create white light. Although perceived as the same white color, a colored object (which absorbs other colors as its own color) may look different illuminated in the different white lights. This will have an influence on the choice of color shades.

Saturation

A fully saturated color has no mix of white. Spectral colors are fully saturated but also other colors, such as magenta (a mix of wavelength), can be perceived as saturated.

Brightness and contrast

The brightness of a colored surface will depend on its illuminance (power of incoming light) and its reflectivity. But the perceived brightness is not in linear relation to the reflectivity.

The contrast of an object or a part of an object, as well as the observer's own contrast sensitivity, will influence the visual acuity. Contrast sensitivity may vary from person to person.

Low contrast and low contrast sensitivity reduces the visual acuity. Often the contrast of object and contrast sensitivity of the observer may be more important than visual acuity for correct perception.

Learning not to see everything

One of the demanding tasks that a newly educated dentist will need to learn is how to suppress all visual information from the peripheral vision not relevant to the task she/he is performing.

This means that only a tiny fraction of the total visual field is in use for a working dentist.

VISUAL PERCEPTION AND REACTION TIMES

Visual perception is the ability to interpret the information from the surroundings from light reaching the eye.

The light sensitive cones and rods in the retina relay their neural electrical impulses to the visual cortex in the back of the brain. The visual cortex is responsible for processing the visual image. From the primary visual cortex, the visual information flows through a cortical hierarchy. Some groups of neurons respond to line and line segments of particular orientation from specific parts of the retina. Others respond selectively to complex objects, and others to human faces or particular objects. According to the "two stream hypothesis" (debated), a dorsal ("the where") stream is involved in spatial attention, and a ventral ("the what") stream involved in recognition, identification and categorization of the visual stimuli.

This description indicates the complexity and high activity of the brain as a result of visual sensory input. For more about visual perception and mental imagery, see Chapter 6.

Reaction times

To answer the question: "What are the reaction times for visual input?"

Reaction time has to be measured under specific conditions. If we are working with unit instruments controlled by the foot controller and we need to change speed or stop the unit instrument, the situation can be compared with the driver's reaction time while driving a car. The reaction time will depend on the degree of "alertness."

The measurements for reaction time in a car from the foot is lifted off the speeder and moved to the brake pedal are as follows:

Reaction time for foot controller:

- alert expected 700 milliseconds (ms)
- unexpected 1250 ms
- surprise 1500 ms
- (all inclusive of foot movements).

Hand movements are about 150 to 300 ms faster. So if only the hands (and not foot) have to react to "something," the following reaction times may be expected:

Probable reaction time for hand

- alert expected 450 to 550 ms
- unexpected 750 to 1,000 ms
- surprise 1,000 to 1,150 ms
- + the "choice effect" time needed for selecting a particular response (choice effect from 500 to 1,000 ms).

Visual feedback takes time, and if a movement with an instrument is controlled by visual feedback, a lot of – or the whole movement – may be made before the visual feedback arrives to the conscious brain.

Do bear in mind that you cannot receive a visual feedback of the outcome of a movement with an instrument before it is done. Also, you cannot base precision work primarily on visual feedback. It is too slow!

Other strategies will be necessary (see Chapter 4).

LIGHT

Light is an electromagnetic radiation, which is visible to the human eye. The wavelength is from 380 nanometers (nm) blue to about 740 nm, red. It has only three definitions, which are all in SI units (Systeme Internationale d'unité), the international unit used in many regions (but not in the USA).

Luminous flux (lumen, lm): the total amount of light from a source of light is measured in lumen.

Illuminance (luminans, lux, lx): The amount of light spread over a given area is illuminance and is measured in lux.
1 lumen is 1 lux per m^2
1 lm = 1 lx per m^2

If a luminous flux of 1,000 lumens is spread on 1 m^2, the illuminance is 1,000 lux, but if it is spread over 10 m^2, the illuminance is 100 lux.

Examples of illuminance

Direct sunlight: 32,000 to 130,000 lux
Full daylight (not in direct sun): 10,000 to 25,000 lux
Overcast day: 1,000 lux
Very dark overcast day: 100 lux.

Reflective factor

When light is spread over a surface, a certain part of it is reflected to the observer. The more white or light the color is, the more is reflected.

Color temperature – kelvin degrees K

Color temperature of an ideal light emitting source is measured in KELVIN, abbreviated as K. Color temperatures over 5,000 K are called cool colors, where color temperatures 2,700–3,000 K are called warm colors.

Examples of color temperatures

- Candle flame, or sunset, sunrise: 1,850 K
- Incandescent light bulb: 1,700–3,300 K
- Daylight: 5,000 K.

Full spectrum light

Full spectrum light is perceived as white light. As described earlier, different balanced combination of colors can also be perceived as white light. But when illuminating a colored surface, the outcome may be different to perception of the color in full spectrum light.

With green, if the color mix perceived as white does not take part, the color of the green object will not be perceived correctly as green. The selection of color by use of a color shade prerequisites full spectrum light, with an even intensity of all colors.

Light sources such as fluorescent tubes emit light with peak values at certain frequencies, which are modified by different phosphor coatings.

These peaks in the spectrum of emitted light are characteristic for LED light sources, and often with only one peak. Phosphor coatings are also developed in order to change the LED light to a more even frequency distribution.

Do not expect that fluorescent or LED light sources emit full spectrum light, which can be used for choosing color shade. Only scientifically controlled experiments will reveal whether a given light source can serve for choosing color shades.

OPERATING LAMP

The operating lamp should give an evenly illuminated area of an area, such as the open mouth of the patient. The illuminance, according to "general experience," should be about 22,000 lux, which will cause the iris of the dentist's and assistant's eyes to be so small that rays of light only pass the middle of the lens of their eyes, which creates the most precise image on retina. A small iris opening allows enough light to pass for achieving maximal visual acuity and contrast sensitivity of the cones of macula in retina.

If the light is too strong it may reduce contrast, which is a part of visual acuity, and furthermore cause dazzling. The color temperature should be about 4,000 degrees Kelvin.

"Shadowless reflector"

In order to avoid disturbing shadows in the visual field, the reflector should be divided into small units, with a computer designed reflection so each unit contributes light to the whole illuminated area. This means that an object intersecting the rays of light will almost not cast a shadow.

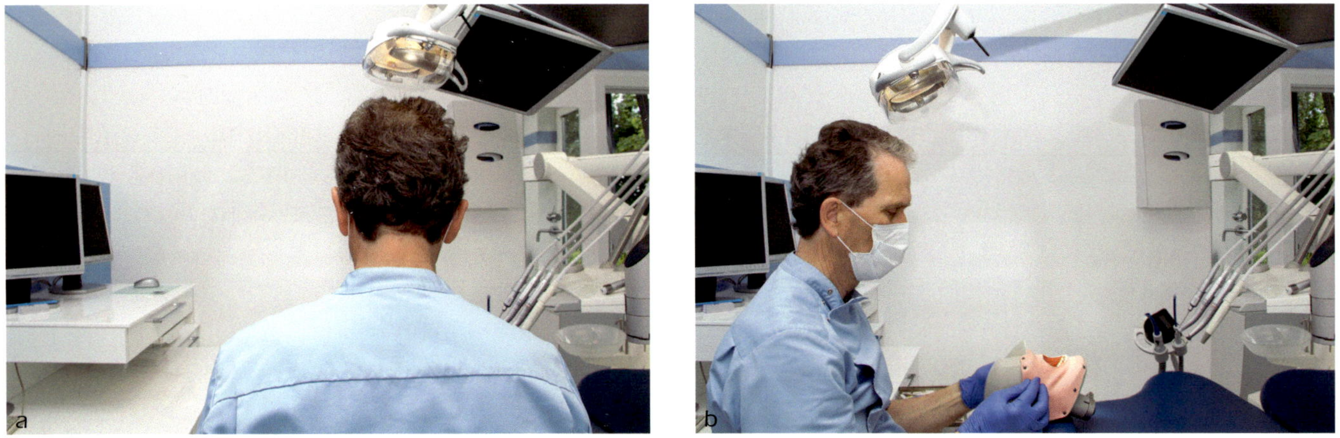

Fig 3–15 (a) Photo lamp close to the dentist's head. (b) Dentist in 12 o'clock position.

The larger the reflector is, the less shadow is casted by objects (instruments, fingers, etc) placed between light and object of vision.

Spotlight lamps, which cast strong shadows, were discontinued for market sale for 30 years, but have since been reintroduced.

The reflector also filters light; so heating rays in the infrared spectrum pass through the reflecting units, and therefore are not reflected into the field of working.

Direction of light

In order to illuminate surfaces or cavities, for which visual access may be limited to a very narrow track or "visual tunnel," the operating lamp must be placed so the direction of vision and line of light are as close as possible.

This means that the head of the lamp must be placed so that the light passes close to the dentist's head, with the light rays passing into the actual "visual tunnel" towards the teeth that need to be seen (Fig 3–15).

The supporting arm for the operating lamp should be so long that the lamp can be adjusted, so that the direction of the light beam can be identical to the direction of vision. This is also important for when the dentist is working in a 12 o'clock position, with a direction of vision inclined 35 degrees from behind the patient.

The supporting arm for the head of the operation arm should be 30 to 35 cm longer than the top of the head support on the horizontal patient's chair. When working with a mirror, the operation lamp should also be placed close to the head of the dentist and the light directed towards the mirror, which reflects light to the bottom of the cavity that the dentist is looking into. The lamp may be tilted sideways for aligning light and direction of vision. This may also be accomplished by swinging the lamp 90 degrees to a side.

The lamp should have full spectrum light and a color temperature as sunlight spectrum. If a Halogen light source is used, a reflector with a filtering effect is needed so that the warm infrared light is not reflected, but passes through the reflector.

The lamp may have a dimmer to reduce the polymerization of composite caused by the operating lamp, and therefore also augmenting the working time from placement and modeling composite.

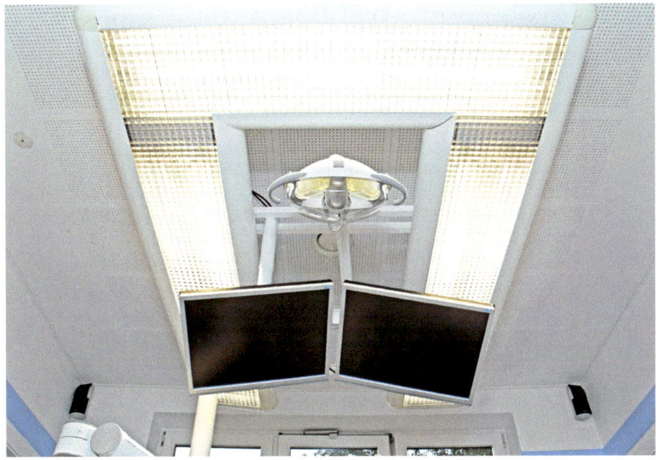

Fig 3–16 A "U shape" armature – in this case with two computer screens for the patient – one for showing radiographs, intraoral photos, etc. The second is for an entertainment program.

GENERAL ILLUMINATION IN THE TREATMENT ROOM

Fluorescent tube armatures provide the best light.

Important

- Use always high frequency (HF) armatures and fluorescent tubes, which emit light without "flittering."
- Fluorescent tubes with five internal fluorescent layers of phosphor provide good daylight color recognition and may be combined with a halogen light.
- Illumination of the patient's mouth surroundings should be intended to avoid dazzling of the eyes of the operator when looking into the patient's mouth, while being highly illuminated by the operating lamp.

The areas primarily seen by the dentist and assistant include the surfaces around the patient's mouth, like the serviette, the clothes of the assistant and dentist, parts of the floor, and the walls. These surfaces should, as a general rule (developed through practice), have a luminance of about 10% of that used in the patient's mouth. The reflective factor of these surfaces should be as high as possible, so the color of the surfaces should be white or very light.

Some of the armatures for fluorescent tubes do not illuminate the walls of the treatment room. If that should be the case, then the walls should be illuminated with separate light tubes. These areas and surfaces should be illuminated so that enough light is reflected, and the dentist will not suffer any visual problems while looking back to the patient's mouth (Fig 3–16).

In order to avoid the patient looking directly towards the fluorescent tubes, the tube armatures can be in a "u" shape, leaving an area in the middle where the patient can relax the eyes. This area should also be illuminated with uplights in top of the armature in order to reduce contrasts in the visual field of the patient. An even distribution of light in the treatment room will give a very dull impression. The illumination can be more vital if walls are illuminated with halogen spotlights. This also applies to the workplace for the assistant.

LOUPES

- Using loupes, your precision vision is improved.
- Your eye-to-object distance may be decreased.
- In combination with a loupe-based light, the object of vision is perfect illuminated.

Health risks for dentists using loupes

Unfortunately, many loupe systems are not sufficiently downwardly inclined. The dentist has to bend his cervical spine 20 to 30 degrees more downwards, compared to what is possible when working without loupes. This may lead to severe discomfort with permanent muscle pain, and in time it can impair the health of the intervertebral discs in the neck region. This may cause a permanent disabling of the dentist.

A large downwards inclination of loupe system is crucial for dentists' health. In most cases the dentist can, after short training, work with 45-degree downwards-inclined loupes. If the loupes are constructed so the direction of vision can be inclined to around 45 degrees, the disadvantage mentioned previously is not present. The dentist's head is therefore kept as high as possible. The weight of the loupes can also be inconvenient.

Loupes provide a magnification with increased visual acuity. In case of presbyopia (see page 42), a magnification of 2.5× will mean that the accommodation width will be inversed proportionally and

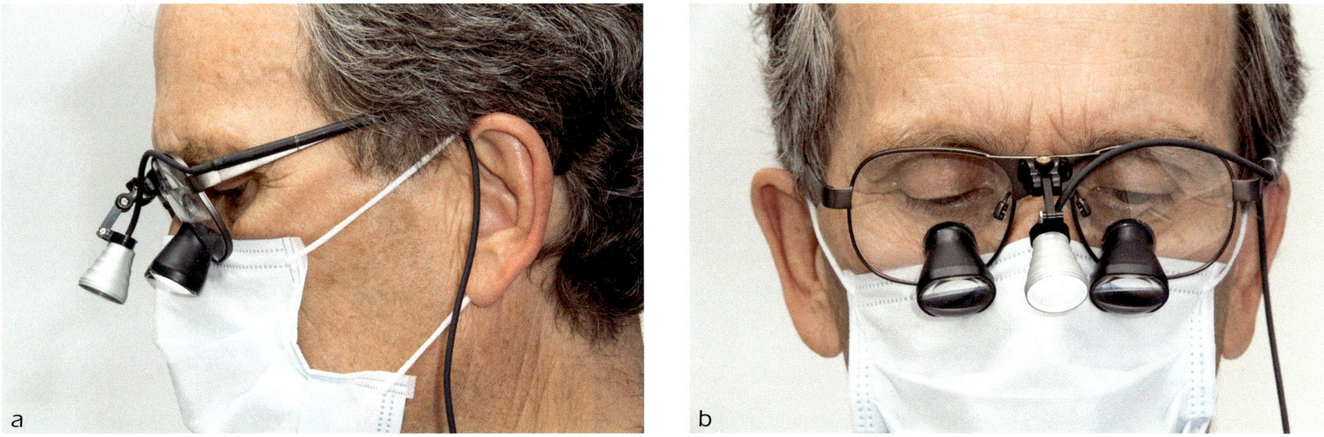

Fig 3–17 (a) Through the lens (TTL)-type loupes, 45-degree inclined. (b) Head up and looking down.

have to be divided by 2.5. The user has to therefore choose eye-to-object working distance.

In case of a reduced accommodation width, the working distance has to be precise. With an accommodation width of 10 cm at an eye-to-object distance of 32 cm for example, the debt of the visual field will now be 4 cm. This is so short that when the eye-to-object focus changes between an incisor to a second molar, the head often has to be moved down. This is inconvenient and may cause muscular tension. A better solution is an adjustment of the vertical position of the patient chair.

There are two types of optical systems used for loupes:

Galiean system

- Built with multiple lenses, consisting of an objective element that is convex and an ocular element that is concave, and acromatic lenses with magnification 1.5 to 3x
- Image sharpest in a central field – the middle part of visual field.

Keplerian system

- A little more long and heavy
- Magnification 4 to 8x
- A compound system of several lenses, consisting of an objective element that is convex, and a ocular element that is also convex (as well as acromatic lenses)
- In between, a so-called Abbe-Koenig roof prism is placed, compensating for a turning of the vision up/down and left/right
- Superior resolution over the whole field of vision.

The loupes may be supported by a frame, positioned in front of spectacles for protection and/or visual correction. The user can adjust these loupes manually.

Alternatively, the loupes may be perforating the spectacles lenses (TTL – through the lens), with or without visual correction. The TTL type of lens allows the ocular (lens closest to eye) to be closer to the eye, which enlarges the field of vision (Fig 3–17). Stereo acuity and depth perception decrease when viewing through a loupe.

The TTL loupes require a very precise measurement of working distance, direction of vision, convergence of the eyes and interpupillar distance. This is done by a specially trained optician.

The Skovsgaard inclined vision loupe system

A new loupe developed by the author allows a much-improved work position. A new internal multi prism system in the loupes allows an internal inclination of the direction of vision, eg, 20 degrees downwards (or more), without cromatic or spheric distortion. This allows the dentist to look into the patient's mouth and keeps the head 20 degrees higher than when working without loupes. This creates an extraordinary improvement for a dentist's working position.

In 2013, this loupe system is at prototype stage – for more details please see www.netergonomie.com.

Loupes and working position

As one cannot look sideways or up/down through loupes, the direction of vision must be made by moving the head. If you look at an object, you can move your head slightly in all directions without loupes, and still see the object. These movements are not possible using loupes. Your head is fixed in relation to the object, which is inconvenient.

This indicates that the use of loupes could be limited to situations where the extra magnification is needed. Therefore the loupes must assure the absolute best working position: keeping the dentist's head up and by inclining the eyes down (as much as possible and comfortably) (see page 17).

Light and loupes

When making a visual inspection at narrow cavities, eg, the opening of narrow pulpal cavities for endodontic treatment, it is often difficult to get light directed to the bottom of the cavity. This is a difficult situation, even if the operating lamp is placed close to the head (and above) the dentist in order to align the direction of vision and light.

A small lamp (LED) placed on the frame of the loupes, and/or close to the loupes, provides excellent illumination, which is precise and always in the direction of vision. Everything seen through the loupes will be always perfectly illuminated. **Loupes and loupe-light is a recommended combination.**

The blind field

Around the visual field, there will be a circular field with a width of about 5 cm, which is invisible. The reason is that the loupes enlarge their visual field to cover a part of the visual field seen around them. Hand instrument transfer and transfer of endodontic instruments is done in this blind field and requires special techniques (see page 212).

The visual field through loupes

The visual field seen through the loupes will depend on their magnification. With 2.5× magnification, the eye-to-object distance will be 35 or 40 cm. With TTL loupes placed very close to the eyes, the visual field may be as large as "the open mouth" area of the patient.

Loupes and concave magnification mirror double magnification

A very cheap solution to double or triple the magnification of loupes, is to look through a concave mirror mounted on the normal mirror shaft.

It can only be used for one eye, and only the central part of the image is completely clear, but for searching for an entrance to narrow root canals, it is an excellent addition. With 2.5× magnification loupes, the total magnification will be 5 to 6 times (dependent on the position of the concave mirror).

When to use the loupes

When to use the loupes will depend on the user's eyes. The visual acuity and contrast sensitivity will be different for each person (page 44).

Some will find it worthwhile to use loupes all the time, and others will restrict their use to specific parts of their work, such as finding openings of root canals for endodontic procedures, as well as for preparations. When the root canal is found and the entrance of the canal opened by a rotating primary file (eg, an initial shaper or other instrument), the loupes can be taken off, because now the openings of the root canals are very easy to find.

Concluding recommendations

Galieian loupe

- Use a through the lens type (TTL) because the loupe eye piece can be placed close to the eye.
- Direction should be 45 degrees downwards.
- The position of loupe should be very carefully measured.
- The loupe ocular lens should be close to the eye for obtaining a large visual field.
- Use a magnification of 2.5×.
- A working distance of 40 cm is recommended (35 cm for dentists with height below about 160 cm).
- The loupes should be fitted with an LED light.
- For larger magnification, the Keplerian-type loupes are used: working distance, inclination etc, as above.

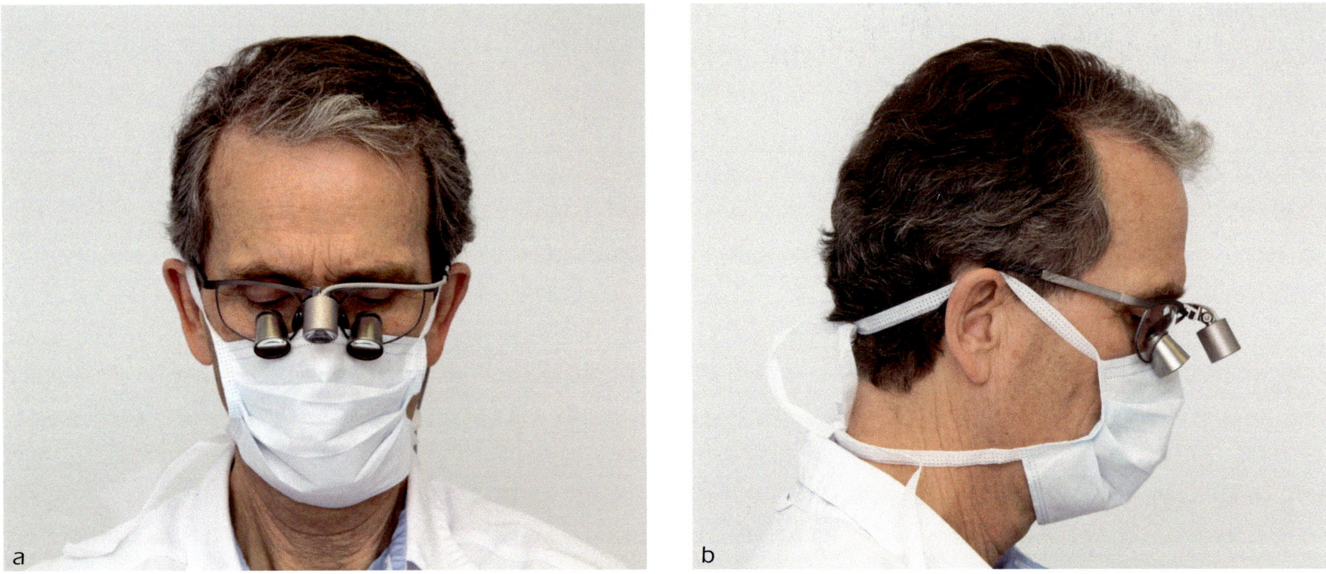

Fig 3–18 (a and b) ExamVision loupes, with 45-degree inclined vision.

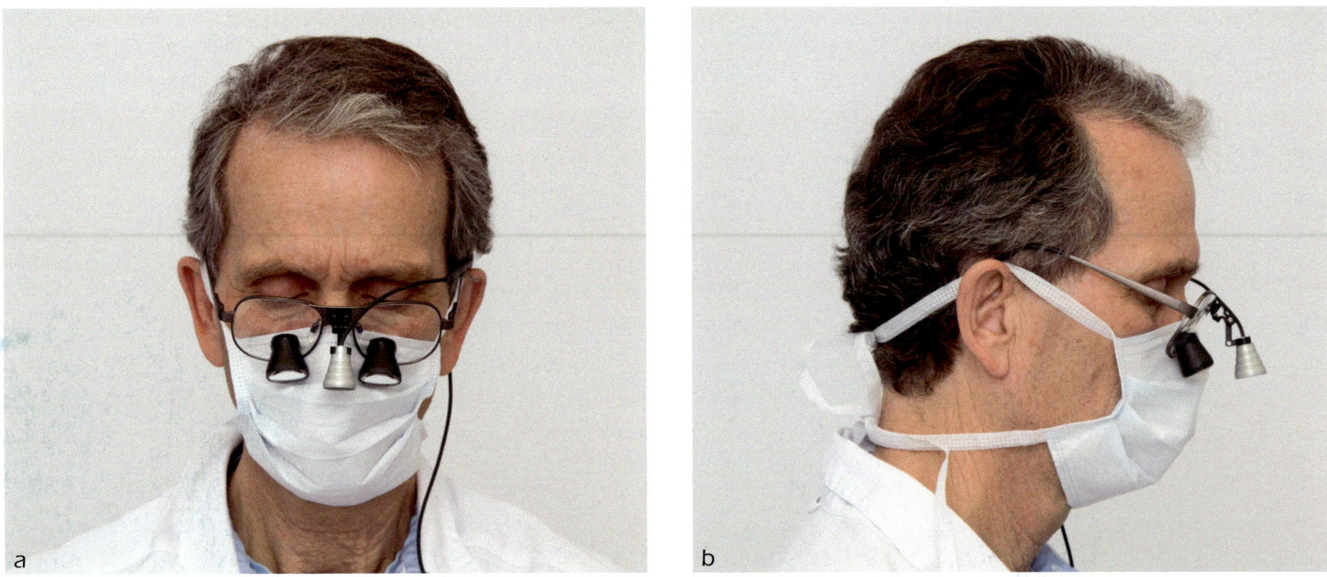

Fig 3–19 (a and b) Orascoptic loupes, with 45-degree inclined vision.

- For an improved working position, an inclined vision system is a solution.

Here are some examples (Figs 3–18 and 3–19):

Chapter 4

QUALITY

INSTRUMENTS' INFLUENCE ON HANDS – MICROERGONOMICS

Some of the most important microergonomic aspects of hand instruments, burs and diamond burs are discussed in this section.

Vision

In axiom number 3 of the 12 basic principles, it is stated that the dentist should be able to see all exterior surfaces of the teeth, and all interior surfaces of possible cavities. This is supplemented by axiom number 1: good working positions.

Working

Now – we combine axioms 1 and 3 with axiom number 5: working with precision dentistry. To perform this work, we use tools in our hands. The shape and form of the tools influence the position and movements of our hands – and arms and body too.

The dentist must have hand instruments and a rotating instrument with angle and shape, so it is possible to perform "work" on these specified surfaces, with visual surveillance and in good working positions. A supplementary condition from axiom number 5 is added.

Minimal invasive methods should be supported

To fulfill these conditions:

- Work with fine vision on all surfaces, and if needed with minimally invasive techniques.
- This will result in sharp demands to the shape, size and direction of hand instruments and rotating instruments.

Terminology of rotating instruments

- rpm: rotations per minute
- Torque: rotation power, cutting power
- Motor model: "motor" means the "motoric movement," eg, of a group of fingers or a hand.

Turbine (air rotor)

The turbine is driven by compressed air and was the first high-speed unit instrument for diamonds and burs. The maximum speed of the turbine may be up to 400,000 rpm idle speed, when the diamond or bur on the turbine is not in contact with anything. This speed is not for practical use and drops much down when the bur/diamond touches the surface of the tooth. The torque is very low and the bur/diamond has very weak "cutting power." Most have a working speed with a reasonable but low torque, which is a speed of about 160,000 rpm. If the air pressure and speed are reduced, the cutting power will fall to a level with little practical use. Due to these characteristics, most turbines are without speed regulations.

The typical sound of a turbine in use is a high tone, caused by low torque at high speeds and idling when not in contact with the tooth. When contact is made with the tooth, the turbine speed is reduced and the sound has a lower frequency.

Because of the low torque of a turbine, many dentists try to increase the cutting effect by lifting the diamond (or other rotating instrument) off the tooth surface until the turbine gains speed again. The inertia of the turbine gives a little extra cutting power until the speed falls again. This produces the typical sound of a turbine in use; a high noise frequency with an idle speed, and a lower noise frequency a second later.

Touch and lift technique

If the turbine does not slow in speed, the amount of pressure needed is so low that many dentists' hands seem to have difficulty in sensing the touch of the tooth surface. When the pressure is increased to give tactility to the dentist's hand, the turbine slows down. After the turbine is lifted off the tooth surface, it gains speed again.

This may be the reason to the use the "touch and lift" technique familiar to turbine users with repetitive inserted visual controls. The touch and lift off working pattern hinders the automation of movements. A continuous three-dimensional planned and trained movement is divided by the repetitive stop–starts.

HIGH-SPEED CONTRA-ANGLES

Basic principle

"The equipment of the treatment room must be adapted to best work methods," and not the reverse.

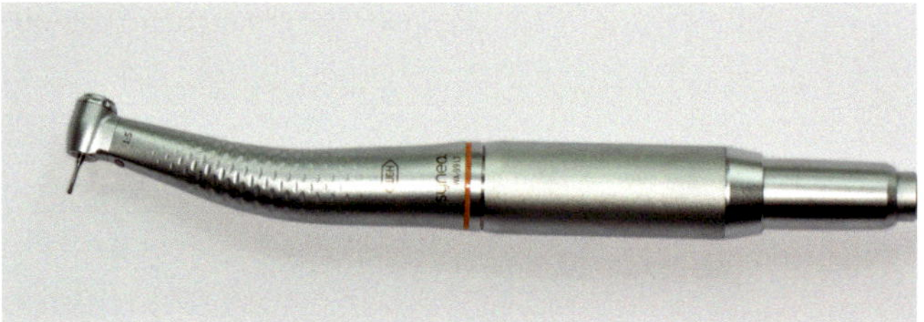

Fig 4–1 High-speed contra-angle on micromotor.

A high-speed 5× multiplication contra-angle (double red rings) on an electric powered micromotor is called a high-speed contra-angle.

Since the 1990s, electric micromotors running up to 40,000 rpm have been used with contra-angles, multiplying the speed by five times (Fig 4–1).

These 5× multiplication contra-angles are normally marked with two red rings, and they use normal turbine diamonds or hard metal (wolfram carbide) burs. Their speed range is dependent on the micromotor, and will run from about 1,000 rpm to a maximum speed of 200,000 rpm. A selected speed is stabilized electronically and does not change if the pressure on the rotating diamond (or other rotating instrument) is increased (within the total power of the micromotor).

Working with a constant speed (adapted to the task) and a constant and low pressure, a preparation can be made by a sequence of connected precise movements. When the speed is unchanged, the cutting ability of the diamond will only be dependent on pressure. The speed can be regulated according to the diamond or bur mounted on the 5× red multiplication contra-angle, as well as to the task and the surface of the tooth.

The torque of the high-speed contra-angle is much higher compared to the weak torque of the turbines. It has not been possible to get an exact measure of the difference, but the torque of the high-speed contra-angle may by more than 10 times higher than the torque of the turbine. The torque for using a diamond (of 1.2 mm diameter, for example) is ideal.

A high-speed contra-angle mounted with a hard metal amalgam cutter may remove a defect "almost amalgam crown" in – maybe – half a minute. A high-speed contra-angle on a micromotor is a much more advanced tool for a dentist than a turbine.

A high-speed contra-angle (5×) on a micromotor compared to a turbine has:

A much higher torque (cutting power)

When needed, the high-speed contra-angle is much more effective than a turbine. Be sure to use abundant cooling.

More speed

The max speed is 200,000 rpm, which is electronically stabilized and independent of the load on the rotating instrument (a turbine in use has a lower speed). A high speed combined with high torque gives excellent efficiency. Sufficient spray cooling is mandatory.

Speed regulation

The speed can be regulated by a foot controller according to the specifications of a task and of rotating instruments. A different task requires different speeds. For example, an ovoid diamond for occlusal shaping of a composite used with a speed of 180,000 to 200,000 rpm. Another example is a 1.4 mm flame-shaped diamond used for the correction of composite at approximal margins, with a speed of 30,000 to 40,000 rpm.

Better tactility

There is much better tactility, because the pressure applied on the rotating instrument may be higher (with sufficient cooling). You can feel the tooth surface much better while working with a high-speed contra-angle. If you need even better tactility because you are working where visual supervision is difficult (eg, distal maxillary last molar), you reduce the speed. The lower the speed, the better the tactility.

It is safer

If the diamond rotates too fast on surfaces with difficult visual supervision, one reduces the speed until it feels "safe."

More centered

The mechanically driven high-speed contra-angle keeps the diamond more centered without lateral micromovements. The hand tactility is very "direct." Thinner and slightly longer diamonds (eg, micropreparation diamonds, see page 60) may be used.

Easy to use

Experience from numerous "hands-on" preparation courses is that it is much more easy to make good preparations using high-speed contra-angles, than it is with turbines. A high quality is easier to obtain.

Supports training

The characteristics of the high-speed contra-angle supports the training of manual motor skills. The burs or diamonds can be used in developing skills using sequences of connected precise three-dimensional movements, which can be automatized.

Compensates for higher weight

A micromotor with a high-speed contra-angle is heavier than a turbine. If the unit instruments are mounted on balanced unit instrument supports, the weight is balanced out and cannot be felt.

The producers of turbines and high-speed hand pieces have experienced that there is no difference between the wear of the two.

Replacing the turbine with high-speed contra-angles

For decades, this is a generally well-known practice in some countries among dentists. In other countries, its advantages are not known.

For working with high-speed contra-angles instead of turbines, two micromotors are proposed. One micromotor should be mounted with a low speed 1:1 blue ring contra-angle, and be close to the assistant to allow the change of burs, stones, polishing disks, etc. The second micromotor, closest to the dentist, is fitted with a 1:5 multiplication (double red ring) contra-angle, replacing the turbine.

THE FOOT CONTROLLER

Speed of the rotating instruments

A great variety of speeds are needed for the different tasks we perform with our rotating instruments, burs or diamonds, disks, etc.

The speed has to be selected taking into consideration the diameter and surface roughness of the rotating instruments, the task, the security of movements, the skill of dentist, the surface of the tooth, the shape of the instruments, and the cutting and the cooling. The manufacturers of the instruments may present suggestions, but the sensitive hand (and foot) of the dentist is probably the best guide for speed selection.

Round burs provide a fine tactile feedback during excavation if they are used with very low speeds down to a few hundred rpm. One can feel the higher resistance of harder dentin, indicating that the actual excavation is about to be finished, before examination with a probe.

Example of speeds:

- 160,000 to 200,000 rpm for preparation.
- 200 rpm for preparing for a dentin pin.
- 300 to 1,500 rpm for excavating caries.
- 140,000 to 200,000 rpm for polishing composite with an ovoid polishing diamond.
- 30,000 to 40,000 rpm for polishing composite with a flame shaped polishing diamond.
- 800 to 2,000 rpm for polishing with a rubber cup, and so on.

So how should the speed selection and regulation be made? A preset fixed speed is not sufficient, because each rotating "instrument" might be used in the lower or higher part of the speed range listed above.

Traditional speed regulation

The foot controller regulates the full speed range of the micromotor. When the micromotor is started, the pedal of the foot controller needs to be moved by the dentist's foot to start the motor, and to gradually find the best speed for the actual task. The speed may be adjusted up or down until the best speed is found.

Now the dentist stops the micromotor, in order to make a visual examination of the surface or cavity where the work is being performed. Then the same speed as before has to be found again, before the micromotor is stopped again for a visual check of the working area.

This procedure may be repeated many times, and every time with the problem of rediscovering the speed. This is a tiring and distracting procedure.

Fixed speeds for each task

One could consider using a program for each rotating instrument with a minimum and a maxi-

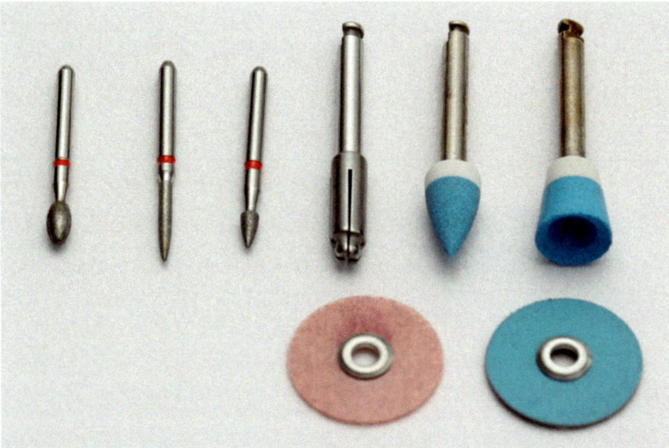

Fig 4–2 Examples of rotating instruments used for polishing.

mum speed. Within each program, the foot controller can regulate speed. For a procedure such as polishing a composite, one might use the following rotating instruments (Fig 4–2):

- Ovoid polishing diamond
- Flame shaped diamond
- Pointed short diamond
- Polishing disk
- Polishing cup and point in diamond abrasive rubber.

Each rotating instrument has its own program with special speeds, eg, for a composite filling, you may need five, six or more! However, that is much too complicated if the program is selected by hand, and especially so if done by foot. Reaction times for a foot are slow – often more than 1 second, so foot controller functions should be as simple as possible. Another type of speed regulation should be considered.

A neuromotoric simplified foot control

The foot controller pedal is pressed down and moved to the side, until the optimal speed for the task and rotating instrument is found (Fig 4–3).

When the micromotor is stopped for the dentist's visual examination of a cavity, the foot is lifted up and the micromotor stops, but the foot controller pedal remains in position. After visual examination of the cavity, the micromotor is restarted by simply pressing the pedal slightly downward. Restarting on the same speed is now done as an on/off function without having to find the speed "from the beginning" each time – an important simplification (Fig 4–4).

In short: the speed is searched and selected by a sideways movement of the foot controller pedal. Repetitive start/stops are made by downwards activation. If one wants another speed, it is selected by moving the foot controller pedal sideways.

Automatic chip blow

The automatic chip blow is a 1970 invention by the author. When the bur or diamond is stopped, the reason is to make a visual inspection (and maybe use a probe) of the working area.

To make this visual inspection, one has to replace the micromotor and use a 3-in-1 syringe to dry the cavity, then replace the syringe, take the micromotor again and continue working. This may be repeated several or many times for each task.

To eliminate (almost) this tiring procedure, the micromotor air spray system is programmed to continue blowing air in the cavity, eg, for 0.8 to 1.0 seconds, after the micromotor is stopped, in order to dry the cavity without having to change to a multifunction syringe and back again (Fig 4–5). The automatic chip blow function provides an important simplification in the work.

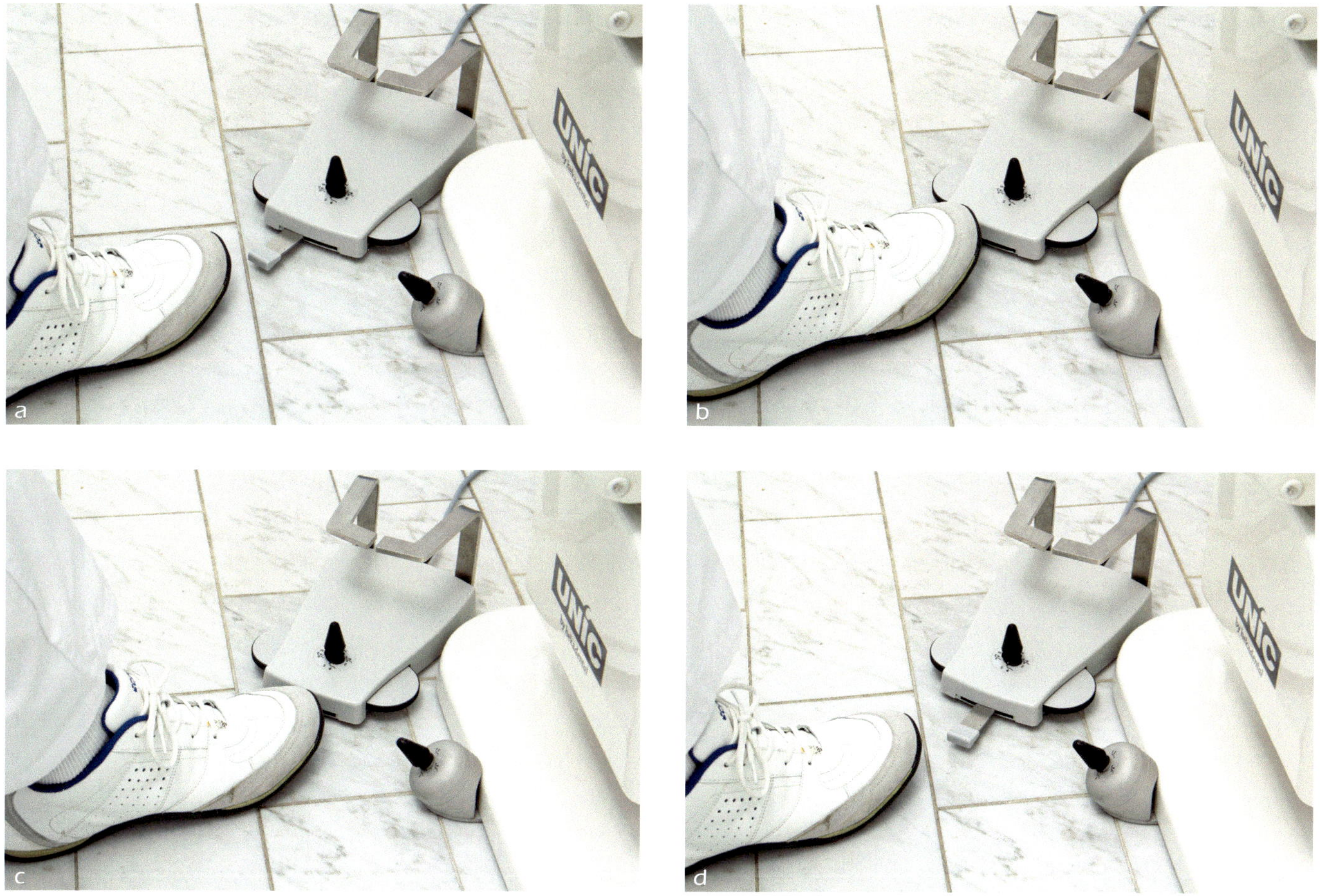

Fig 4–3 (a) Foot controller pedal. (b) Moving foot controller pedal to the right for speed selection. (c and d) Pedal stays in the selected position.

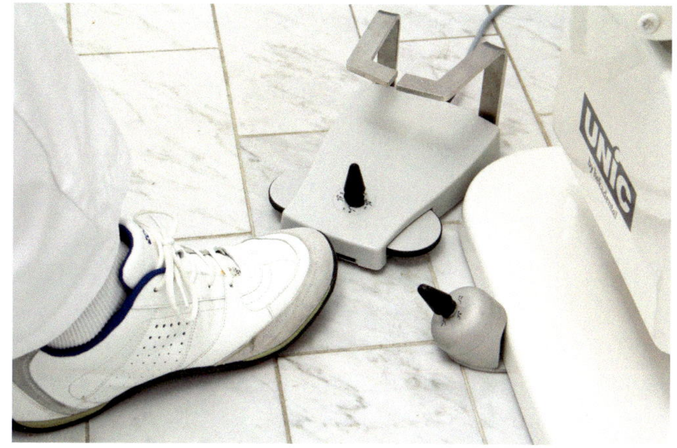

Fig 4–4 The foot controller pedal can now be activated with a vertical movement to on/off start on selected speed.

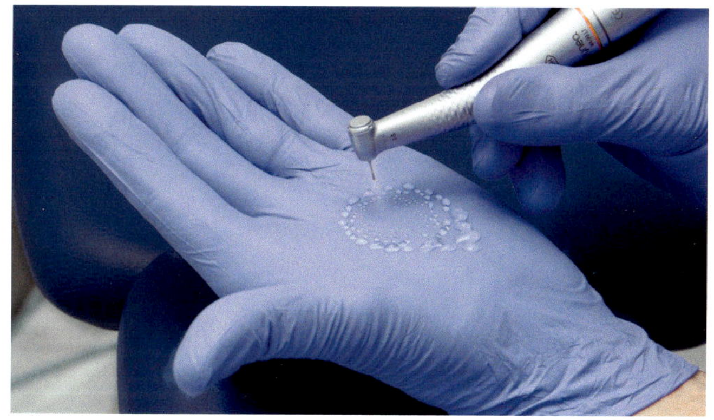

Fig 4–5 Automatic chip blow.

THE TOOLS – BURS AND DIAMONDS

This section puts forward some examples of microergonomics and minimally invasive aspects that can be proposed for integration in the preparation protocol.

Removing an amalgam filling – very fast – with a high-speed contra-angle

A hard metal bur for amalgam, an amalgam cutter, removes a defect amalgam filling very fast. A special cutting geometry cuts the amalgam into small pieces rather than a diamond, which grinds the amalgam to fine powder. It is believed that this method reduces the release of mercury vapor. As a result of the high speed and excellent torque of the high-speed contra-angle, the initial movements are calm and continuous until 0.2 mm from the tooth substance (Fig 4–6).

The amalgam cutter induces small vibrations, removing amalgam often without touching the walls of the cavity. The remaining amalgam may be removed with a round bur or a 0.9 mm micropreparation diamond.

Do you have round burs?

The most of the so-called round burs used in the blue 1:1 contra-angle are in fact not burs at all, because it cannot "bur" in that area (to "bur," meaning that it can remove tooth substance while working in an axial direction).

With a standard round bur, the cutting edges meet each other in a point (Fig 4–7), which means it cannot work in an axial direction. It cannot act as a bur. Technically, the instrument is not a bur, but a round miller.

When needing to excavate caries in an axial direction, one has to use the round bur in zigzag movements. This is to try to let the instrument cut on lateral cutting edges, even when wanting to excavate a small cavity, eg, in the direction axial to the bur. This means that for smaller cavities, the round miller tends to "create" larger cavities than necessary.

If you use a 1.4 mm round miller, your minimal cavity diameter may be 1.6 mm or more. This is seen very often. Fillings in molars with fissure caries tend to be what we could call "large," or unnecessarily large.

Narrow shaft end cut round bur

A new round bur (Komet H1SEM, Komet Dental) is used on a blue 1:1 contra-angle. In order to use the bur in the axial direction, there are transversal cutting edges at the end of the bur. This means the round bur can now be used in an axial direction without zigzag movements. With abundant cooling, it can be used directly axial down into small caries attack areas.

As in the case of the hard round metal bur shown in Fig 4–8, the shaft of the bur is very thin, so the cutting parts of the bur for sideways use are larger. This means it cuts very well, both lengthways and sideways.

The small diameter shaft of the bur leaves room for visual examination when working in narrow cavities. It also provides a larger cutting effect for sideways use. The narrow shaft end cut round bur is used without zigzag movements (Fig 4–9), and is simply moved straight in the direction in which you want it to work. It is an astonishing improvement of one of our basic tools. It also supports a minimally invasive technique.

Deep cavities

If a cavity is deep, the head of the contra-angle is close to the tooth, which either disturbs or hinders the vision into the cavity.

Instead of either working blind in short moments followed by visual examination, or widening up the entrance to the cavity in order to see what the bur is "doing", there is a third solution.

With a 5 mm extra long bur, eg, 26 mm length (standard bur length 21 mm), then it is possible to view the working part of the round bur while it is being used.

Diamonds and microergonomics for composite preparations

In the bur stands beside many dentists, one finds a variety of cavity preparation diamonds. Most of them are thick, around 1.4 mm or more (Fig 4–10a), and many of them are quite short (Fig 4–10b).

Large diameter

When the diameter of the used diamond is large, the minimal width of a cavity will of course be as

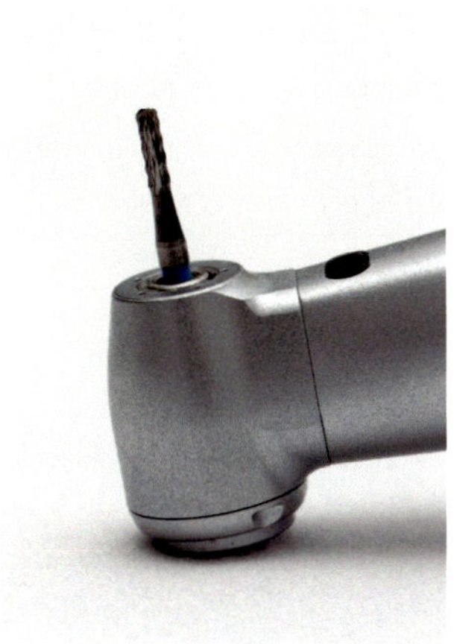

Fig 4–6 Amalgam cutter on contra-angle.

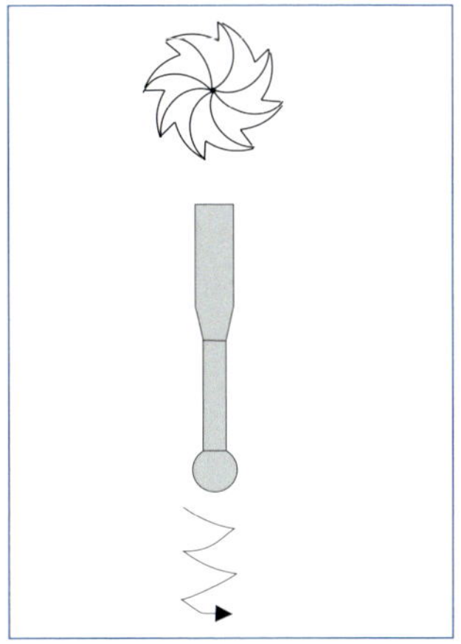

Fig 4–7 A round miller, with a downwards zigzag movement.

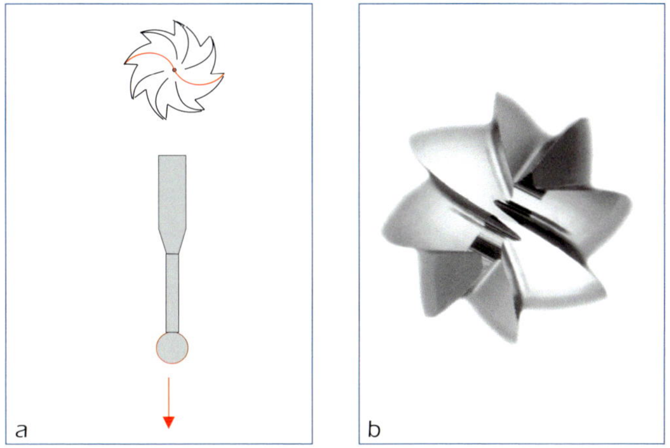

Fig 4–8 (a and b) A round bur, which works in an axial direction.

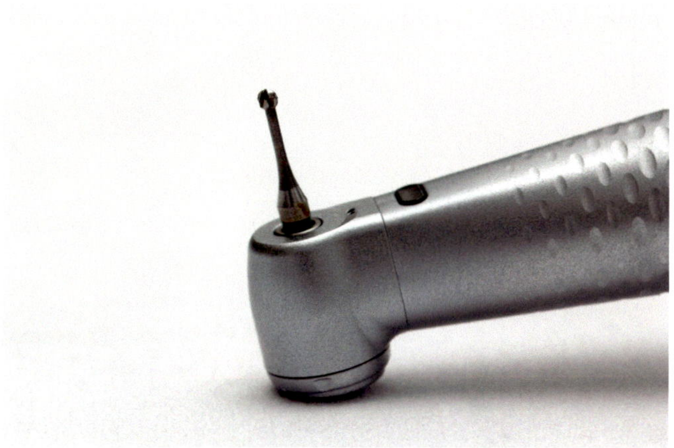

Fig 4–9 Side vision of the narrow shaft bur.

large or even bigger. But if the carious attack is small – in all or in a part of the cavity – the bur should not expand the preparation unnecessarily. Therefore, a smaller diameter of the diamond would be an advantage.

- Large diameter diamonds produce larger cavities.
- Small diameter diamonds produce smaller cavities, but can make larger preparations when needed.

Short diamonds

Short diamonds mean that the head of the contra-angle is closer to the tooth and the contra-angle disturbs the visual supervision of the rotating diamonds (Fig 4–10b). The deeper the cavity, the more the vision is disturbed. In order to improve

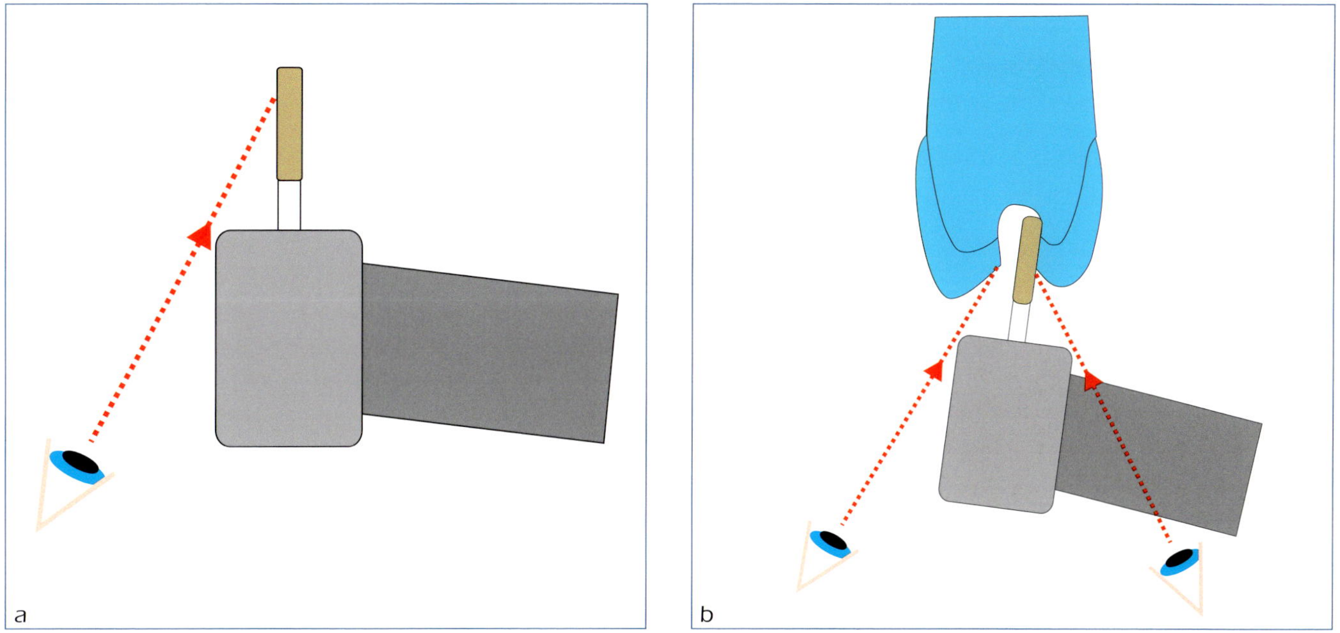

Fig 4–10 (a) A standard cavity prep diamond. (b) A short diamond in a standard cavity contra-angle head disturbs vision.

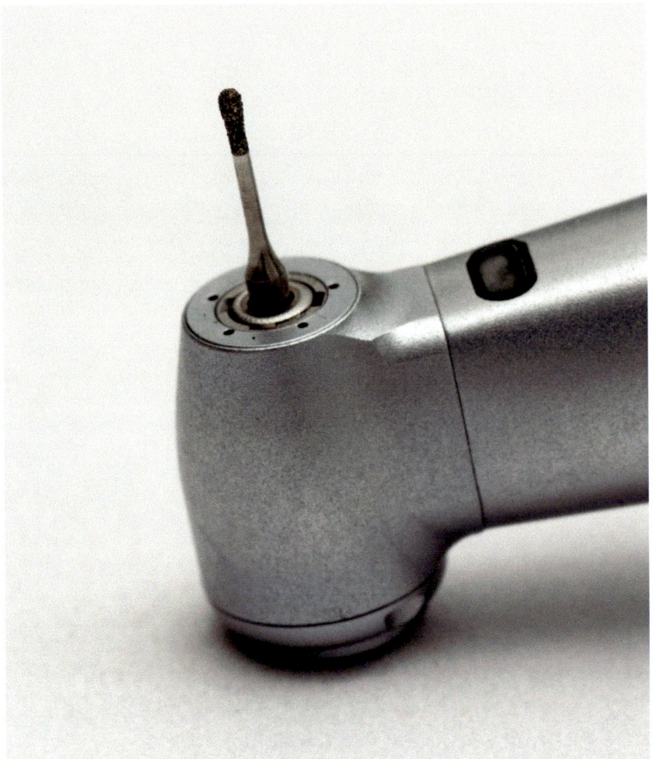

Fig 4–11 A 0.9 mm micropreparation diamond.

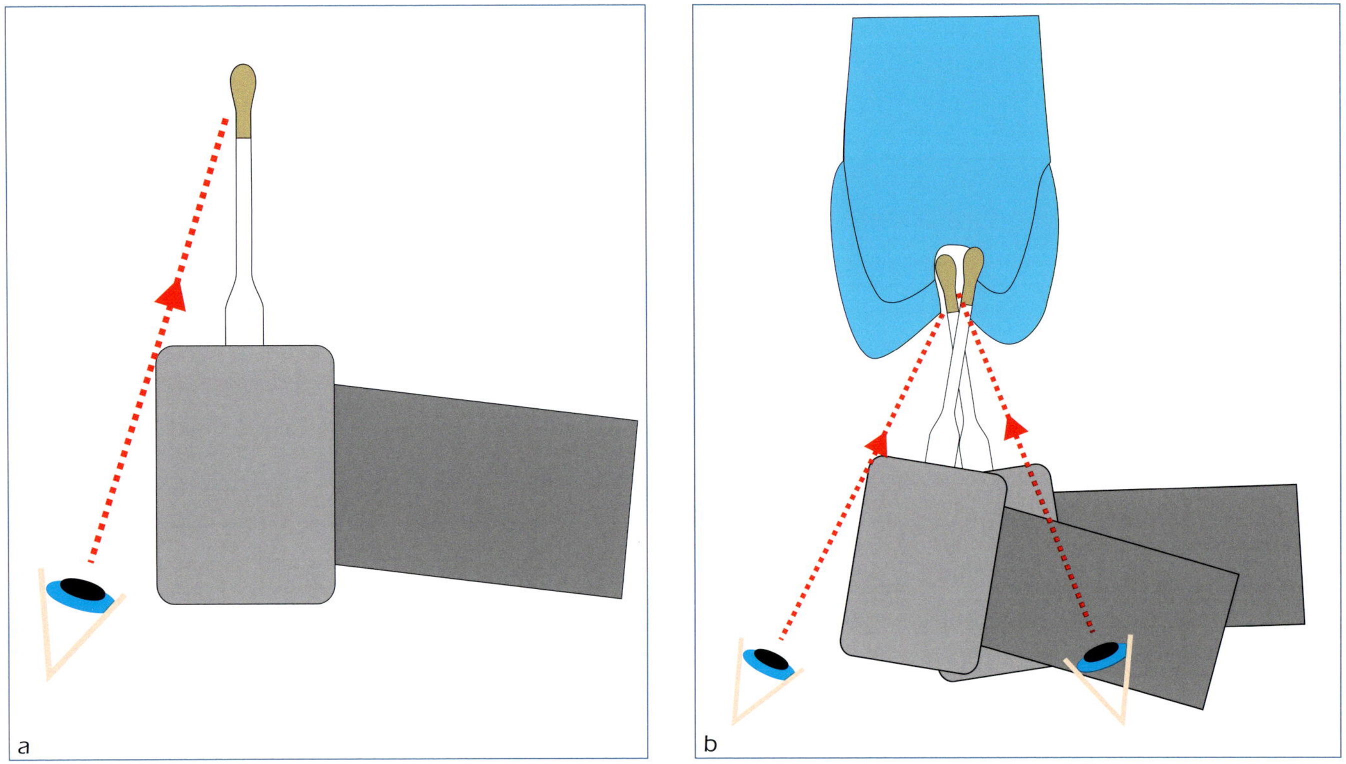

Fig 4–12 (a) Vision from side of the narrow and long shaft. (b) Inclined with a deep cavity.

vision, one has to tilt the contra-angle to the side, with the resulting effect that the cavity opening is increased.

Short diamonds for cavity preparation tend to cause larger cavity openings. This often happens when working in deeper approximal cavities.

A new design – micropreparation diamonds

Micropreparation diamonds (or rather mini-preparation diamonds!) create smaller cavity extensions, and could be used if a carious attack is small. They are 21 mm long, longer than traditional cavity preparation diamonds and have a very thin shaft (Fig 4–11).

The visual supervision of the working part of the rotating diamonds is therefore much better because the contra-angle is a little further away from the cavity, and the contra-angle does not need to be tilted more than slightly to the side for vision, reducing the unnecessary expansion of the cavity (Fig 4–12).

The cutting edge is 2.2 mm long, shorter than on most preparation diamonds. This has a specific advantage. Working in deeper cavities, eg, approximal cavities, the cutting part of the diamond can

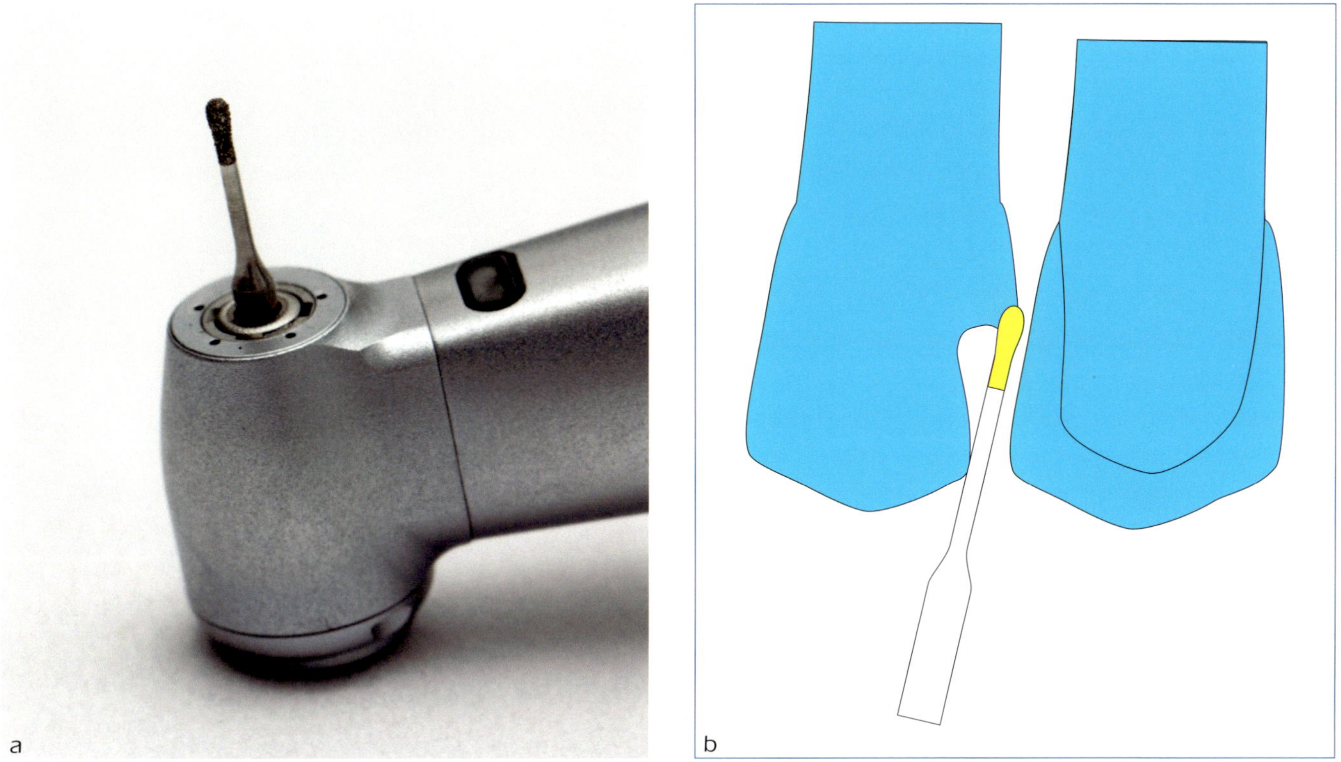

Fig 4–13 (a) A 0.9 mm micropreparation diamond. (b) The micropreparation diamond can be used even where the approximate space is minimal without touching the neighboring tooth. (If the space is closed, a proximal protector metal strip can be used.) As the shaft is smooth, no harm is done to the neighboring tooth, should it be touched.

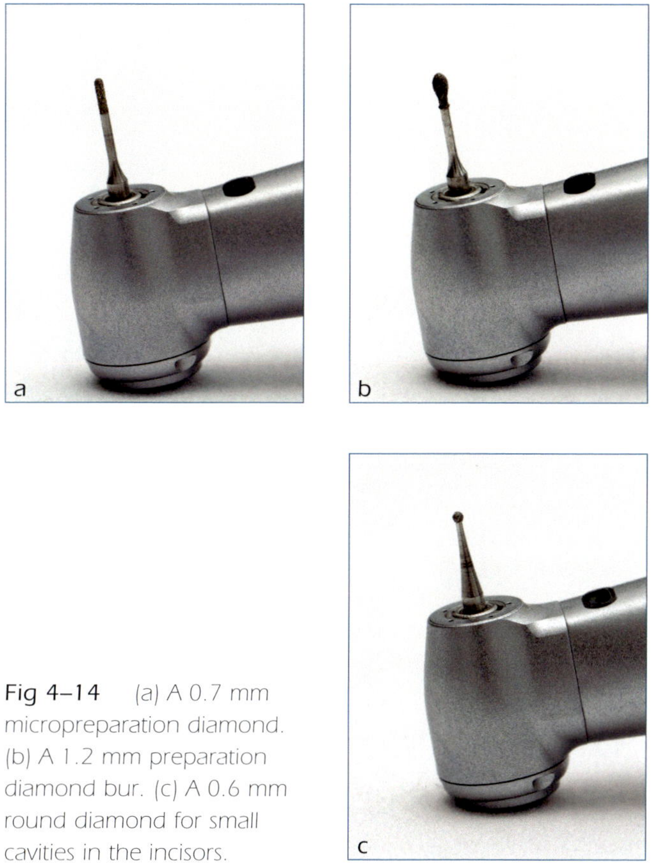

Fig 4–14 (a) A 0.7 mm micropreparation diamond. (b) A 1.2 mm preparation diamond bur. (c) A 0.6 mm round diamond for small cavities in the incisors.

work in the bottom 2.5 mm of the cavity and if touching the cavity entrance nothing happens here, because the shaft is smooth without a diamond layer. This means that unnecessary and unintentional enlargement of the cavity entrance is avoided. The risk of touching the neighboring tooth is reduced. A 0.9 wide micropreparation long shaft diamond (Fig 4–13) is suggested for use as the “diamond of choice” for primary caries (and a 1.2 mm wide micropreparation diamond for very large cavities).

For very small cavities, a 0.7 mm micropreparation diamond is proposed (Fig 4–14a). For incisors, a 0.7 mm round diamond on a thin shaft is the appropriate choice. For very large cavities, use a 1.2 mm micropreparation diamond (Fig 4–14b).

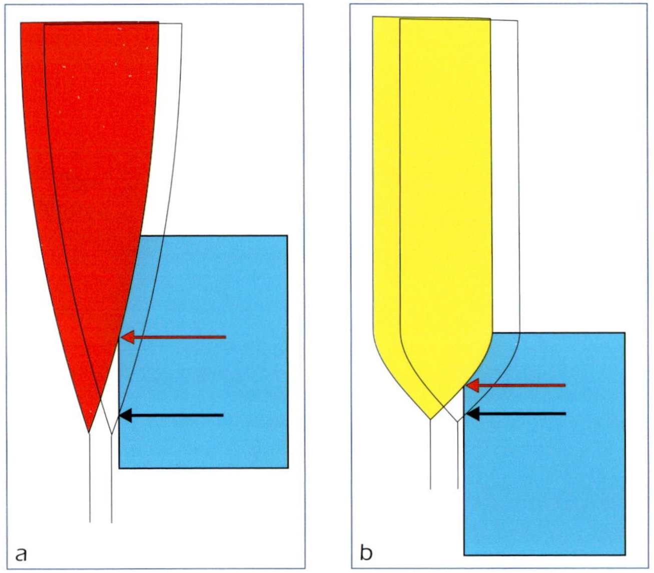

Fig 4–15 (a) A flame-shaped diamond moved 0.1 mm sideways (the vertical displacement is about four times larger). (b) Chamfer diamond.

MICROERGONOMICS

The shape of the diamond and the preparation margin

A preparation is a geometrical 3D structure made by geometrical 3D instruments moved by geometrical 3D movements. Meanwhile, the hands of the dentist cannot be completely controlled precisely. Micromovements will be made as a result of the neuromotoric activity of the muscles. If these micromovements are smaller than about 0.1 mm, they are not visible to the naked eye (without using loupes or a microscope).

However, the effect of these micromovements can be magnified. This will happen when a margin for a crown is prepared with a flame-shaped diamond. This margin, which is sometimes called the "knife edge," may be used with metal margins, eg, porcelain fused to metal crowns.

As a result of the angle of surface of a diamond, a 0.1 mm micromovement to the side will induce a four times larger 0.4 mm axial displacement of the preparation margin (Fig 4–15a). This will make it very difficult to create a precise marginal preparation, in particular when refining the margin a second or third time. It is almost impossible to see, feel or reproduce the margin in the axial direction of the tooth.

Either the margin is undefined (can be identified by its roughness) or the diamond is inclined to produce a better-defined margin, but then the angle of convergence is larger than the ideal of about 12 degrees.

If the diamond has an angle of 45 degrees at the tip, a micromovement of 0.1 mm will result in an axial displacement of margin of only 0.1 mm.

This is the so-called chamfer diamond, producing a 45-degree chamfer for the porcelain to metal fused crown, without shoulders (Fig 4–15b). The chamfer is easy to feel with a probe and to see from the axial direction of the tooth, and also quite easy to reproduce. The depth of the chamfer will depend on the type of preparation. Training courses have shown that most dentists have difficulties making a chamfer preparation, if the diameter of the diamond is less than 1.0 mm. A chamfer diamond with a cylindrical part diameter of 1.2mm is easy to use for almost all dentists.

Dentists are different

The amplitude of the micromovements is different, as is the visual acuity (the ability to see the micromovements).

Microergonomics of shoulder preparations

Often shoulder preparations are made by diamonds with a rather large diameter, that when used harm the gingival surfaces because the diamond surface touches/work in the gingiva. The dilacerations in the gingival area may induce a gingival retraction.

A non-invasive gingival shoulder preparation

The following describes a gingival non-invasive shoulder preparation:

- If the shoulder needs to be 1.4 mm deep, make the initial preparation with a 1.2 mm diamond, rounded like a sphere at the end (Fig 4–16).
- Create a gutter preparation 0.2 mm from the external surface without touching the gingiva. The direction of the diamond is almost parallel to the tooth axis.
- Follow the gingiva in an external curve (if involving a retraction of gingival tissues) (Fig 4–17).
- Refine the margin with a slightly curved-end cutting diamond (Fig 4–18).
- Direct the diamond perpendicularly to the periphery of the curve (if there is a curve) of preparation.

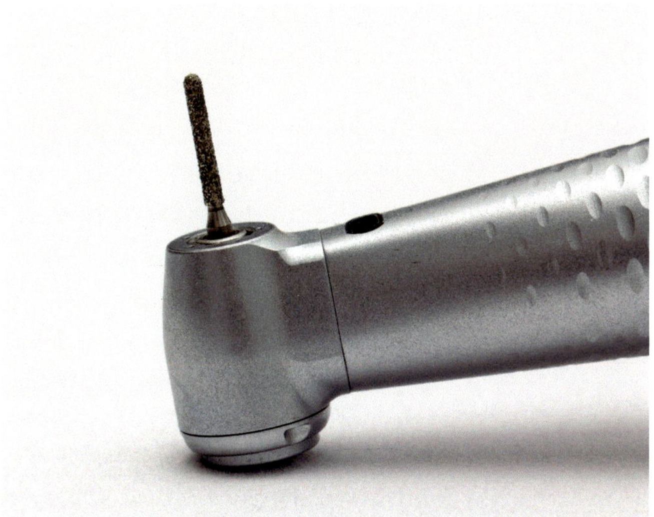

Fig 4–16 A cylindrical diamond with a rounded end is used.

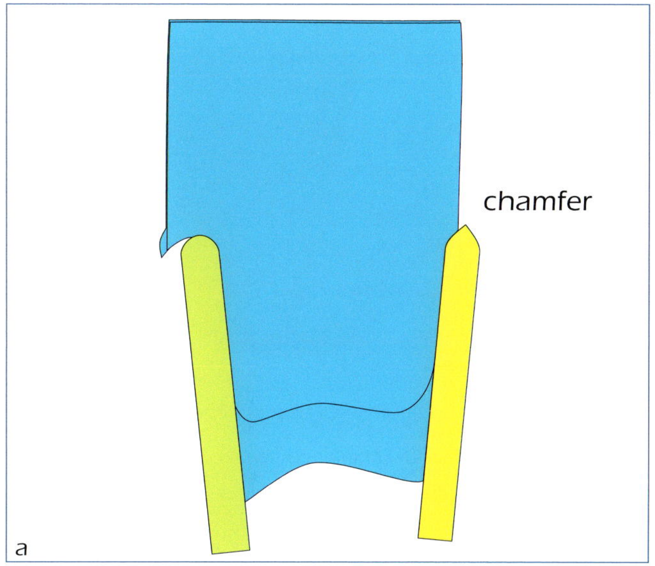

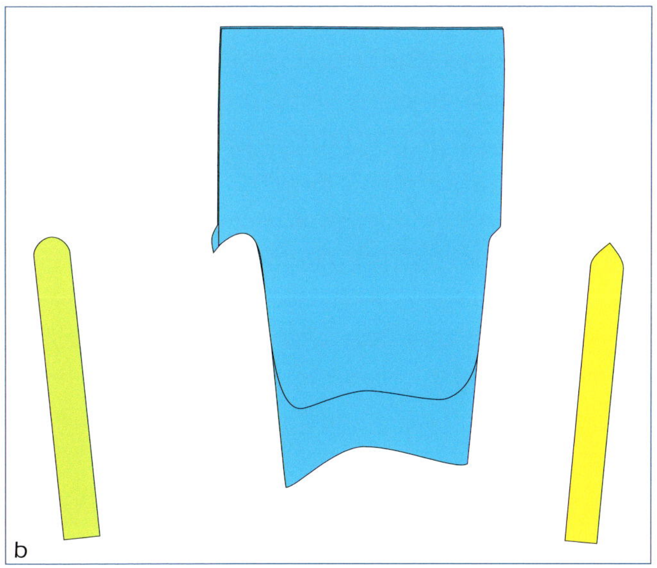

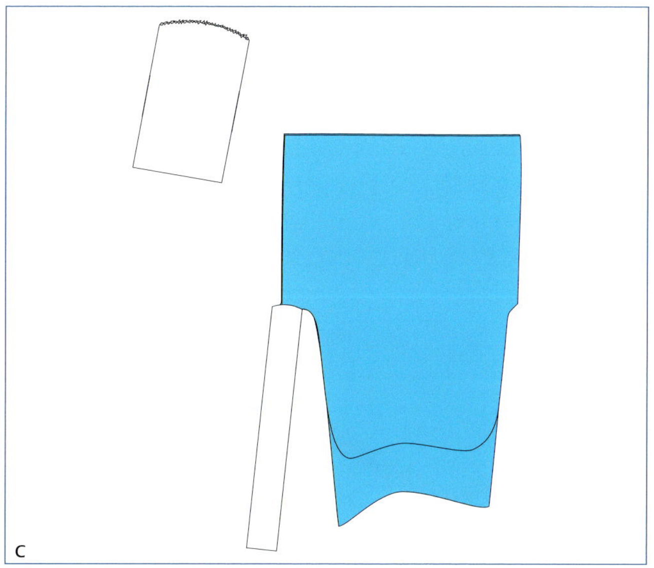

Fig 4–17 (a and b) Initial "gutter" preparation. The rounded shoulder is prepared 0.2 mm from surface. The gingival area is not touched. (c) The margin of the "gutter" is refined with a slightly curved end cutting diamond. As the sides are completely smooth, the gingiva is not dilacerated if touched (a thin retraction cord may be placed before the preparation).

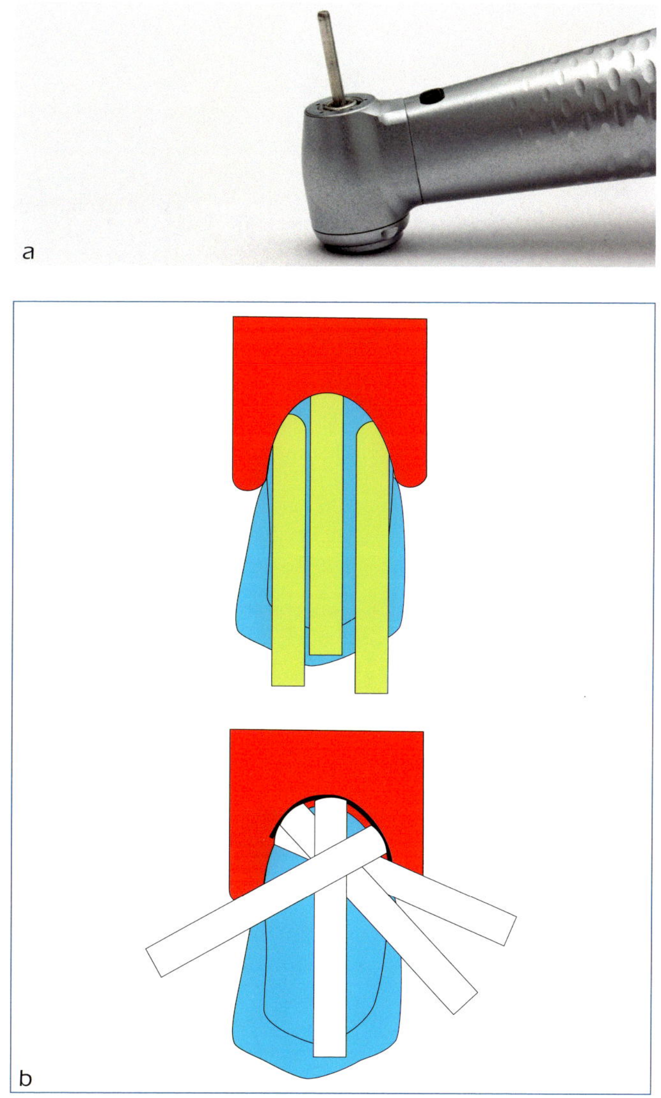

Fig 4–18 (a) The initial preparation is made parallel to the tooth axis, corrected to slight convergence. (b) The exterior margins are finished with the end cutting diamond and made perpendicularly to the preparation margin. This results in a perfect internal rounded and external curved (stepfree) preparation.

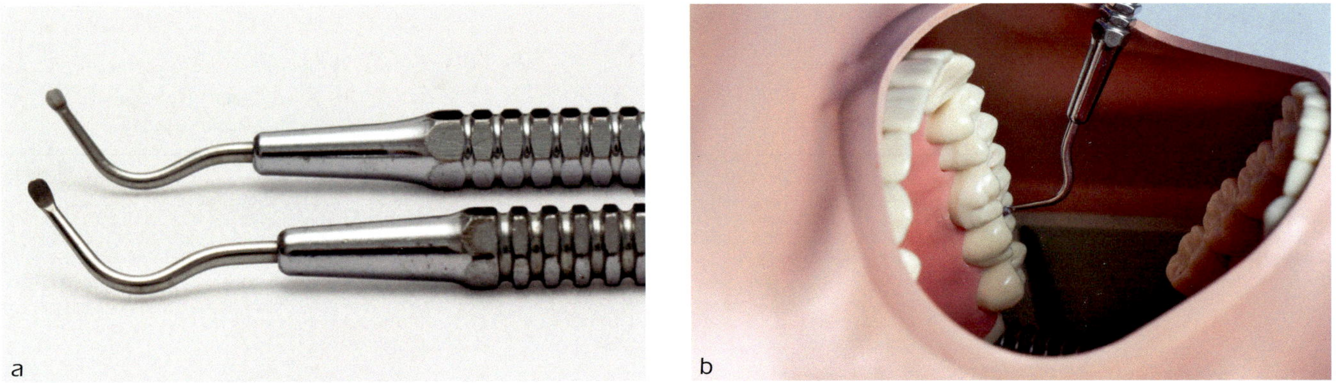

Fig 4–19 (a and b) Hand excavators from Maillefer have a sufficient angle (45 degrees in relation to shaft) and shape designed to be easy to use, even in distal cavities.

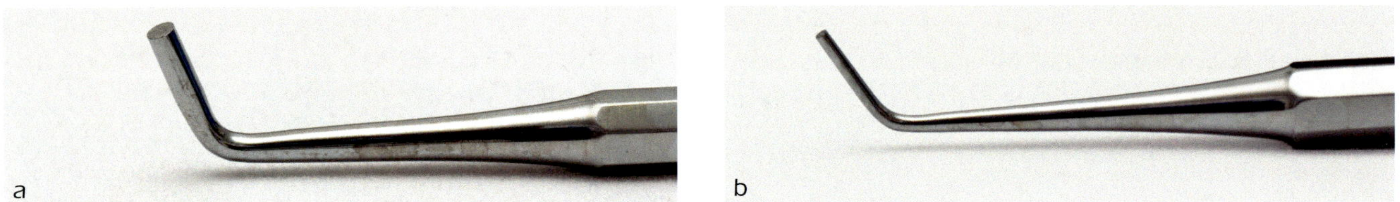

Fig 4–20 (a) Composite and adapting instruments must be angled (110 degrees in relation to shaft) so they can be used in a distal cavity. One end of the instrument must fit into minimal cavities of 0.9 mm. (b) The angle between the shank and the working part of the instrument must be about 110 degrees.

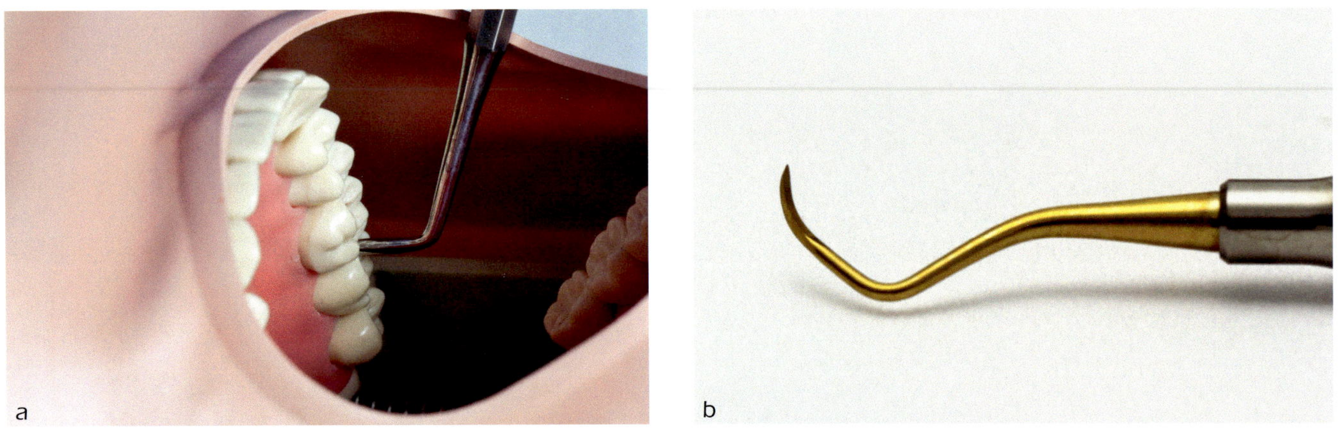

Fig 4–21 (a) Composite instrument in a distal cavity. (b) Hand scaler angled 45 degrees sideways.

IMPORTANCE OF ANGLE AND SHAPE

Hand instruments must have a shape and angle so they can be applied on all external or internal surfaces, with the dentist in a good working posture. Some examples will follow in the sections below.

Hand excavator

A hand excavator is an excellent tool for removing dentin caries. At the same time as carious dentin is removed, the dentist has a fine tactile feedback. One can feel when the softer carious tissue is removed, and the instrument touches hard dentin. A hand excavator is a very fast, careful and simple instrument to use.

Unfortunately the working part of most hand excavators has a length and angle that makes it very difficult to gain access in deep cavities, especially distally located ones. This seems to be the reason why many dentists do not use hand excavators.

Hand excavators from Maillefer have an angle and shape, so they are easy to use even in distal cavities (Fig 4–19). Composite and adapting instruments must also be angled so they can be used in a distal cavity (Fig 4–20).

One end of the instrument must fit into minimal cavities of 0.9 mm.

The angle between the instrument grip and the working part of the instrument must be about 110 degrees.

Handscaler

The sideways angle of the working part of a supragingival handscaler must be 45 degrees. This is so that scaling in the lingual side of the incisal area of the mandibular jaw can be instrumented from an 11 o'clock position (and with sufficient space between the patient's nose and the instrument to the dentist's thumb!) (Fig 4–21).

Few handscalers comply with these guidelines, however. Using these lingually on the mandibular incisors will especially guide the dentist into a bad working posture.

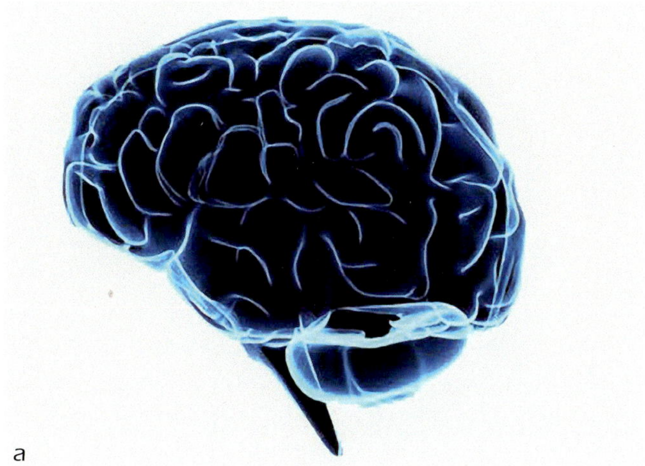

a

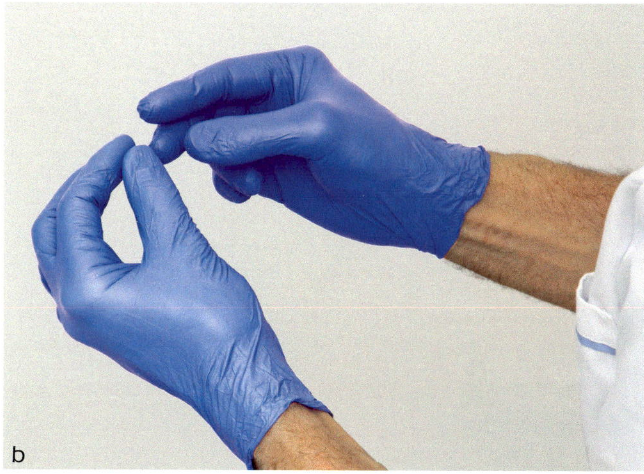

b

Fig 4–22 (a) The brain is the control center for all motor functions. (b) When you are training your hands, you are training both hands and brain together. By using mental animation of movements, you can even train your hands without using them.

TRAINING HANDS AND BRAIN

Few are fond of challenging their basic habits. Our arsenal of habits forms a secure base for our professional life. If habits are questioned, it may question our confidence and competence, and cause us to be insecure about what to do, and how to learn new motor patterns. It can feel like it may be better to keep on the known track.

Can you learn while you are treating your patients? That is difficult, unless you have some definite learning objectives. The attention required by the patient demands your mental presence, and may disturb your attention to training.

The patient may also easily realize that undefined searching movements replace the routine movements that reassure the competence of the dentist. That will not create a good experience either for the patient or for the image of the dentist. Furthermore, the training of new manual movements needs many repetitions, which will not be possible while treating a patient.

A "skill" is a sequence of movement. The training of skills could be practiced on a phantom head in the patient chair, or with simulated treatment on a family member, a friend or one of the practice staff.

For a start, a skill should be defined as a sequence of precise movements. The number of movements should not be too large – normally 5 to 10 or maybe 15. Then one starts to train the skills slowly, and in the beginning correcting details by looking in the illustrations of this book. The skill is repeated, while assuring every detail is correct.

When the skill has been performed correctly around 10 times, the speed is increased, and often a bit of confusion or mistakes result after 15 to 20 repetitions and one starts to relax a little. Then the skill is continuously repeated, say 50 times. This may take 10 to 15 minutes altogether. After 1 hour, the skill is repeated again, 50 to 75 times. The skill is repeated the next day, until the beginnings of automatization is learned. Skill-based professions like musicians, dancer or athletes spend much of their time and energy training their skills.

So can dentists. The outcome may be extraordinary.

This training is called manual training, but in fact it is probably more a training of the brain than of the hands (Fig 4–22).

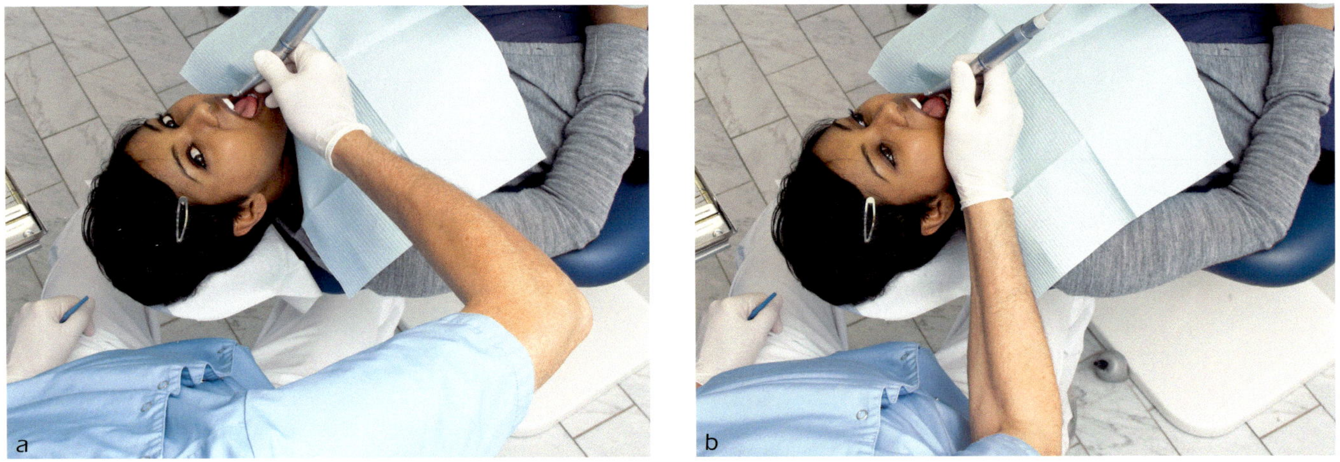

Fig 4–23 (a) A dentist using an elevated elbow caused by the instrument grip. (b) The elbow can be kept in close contact with the body, because the instrument grip is more angled.

Mental manual motor training – brain training!

Manual training programs of skills can be supplemented by "mental manual motor training" – a method used by athletes. You imagine or animate in your mind (see page 73) all movements of the skill one by one and later in sequence, but you do not move. It seems like the neural activity in the brain controlling the mental motor training is the same as that performing the real movements up to and including the premotor gyrus in the brain. Meanwhile, the motor gyrus is not activated. You can even perform the mental motor training of dentists' professional skills at home in your armchair! A mix between hands-on and mental motor training is beneficial.

HANDS FOR PRECISION

When using hand instruments, eg, contra-angles, in the mouth of the patient, several elements are interacting:

1. The dentist's "clock" position is decided by the direction of vision, whether direct or with a mirror. The direction of vision is decided by the direction of the external or internal surface to be observed.
2. The position of the patient's head is dependent on the visibility of the surface (external or internal) where the task is performed (see page 78).
3. The eye-to-object distance is related to the eye-to-elbow distance, which defines the angle of lower arms (see page 67).

Together, the following points determine the direction of the instrument shaft:

4. The correct position and direction of the working part of the instrument (hand instrument or rotating instrument on contra-angle, or inserts of ultrasonic or sonic scaler handpieces) in order to perform the actual task allowing a simultaneous visual control.
5. The shape and angle of the working part of the instrument in relation to the part of "instrument shaft," which the dentist grips.
6. The access to the mouth in general, and the area where the task is performed – and soft tissue retraction.

These positions are specific, eg, the surface of the tooth, see section later, page 217.

The following elements determine together the position of dentist's fingers, wrist and lower arm:

7. The instrument grip, including the angle of grip.

As described in Chapter 10, the dentist's elbow should be kept in slight contact with the body, and therefore the right shoulder is relaxed and kept down. This is accomplished by an instrument grip that allows a lowered position (Fig 4–23b) (see Fig 4–24 for some examples of instrument grips).

The instrument grip is essential for positioning and using the instrument in a correct working position, AND at the same time achieving a fine work posture. The angle of the instrument grip compensates for the inclination of the lower arms upwards,

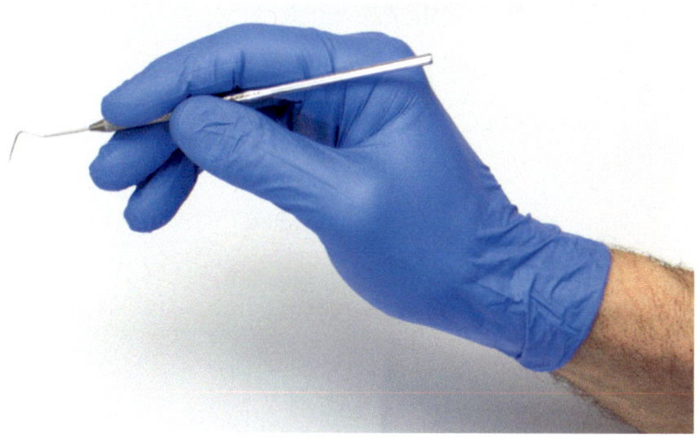
a

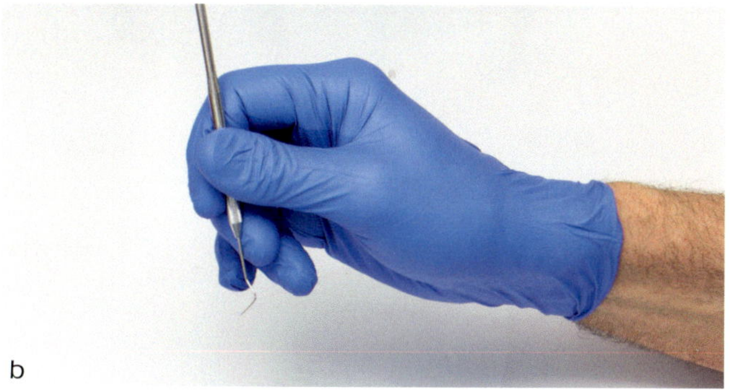
b

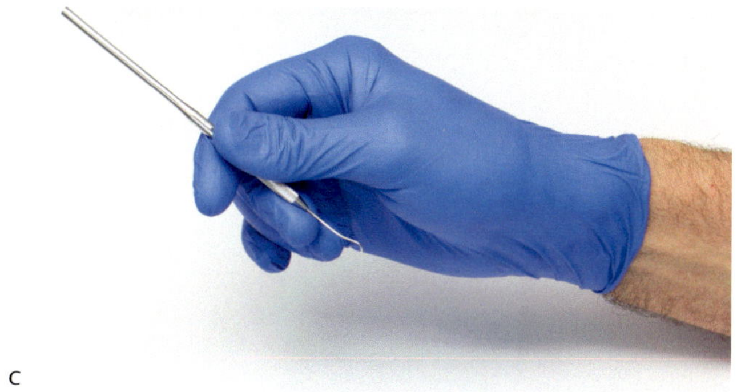
c

Fig 4–24 (a to c) Different examples of instrument grips.

and therefore reduces/eliminates the risk of elevating the shoulders.

8. The forearms are angled upwards in order to obtain a distance for precision vision (about 32 cm, less for young dentists). The taller the dentist is (or more precisely, the longer the eye-to-elbow distance is for the dentist), the more the lower arms are inclined upwards. The less tall the dentist, the less the lower arms are angled.

The forearm is the stable support for the dentist's hand. If the support for the hands or the fingers is not stable, then the arm muscles must try to create stability. This is achieved by creating tension in the muscles, so that the large muscle groups connected to the shoulder, upper arm and lower arm contract simultaneously with their antagonists to create stability. However, the groups of muscles elevating the scapulae (shoulders bones) are not only tense for creating stability; they also have to carry the weight of the whole arm, so these muscles are a high risk for causing pain. The better the support for hands and fingers, the smaller the risk.

9. Finger and/or hand support – it is strongly recommended to always work with a secure and stable support for the right-hand. Support for the right hand (for right-handed dentists, of course) is a very important and necessary condition for performing precision work. Also for dentists, the hand/finger support for the left hand is important in order to relax muscles in and around the left shoulder that "carries" the left arm. Creating a support that allows the relevant and correct movements of the instrument is more complicated. The type of "mobile support" will depend on these factors.

Three types of hand support

Support for right hand on a tooth with a finger

The photos show the finger support using the right hand's ring finger. The left hand's index finger simulates the supporting tooth (Fig 4–25). While working at the cavity preparation at the maxillary right molars, the ring finger of the dentist's right hand can be supported by a cotton roll (the best are the parotis type – long and thin) placed in the vestibulum (Fig 4–26).

Extraoral support on the patient's face/skin of the patient

Extraoral support on the patient's cheek using the back side of fingers (Fig 4–27).

Support of the dentist's right hand on her/his left hand, which again is supported extraorally on the face/skin of the patient.

This support is specific for working parallel to maxillary right vestibular surface. The left index finger's back side is supported on the alveolar process. Meanwhile, the right hand's middle finger is supported on the left index finger (Fig 4–28).

The left hand's small finger is supported on right cheekbone of the patient, and retraction is done

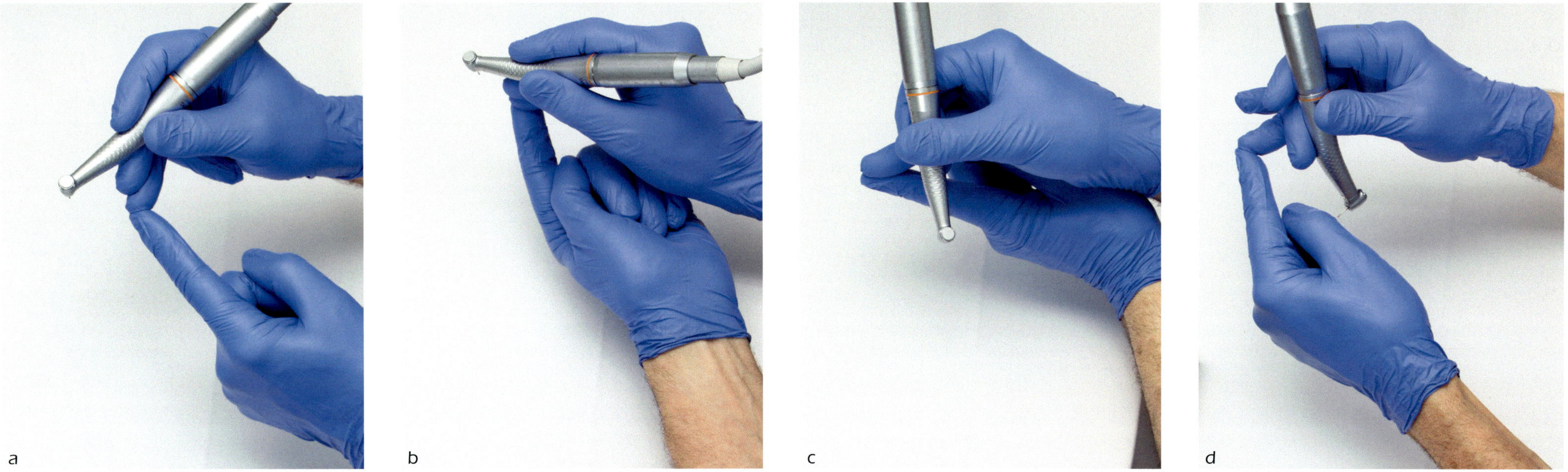

Fig 4-25 (a and b) Finger support using the right hand ring finger. (c and d) The index finger of the left hand simulates a tooth support.

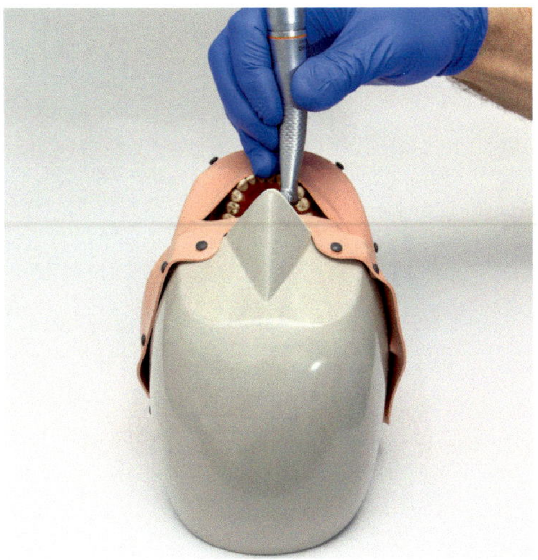

Fig 4-26 Support by a ring finger on a tooth.

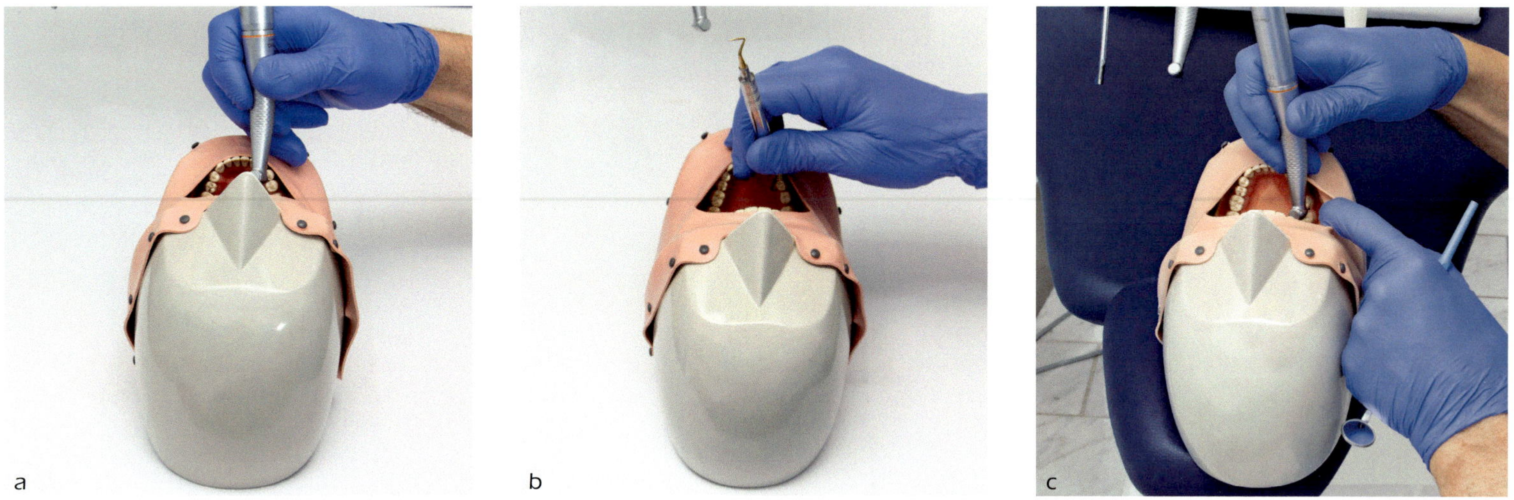

Fig 4-27 (a to c) Extraoral support.

with a mirror (see Fig 4–29 for correct positioning of contra-angle and right hand support).

10. Biomechanics of movements to perform the task (see Chapter 4)

We will return to finger and hand support, when the biomechanics and neurophysiology of precision movements are analyzed and described. It is quite normal to find this all quite complex – manual performance has complicated elements one needs to understand and to train in. For some dentists, "manual intuition" can lead to excellent solutions, but most dentists will benefit greatly from conscientious, knowledge-based understanding and decisions.

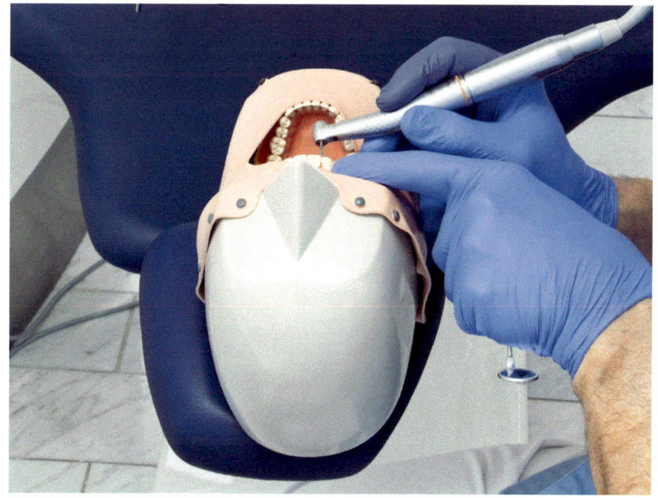

Fig 4–28 The left index finger is supported on the alveolar process.

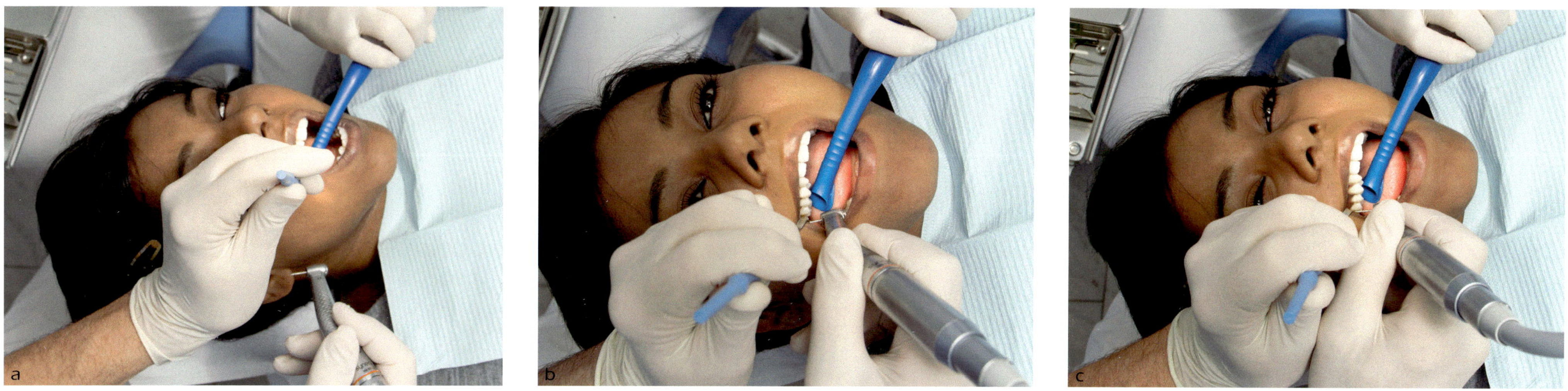

Fig 4–29 (a) The dentist's left hand is supported on the right cheek of the patient. (b) The contra-angle is placed in the correct position. (c) The left hand is moved to right side so the right hand is supported at left hand with several contact points.

MOVING THE INSTRUMENTS

When observing dentists working with their hands, it is noticeable that the movements for the same task are performed quite differently – but well – with different outcomes, different uses of time and developing different levels of fatigue.

Motor output and sensory feedback

Movements are performed by an interaction between motor nervous control and the corresponding sensory feedback system.

The feedback system is the controlled by the proprioceptive system with the following elements:

- Muscle spindles register how much the muscles are stretched, their length, which indicate the relation (angle) between the bones to which the muscles are attached. The velocity of movement and acceleration of movement are also registered.
- Tendon spindles (Golgi sensors) register the tension in the tendons, and which force the muscles are applying.
- The kinesthetic system ("sense for movements"). This term is sometimes used for the proprioceptive system and the sensors of skin for tactility and pressure. Sensors in subcutis provide a tactile and pressure feedback.

Feedback arrives after the movement, or part of the movement is done. The kinesthetic system provides us with a feedback from our movements. The proprioceptive feedback time is 80–120 milliseconds. However, visual feedback is slow.

We will first have a visual system feedback after the movement is performed. You have to make the movement before you can see it. The visual reaction time is about 150 to 180 ms, and time for manual reaction must be added to this, which together is more than 500 ms. Selecting a particular response is called the "choice effect," which adds 500 to 1000 ms. **In fact, visual feedback is so slow that a fast movement may be way out of track before a new visual signal is updated.** This indicates that relying on visual and proprioceptive and tactile feedback is not sufficient for effective motor activity. It is too slow. The movements have to be planned by the brain before they are done. This is described as **feed forward control,** or **anticipatory control**.

Feed forward control relies on information acquired before the feedback sensors are activated. This mechanism is essential for rapid movements.

Movements by fingers – a complex matter

The following is an attempt to describe a very frequent practical experience from courses. Fine motor movements for using rotating or non-rotating instruments are performed by some dentists by only moving the fingers that are supporting the instrument.

However – movements of instruments made by finger movements are questionable! These movements are three-dimensional, complex, compound movements. The position of the fingers is continuously changed. The number of muscles and articulations with proprioceptive sensors for muscles and for tension is very high. Every time the fingers are moved, a new proprioceptive and tactile feedback is transmitted to the brain of the dentist.

An overwhelming stream of feedback seems to widely overflow the "bandwidth" of the neural sensory "transmission" system, with a resulting loss of tactility and proprioception.

Furthermore, if using a crown preparation diamond, the direction of the axis of the diamond is very difficult to maintain throughout the movement. It has to be done visually. This makes it very difficult to train and automatize the movements. The movements are much too complex to create a specific standardized sequence of movements (a "skill"), which can be trained and automatized.

Visual feedback and step-by-step control is needed. The delays for proprioceptive and for neural, as well as for "choice delay" of visual feedback, is easy to observe as small, very frequent repeated pauses. The movements tend to run step-by-step, instead of in smooth, well-defined and connected pretrained movements. This technique could be called **"stop and go,"** where the continuity of movement (the skill) is divided into small sections.

Movements of an instrument made by finger movements can be replaced by a biomechanical simplification, which is more precise, faster to perform, less tiring, and can be trained as a skill.

MOVEMENTS BASED ON BIOMECHANIC SIMPLIFICATION AND SKILL TRAINING

Instead of using complex three-dimensional micro-movements of the fingers, the movements can be simplified using biomechanically guided continuous movements.

- Hold with the fingers
- Feel with the fingers
- Move with the "instrument-finger-hand-lower arm complex" with paralellometer-like movements
- Movable support on flexible ring finger supported on teeth or extraoral hand/side of finger support on the patient's skin using its mobility.

This important aspect is difficult to imagine so it will be described several times on the following pages. It is, however, easy to take into practice.

Fingers provide tactility

The movements of the fingers are limited to a primary grip, which places the working part of the instrument (bur, diamond etc, of the contra-angle insert of the scaler or the working part of hand instrument) in the correct position for the action planned.

After this primary grip, the fingers holding the instrument and wrist do not move. This means that brain does not receive a cascade of proprioceptive and tactile input from moving the fingers, as described in the previous example.

As the finger grip remains in an unchanged position, the tactile sense of the fingers do now refer only to the "touching" of the involved surface with the instrument. The instrument is now under tactile control, undisturbed by other sensitive inputs. Fingers are used to find and maintain a grip for best vision, working posture, and precision work. If fingers are not moved in relation to the hand, then sensitivity is improved.

The following method is intuitively used by many dentists:

- Place the instrument or contra-angle perfectly, and hold with the fingers.
- Do not move the fingers, or move the hand, but instead move the "instrument-finger-hand-lower arm" together as a fixed unit.

Using flexible support to create precision movements

- Support for right hand on a tooth with a finger
- Extraoral support on the face/skin of the patient
- Support of the dentist's right hand on his/her left hand, which again is extraorally supported on the face/skin of the patient.

PARALLELOMETER-LIKE MOVEMENTS

When neither the fingers nor the wrist are moved, how are the movements performed?

As an example, consider an amateur's use of a saw. The hand is closed on the handgrip of the saw, and the sawing begins. While sawing, the handgrip and/or the angle of the wrist may change, which will cause the saw to change direction. When the direction of the saw changes, the saw cut begins to be oblique.

Now this is discovered visually, when the mistake is visible and leads to attempts to correct the cutting direction of the saw (which is sometimes too late to make).

The professional use of a saw prevents oblique sawing by adhering to the following: the fingers of the hand are closed on the handgrip and is parallel to the upper arm. Now the fingers and wrist are not moved in any way, and the saw is moved only by the forearm and upper arm, which form a parallelometer and create a straight cut. The sawing movements remain perfectly unchanged, on the condition that the grip and wrist position (angle and torsion) is not changed. We could call these "parallelometer movements" (Fig 4–30).

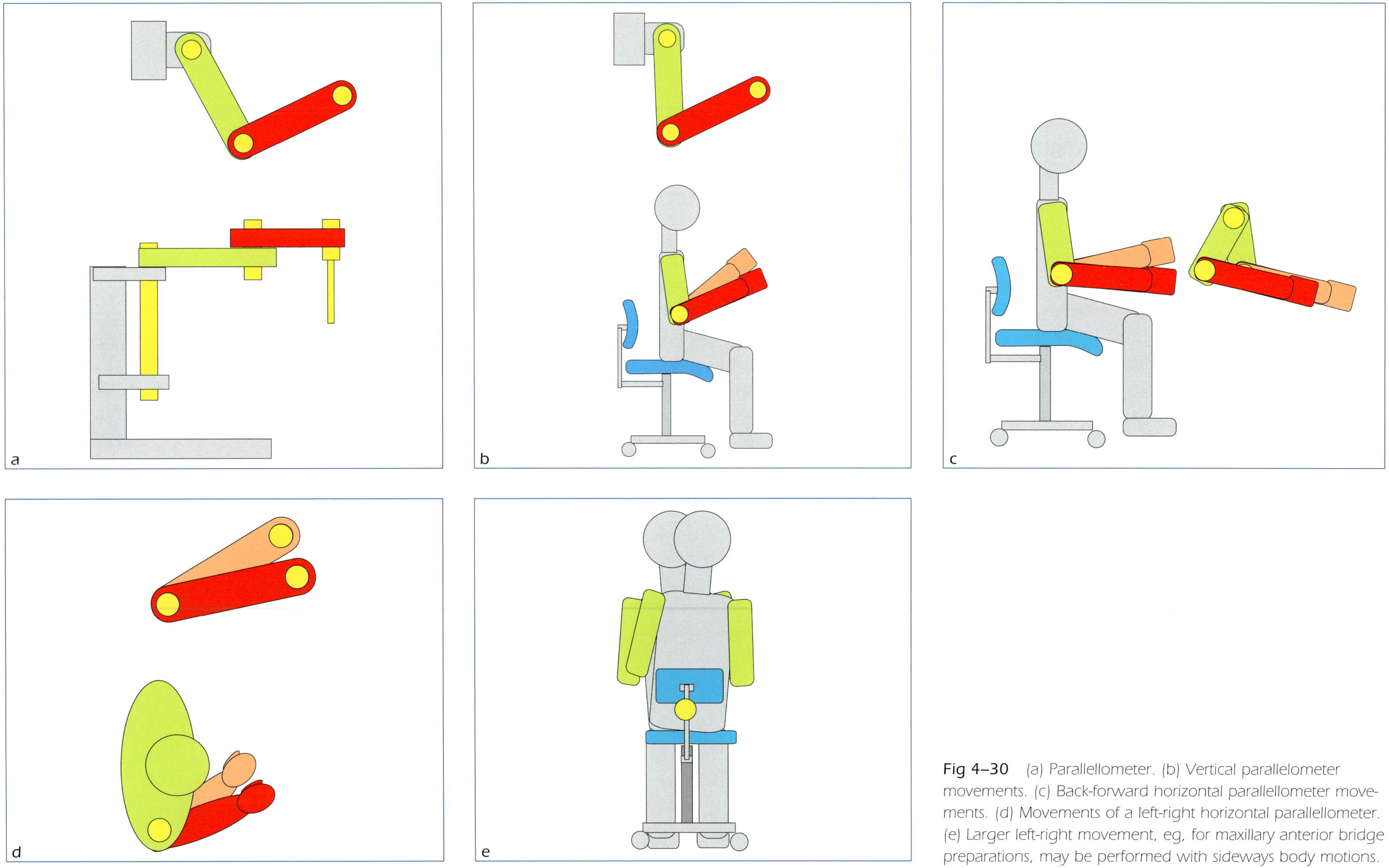

Fig 4–30 (a) Parallellometer. (b) Vertical parallelometer movements. (c) Back-forward horizontal parallellometer movements. (d) Movements of a left-right horizontal parallellometer. (e) Larger left-right movement, eg, for maxillary anterior bridge preparations, may be performed with sideways body motions.

Crown preparations with parallelometer movements

The diamond for a shoulder or a chamfer preparation is placed in the correct position by the instrument grip in the relevant angle. Then neither the fingers or wrist position are moved, nor is the wrist position changed by angling or twisting. The movements are now made by parallel movements controlled by the upper arm and forearm, supported by a flexible ring finger or a flexible support on the patient's face.

The biomechanical model of movement planning relieves stress on the dentist. Biomechanical training controls the movements. The tactility of the dentist's fingers is used for sensing the touch to the task object. The dentist overlooks the movements, paying extra attention to the position of the instrument tip.

Parallelometer movements are relevant for the crown and bridge preparations (with final correction to the angle of convergence), inlay preparation, composite preparation, polishing of surfaces of composite fillings or amalgam. The type of movement will of course depend on the task in hand, eg, to use a hand excavator, a small rotating movement of wrist is required.

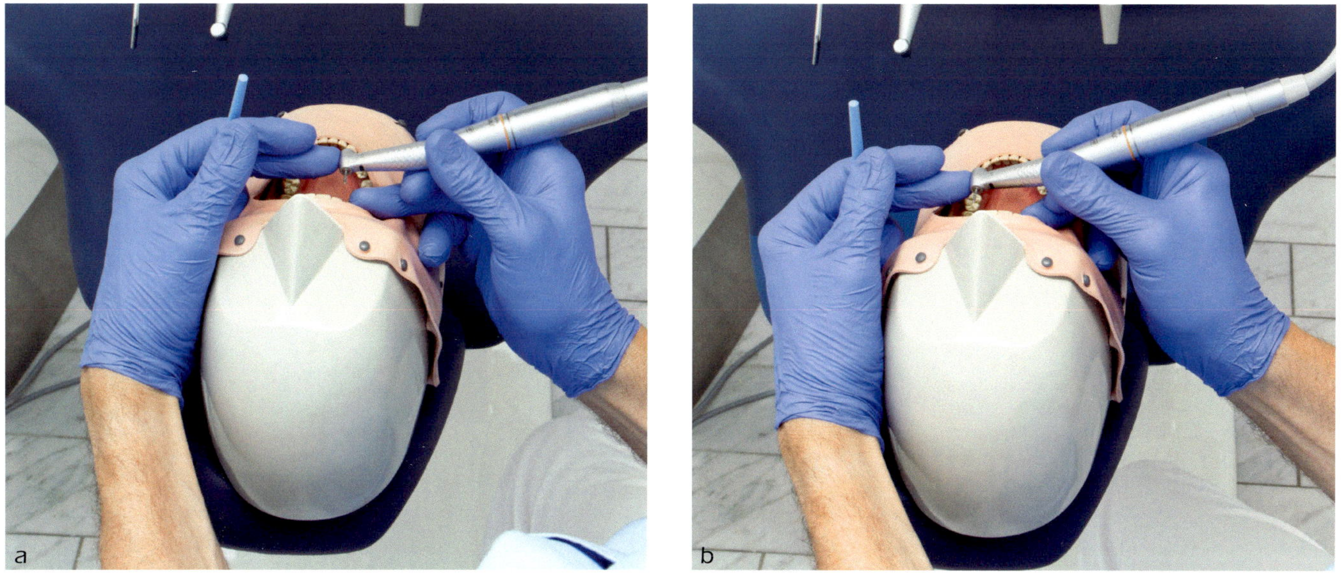

Fig 4–31 (a) The contra-angle stably supported without movement, while (b) 5–6 cm right-to-left sideways movements are accomplished.

Knowing the result of your movements before you have performed them – feed forward

A detailed planning of movements involves a primary visualization of the movements to be performed later in a three-dimensional space. This is the first step.

Visualization, however, does not mean you are "ready to make some movement" – to do this you must mentally envisage the movement you are going to perform. The word "imagine" is not correct, because "imagine" means making a mental image of. And this is not the case, because you in your mind will have to create a **mental representation of the movements you are about to perform**. We will call this "mental animation in a 3D space," to separate it from the visualization and from the real performance of the animated movements. Mental animation of movements in a 3D space before you perform them is essential. One could call it mental planning of the movement. All movements need to be planned before performing them. When repeated sufficiently, they can be learned to automatization level. You can even train your hands by frequent repetition of the mental model for performing the sequence of movement involved in a specific skill.

Visual input also disturbs mental animation

As visual sensory input tends to dominate other sensory inputs, visual imagination or visualizations must be consciously separated from the mental animation of the movement process.

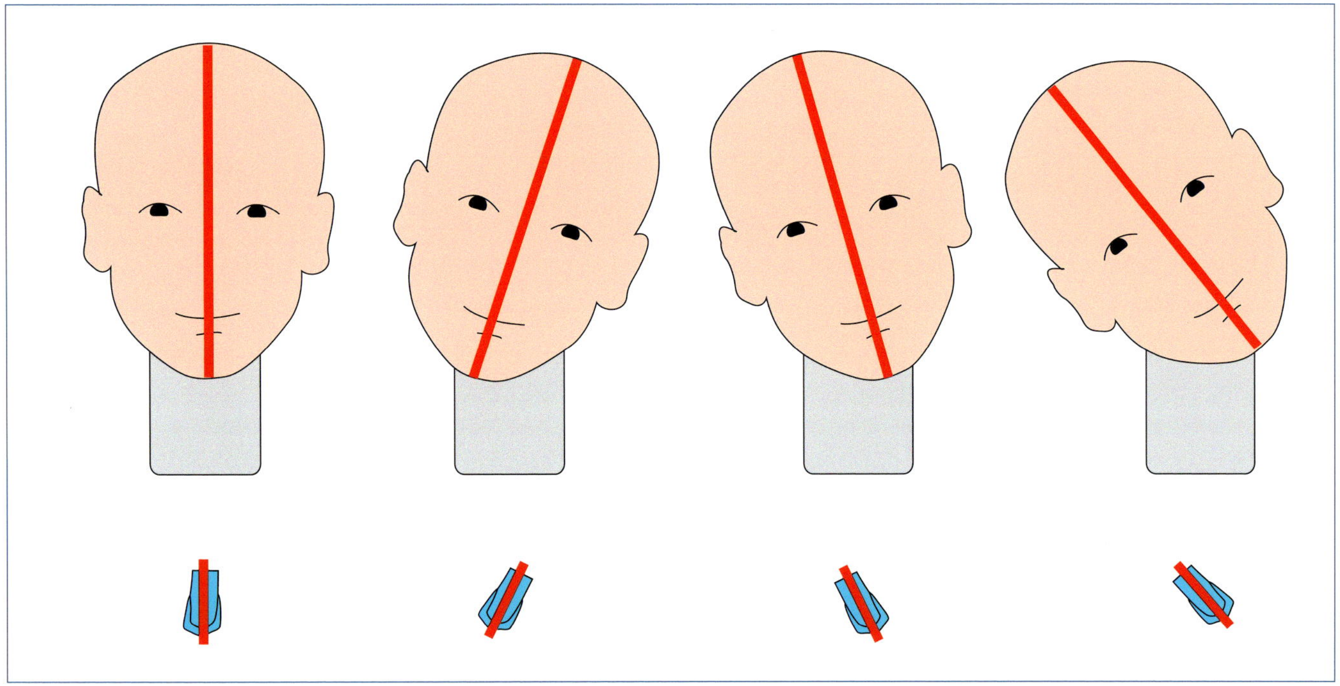

Fig 4–32 A habit of making a physical alignment with the head to the axis of the tooth often will very often lead to poor work positions. Biomechanical guided mental training can help for performing the movements as described above.

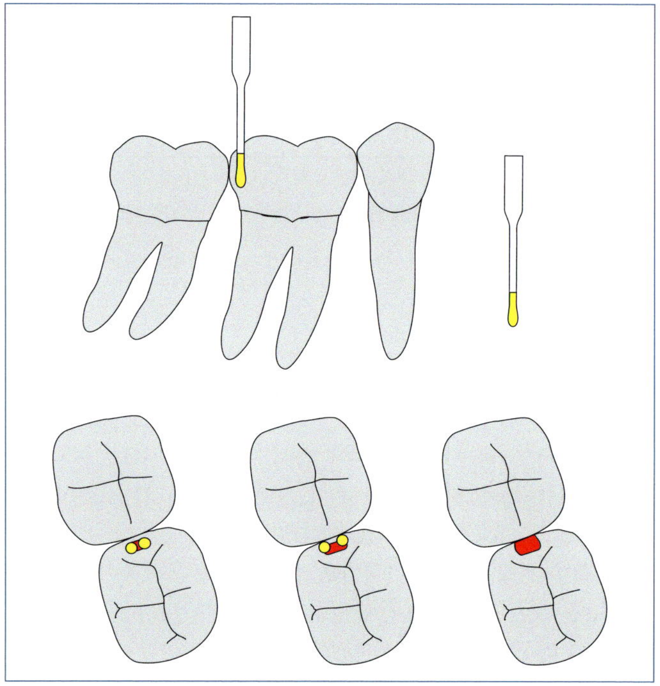

Fig 4–33 Opening a carious cavity with a minimally invasive preparation.

In order to perform movements, one must first visualize a three-dimensional space and then mentally animate the movement in 3D. The biomechanical simplification, together with simplified sensitive feedback makes pretraining of skills, as well as preplanning of movements possible.

Mental animation is essential

Mental animations of an object in a 3D space is difficult to do for some people and easy for others. It seems like there may be a genetic reason for this.

Some can, without trouble, imagine a house in 3D from a 2D plan, and others have difficulty doing it. Some people can easily move around in a city and maintain their orientation, whereas others have difficulties. However, problems with 3D manipulation can pose **"the alignment problem."**

Some dentists have the habit of aligning her/his head to the axis of the tooth where a crown preparation is made (Fig 4–32). This often leads to bad working postures. This habit can be difficult to unlearn. But by using the biomechanical simplification model, the direction of the actual tooth is now controlled by instrument grip and the finger/hand support alone. This gives the dentist the freedom to place her/his head in a convenient position.

- Vision and visualization tend to dominate the mental animation.
- Thinking also disturbs mental animation.
- Both thinking and visualization activate the same parts of the brain as mental animation, and the real time performance of movements.

This is why the introduction of this book encourages the reader to "STOP THINKING and enjoy your 'dancing' hands." Biomechanically simplified movements where the fingers are not moved when the grip position is found, and using parallometer movements, can be easily learned because they are simple to do.

Making a mental model

Vision is slow – you cannot see movements and the outcome of the movements before they are performed. A skill is a sequence of movements, which can be trained by repetition. You initiate a manual task by a visualization of the outcome, and you shift the function of your brain in order to plan the movements. This has been described as making a mental model of the movements or a mental animation of the movements. This allows an anticipation or "feed forward" of the real time movements. Then the movements are performed under visual supervision with ad hoc adjustments.

The minimal standard cavity preparation

As an example the reader may imagine the following:

- Bitewings have showed an approximal carious attack needing treatment by means of a composite filling. The occlusal enamel is still intact.
- In order to simplify (and almost automatize) the preparation procedure, the following technique is used. It can be described as the "minimal standard cavity preparation."

A micropreparation diamond with a diameter of 0.9 mm, reverse pear shape, and a 2.5 mm long cutting diamond surface is mounted at the high-speed contra-angle on a micromotor. The objective is to open the cavity in a minimal (but not micro) preparation (Fig 4–33).

A "groove" is prepared, with a 1 mm width in the mesiodistal and a 1.5 mm width in the buccal oral direction, with a depth of 1.5 to 2 mm. With a security distance to the neighboring tooth of about 0.2 mm. A protection shield-like fence may be placed in the interproximal space. Using two small movements with the diamond, the 0.2 mm of enamel close to the neighboring tooth is removed, the cavity inspected visually and with the probe. The round bur or the hand excavator removes the remaining caries. The gingival enamel margin, as well as the lateral and occlusal, is finished. The cavity entrance is enlarged if necessary to assure proper excavation. The short cutting edge of the diamond makes it possible to finish deeper preparations without unintentionally widening the "entrance" to the cavity. The cavity preparation is refined and finished.

Using "the minimal standard cavity preparation," it is possible to train and automatize the first steps in the preparation for a primary caries attack – performing it precisely, quickly and with minimal invasiveness.

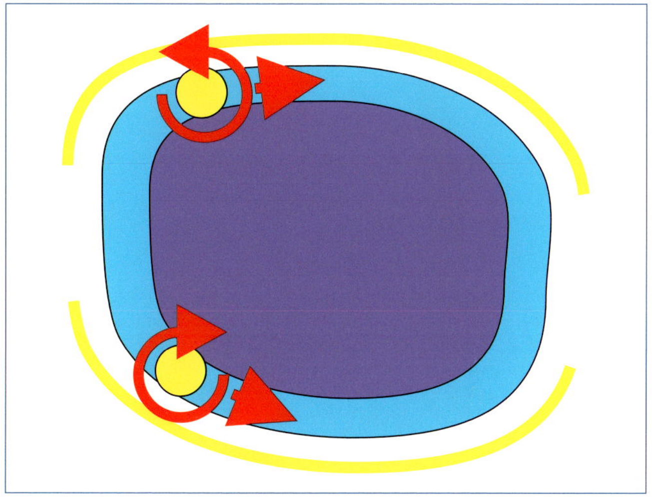

Fig 4–34 Enamel dissection preparation.

Preparation for a porcelain fused to metal crown with buccal shoulder

As another example, let's look at the preparation for a porcelain fused-metal or zirconium dioxide-based crown, with a buccal shoulder.

Initial preparation

The preparation is accomplished using the parallellometer technique, modified for creating a 12-degree angle of convergence. Two types of movements are used.

The initial preparation at the inner side of tooth involves a coarse diamond (150 mm diamond grains chamfer diamond), used with one slow precise movement while the diamond is working in the dentinoenamel junction. Maximal spray cooling is used. This is the "enamel dissection movement."

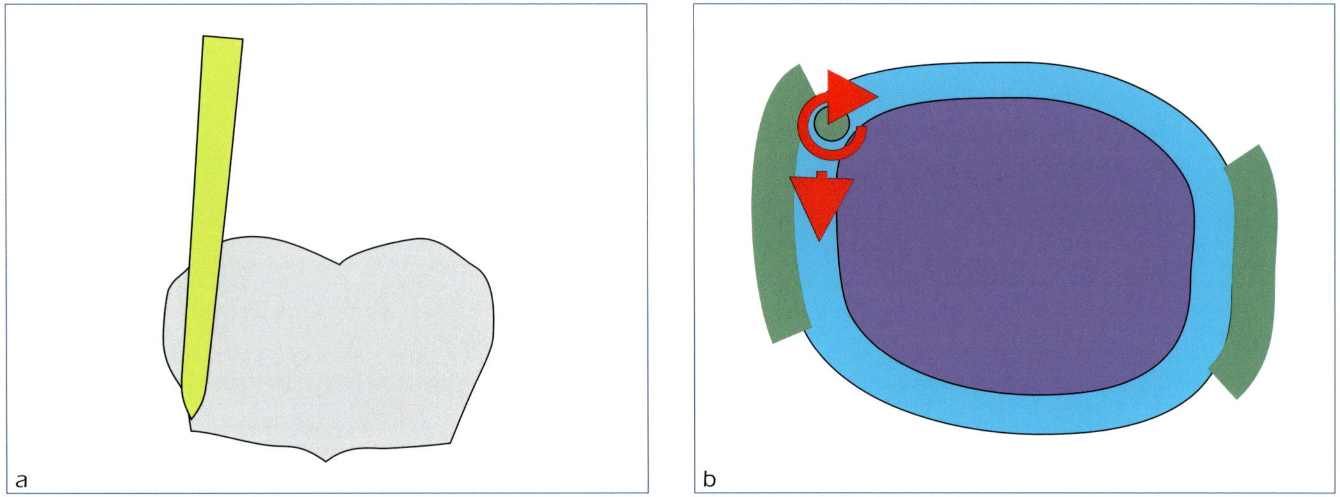

Fig 4–35 (a and b) Initial slice cut with a thin rough chamfer diamond in 0.2 mm security distance from neighboring tooth.

This movement is performed with a pulling movement, and the depth of the preparation is stabilized by the direction of rotation of the high-speed contra-angle, as shown in Fig 4–34.

On the buccal side, a first initial preparation with a 1.2 mm shoulder diamond is performed (see page 62), gingivally with an angle of convergence of 12 degrees, in relation to the inner side preparation. In the mandibular jaw, a second initial preparation is made at a longer distance from the gingival margin, and inclined like the maxillary buccal side of the molar. A thin coarse 150 mm (approximately) diamond grain diamond is used for a slice cut of 0.2 mm from the neighboring tooth, before the 1.2 mm chamfer diamond is used.

Final preparation

A finishing diamond producing optimal roughness (and not optimal smoothness) is chosen for bonding (estimated to 25 mm roughness obtained with diamond grains of 75 to 100 mm).

A fast, slight touch with a forward and backwards smoothing motion is made using perfect parallelometer-like movements. The critical connection between the approximal and buccal or oral side is made with a finishing diamond. These movements are mentally rehearsed (and exercised "in the air" without touching the tooth) several times, before contact is made on the tooth (Fig 4–35).

VISION FOR PRECISION – WITH OR WITHOUT A MIRROR

The patients seen on the photos below were selected because their mouths are rather small, and the access to the working area is not easy.

Basic conditions for quality dentistry

- You must be able to see all external surfaces of all teeth, and all internal surfaces of a given cavity wherever it may be placed on any tooth – and in a good working posture. It is not enough just to see a tooth, you must see the surface of the tooth or inside surface of a cavity, where work has to be done. Therefore, in Chapter 10 there is a detailed description showing how this is done.
- Furthermore, the dentist needs to know and learn to use many instrument grips and finger supports, which are necessary to work on any tooth surface or in any cavity surface. This requires a meticulous analysis. Direct vision is preferred when possible, with a good working posture for the dentist. Otherwise indirect vision with a mirror is used (lacking vision of certain surfaces or only having vision in bad working postures, not an acceptable option).
- It is necessary to learn the methods and routines for working with a mirror in the maxillary jaw and to learn to work inversed, with a reversed way of working with the mirror in distal cavities in molars, and premolars in the mandibular jaw.

To read, understand, see, imagine and learn these concepts, is complicated.

Direction of vision and sitting position

The direction of vision in the mouth of the patient is decided by the direction of the surface, exterior or "interior" of the tooth where you work.

The different directions of direct vision without a mirror – in good working postures – will depend on:

- the clock position of the dentist
- the position of the patient's head
- the mouth opening and visual access to the mouth of the patient and of the retraction of soft tissues done by assistant on her side, and sometimes at dentists side, and retraction done by the dentist.

Clock positions of the dentist

Direct vision (without the dentist twisting or bending her/himself) is a result of the clock position of dentist and the position of the patient's head.

In order to look at different surfaces of the patient's teeth, the dentist needs to look from different directions. And to do this without twisting the spine or turning the head, the dentist needs to sit in different "clock" positions. The initial short conclusion is that the dentist must be able to work in different postures between 9 and 12 o'clock.

This is possible if the base of the patient chair is small, so the foot controller can be placed as shown in Fig 4–36. Here the pedal of the foot controller and also the joystick can be activated with both the

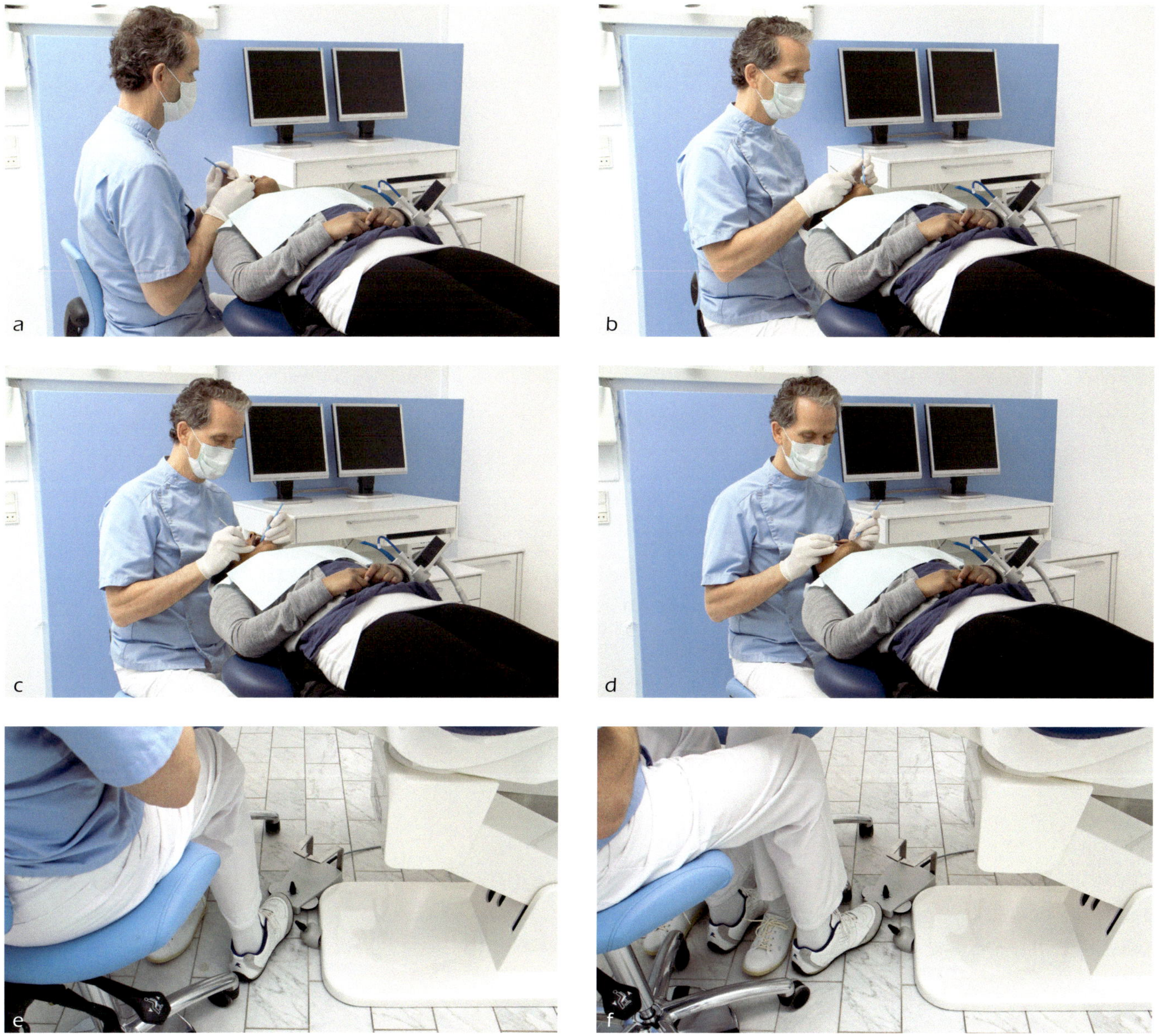

Fig 4–36 (a to d) 9, 10, 11, 12 o'clock position. (e to h) Position of the dentist's foot activating the foot controller, when working in a 9, 10, 11, or 12 o'clock position.

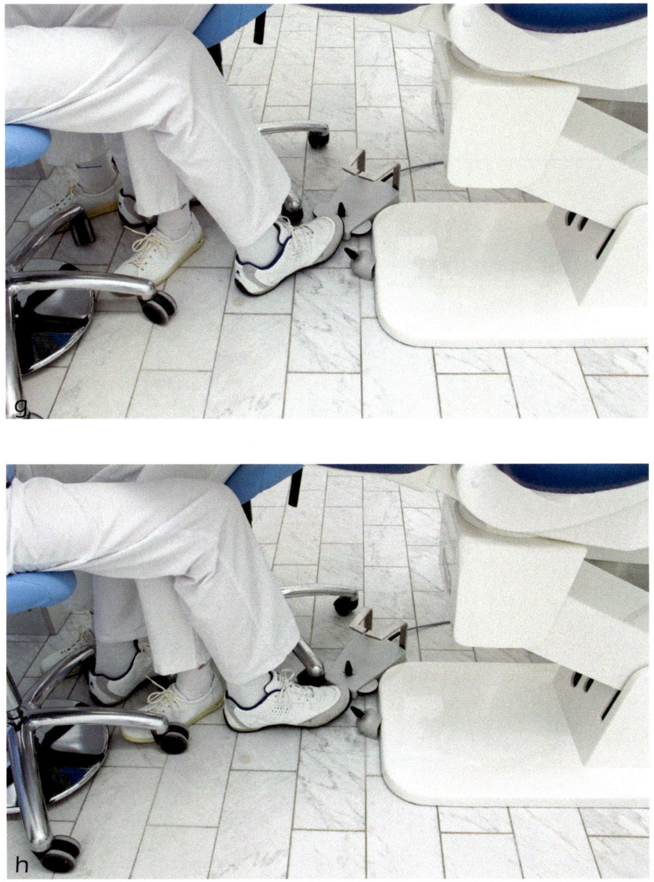

Fig 4–36 (a to h) The foot control in different positions.

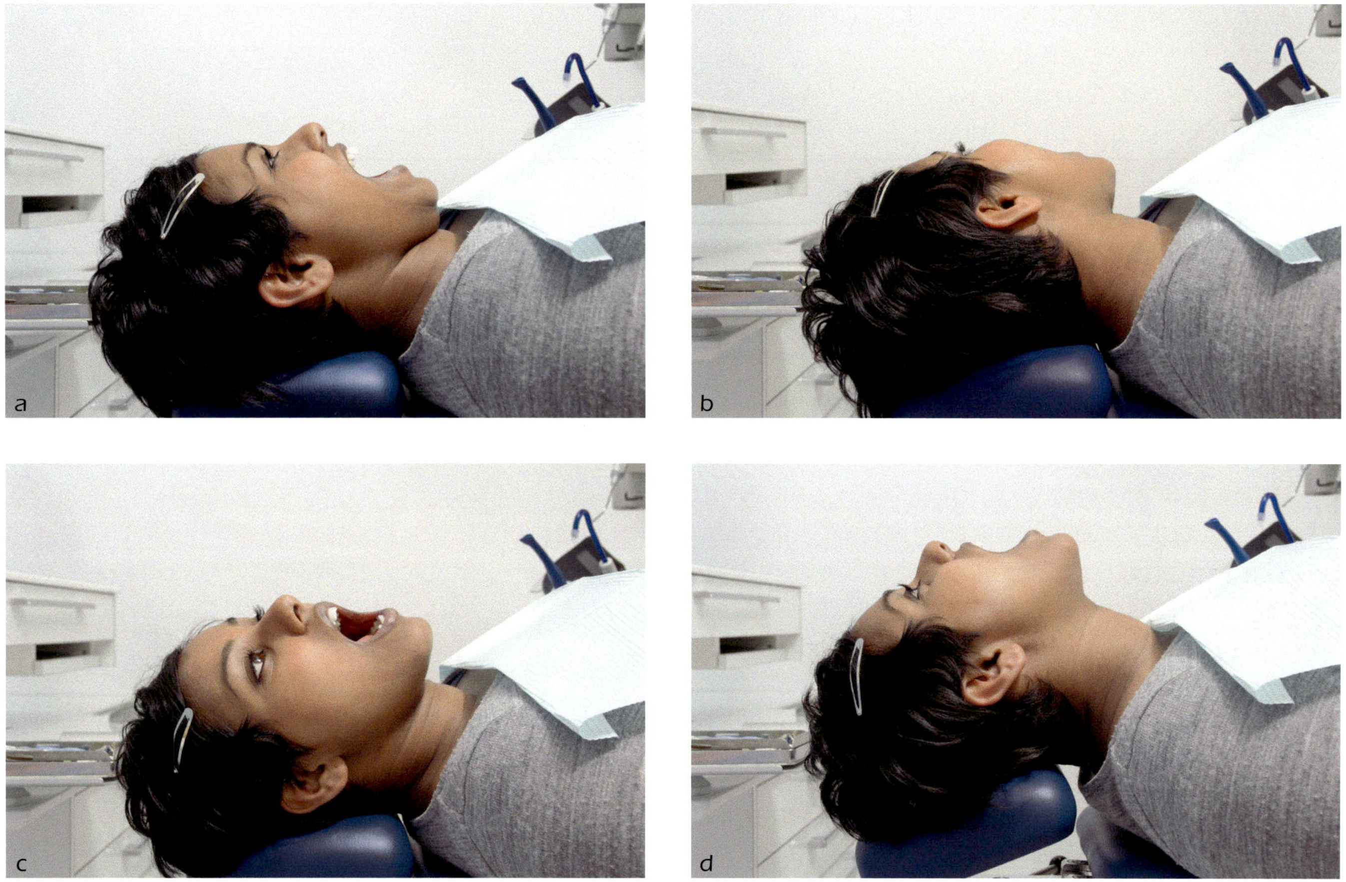

Fig 4–37 The head of the patient can be inclined forwards (a), to the left (b), to the right (c) and backwards (d).

dentist's right foot in 9,10, 11 and 12 o'clock positions, or with the left foot in the 12 o'clock position.

When the dentist and assistant sit with inclined upper legs in a balanced sitting position, it is possible to sit together in all positions with legs "intercrossed."

Horizontal position of the patient

The horizontal position of the patient is necessary in order to access what needs to be seen in the patient's mouth, with the dentist in a good working posture.

The position of the patient's head

The patient's head can be inclined forward, to the left, to the right and backwards (Fig 4–37).

Supporting the patient's head

In the case of a flat headrest, the flexible support is created with a combination of pillows:

a. a very soft base rubber foam pillow (like "Tempur" (red))
b. an additional 4 cm pillow of polyether foam (yellow)
c. a 8 cm thick polyether foam pillow (orange).

To see "everything" and have a good working position in the midline of the body, the dentist's positions and the patient's head are combined specifically for each surface of each tooth (or group of teeth).

Surfaces of the right side of the teeth

- Buccal right side, palatal and lingual left side
- Left front teeth mesial side
- Right front teeth distal side
- Dentist: direct vision from a 9 to 10 o'clock position (Fig 4–40). Patient turns head more or less to the left side (how much depends on space for visual access).

Surfaces on the left side of the teeth

- Buccal left side, lingual and (maybe) palatal left side
- Front teeth left, distal side
- Front teeth right, mesial side
- Dentist: direct vision from the 11 to 12 o'clock position (Fig 4–41). Patient turns head more or less to the right side (how much depends on space for visual access).

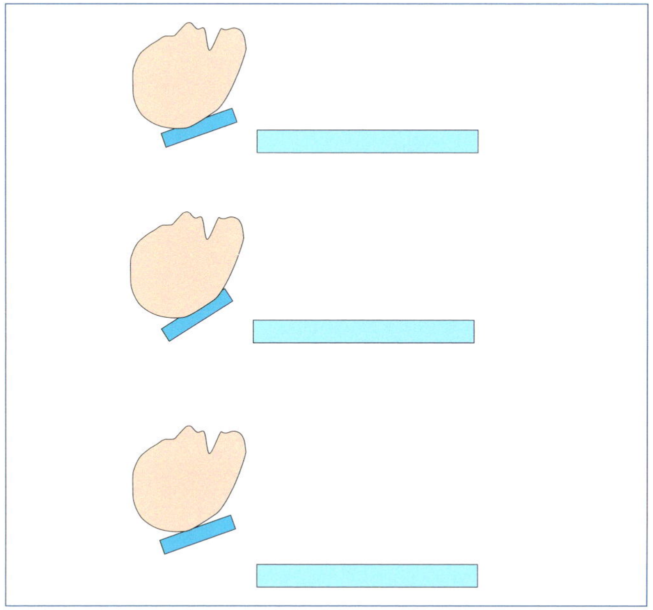

Fig 4–38 The headrest is more or less inclined, depending on the length of the back of the patient's head. If the back of the patient is rounded or the neck is bend forward, the headrest is elevated, in few cases even up to 12–15 cm. A double articulated headrest provides these positions.

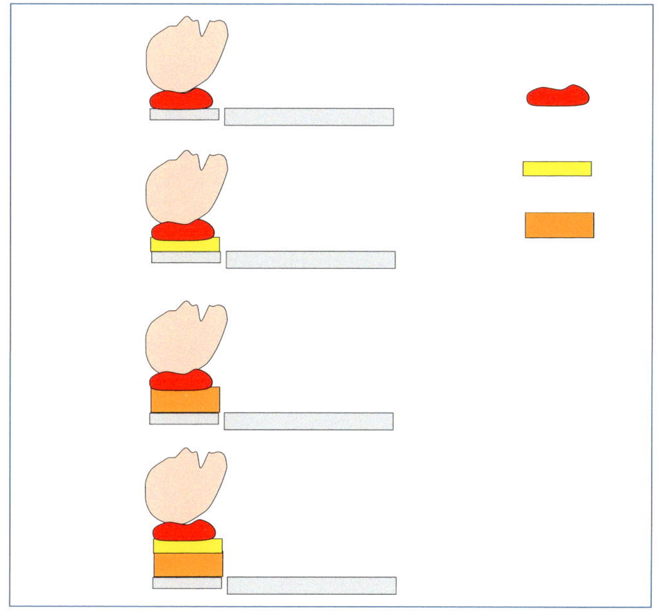

Fig 4–39 If a headrest is rather flat, then the flexible support is created with a combination of pillows. (a) A very soft base rubber foam pillow (like "Tempur" (red). (b) An additional 4 cm pillow of polyether foam (yellow), (c) and an 8 cm thick polyether foam pillow (orange).

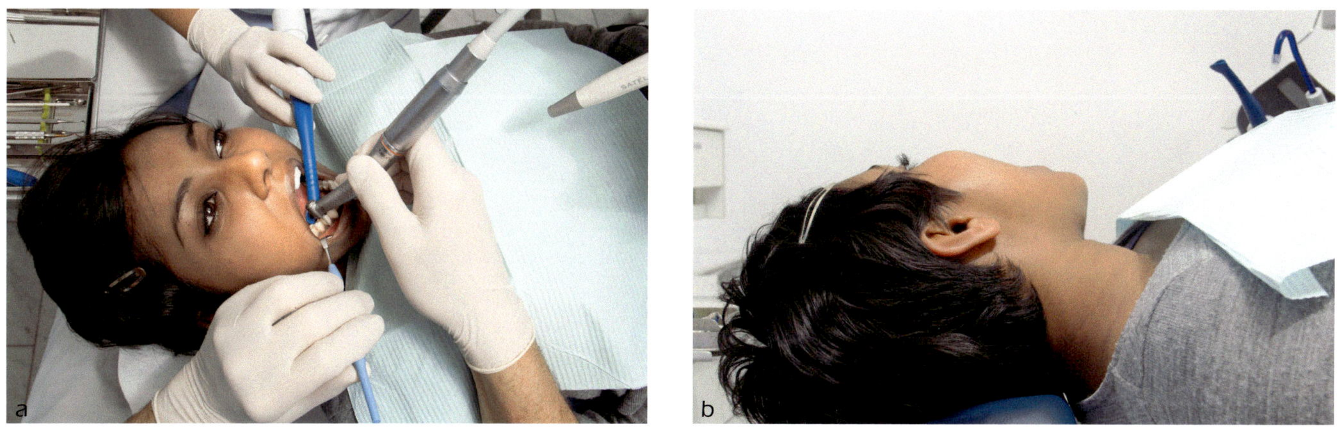

Fig 4–40 (a) Right side of the teeth, with the patient's head turned to the left. (b) Dentist at the 9–10 o'clock position.

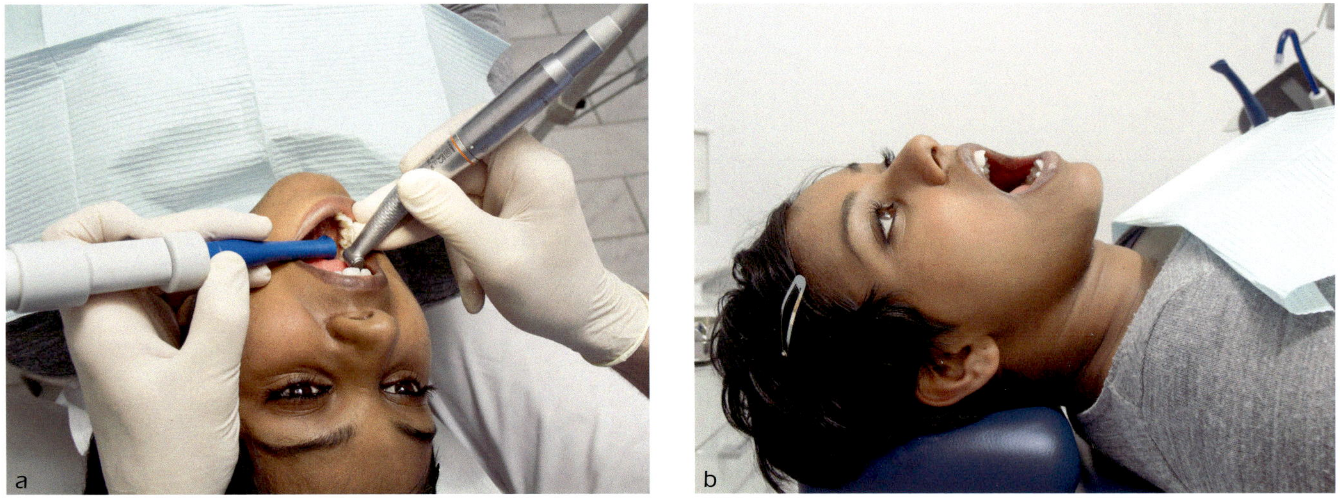

Fig 4–41 (a) Left side view of patient's teeth. (b) Dentist at the 11–12 o'clock position.

Maxillary jaw – occlusal and mesial surface

- Offers direct vision in molars and premolars
- Patient head is backwards (Fig 4–42)
- This is possible if the patient can tilt their head quite far back.
- This is often possible with younger patients and is less so when the patient exceeds about 25 years of age.
- This means that it is not possible to count on direct occlusal and mesial vision in the maxillary molars. However, when it is possible, it is a good solution.
- Dentist: direct vision in a 9 o'clock position.

It is only possible to see all the internal walls of a cavity here with direct vision if the cavity is not too narrow. If the cavity is narrow and deep or placed distally, then a mirror should be used.

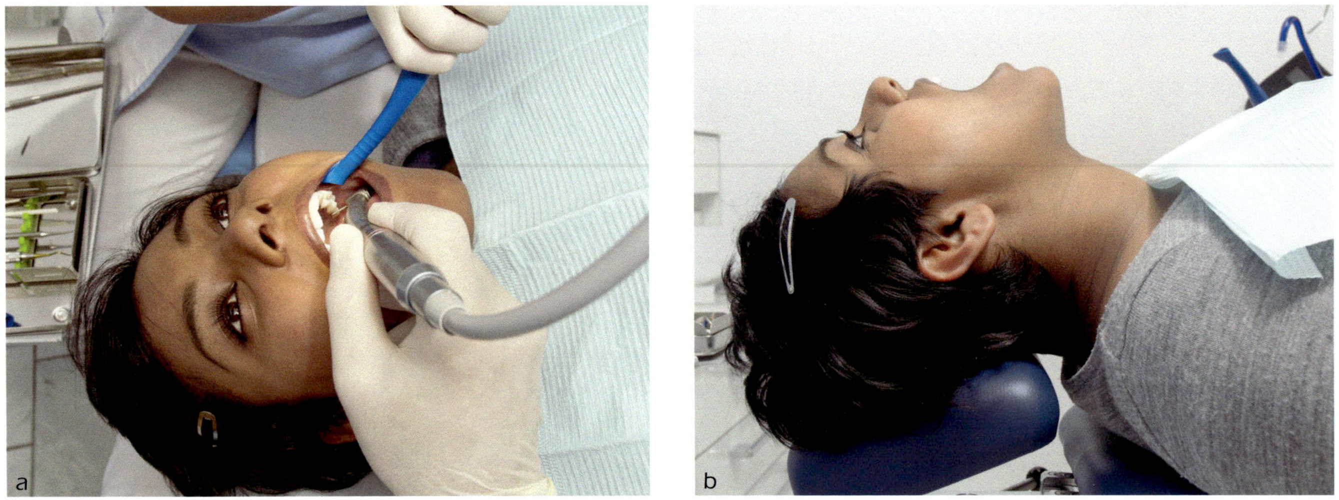

Fig 4–42 (a) Patient's head back. (b) Dentist at the 9 o'clock position.

Maxillary jaw – working with mirror

The mirror is placed as far away from the maxillary teeth as possible (so it is almost touching the mandibular teeth), and slightly in front of the maxillary tooth where a task has to be performed. The patient's head is facing upwards.

- Dentist: mostly positioned at 11 o'clock, but positions 9, 10, 11, and 12 can be used (Fig 4–43).
- Maxillary jaw, occlusal, distal and mesial view, mirror placed in an occlusal direction.
- Maxillary jaw, lateral view, mirror placed in a lateral direction.
- Maxillary jaw, palatal, incisors and cuspids, mirror placed in an incisal-palatal direction.

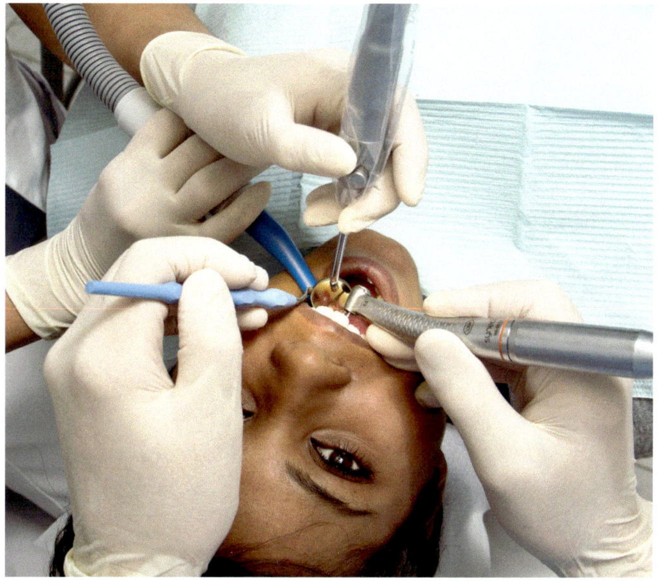

Fig 4–43 Mirror placed for working maxillary left.

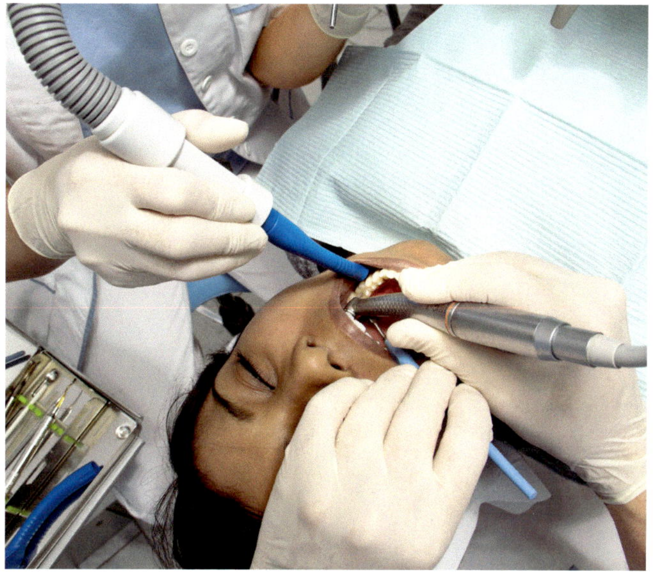

Fig 4–44 Working with direct vision on the mandibular left side.

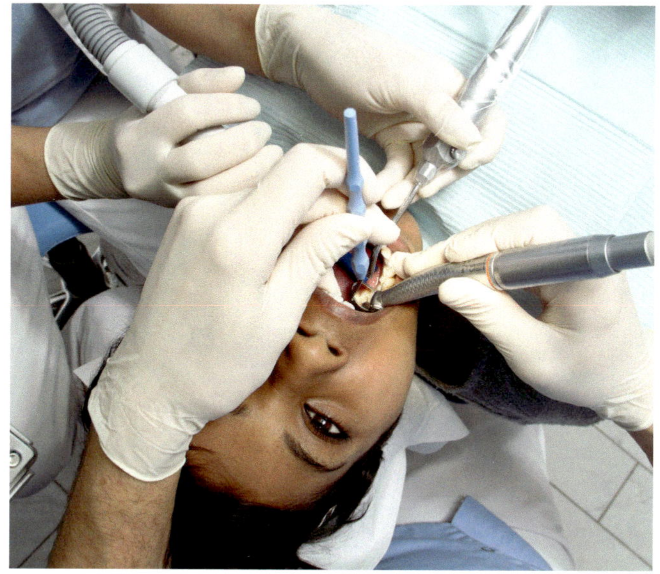

Fig 4–45 Working with a mirror at a distal cavity, mandibular right jaw.

Mandibular jaw – working directly

- Access to surfaces both occlusal and mesial.
- Dentist is in an 11 o'clock position.
- Patient turns slightly forward for working at premolars – and backwards when working at the molars (Fig 4–44).
- Internal surfaces of rather narrow cavities cannot be seen directly in molars (and may be premolars). Here a mirror must be used.

Mandibular jaw – working with mirror

- Using a mirror in the mandibular jaw is fundamentally different to using a mirror in the maxillary jaw.
- To see internal surfaces in narrow cavities in the mandibular premolars distal, occlusal and sometimes mesial it is necessary to use a mirror.
- The mirror is placed distally to the cavity and in order to look at the mirror, the patient has to move his or her head backwards. The optic system of vision in a mirror turns the vision of tooth/cavity upside down (compared to vision directly or in a mirror in the maxillary jaw).

Most dentists need focused brain–hand training to learn to work with their vision turned upside down.

When working in the mandibular jaw, it is also necessary to have the patient in a horizontal position in order to see what needs to be seen in the patient's mouth, while still maintaining a good working posture (Fig 4–45). When working in the mandibular jaw, the mirror is placed disto-occlusally for the tooth.

Note: When the mirror is used for the mandibular molars, the direction of vision is almost vertical and downwards.

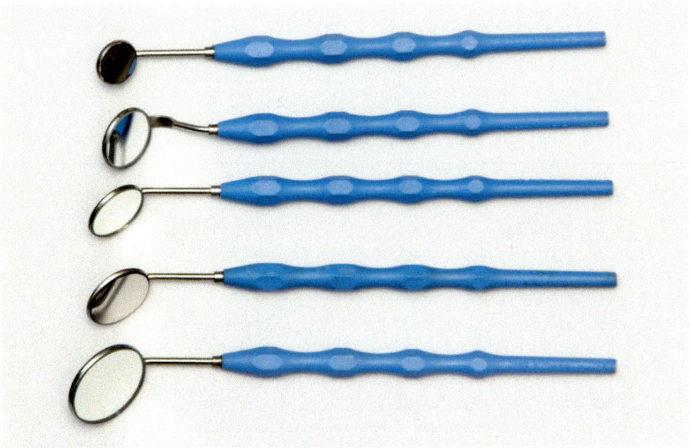

Fig 4–46 Different types of mirrors.

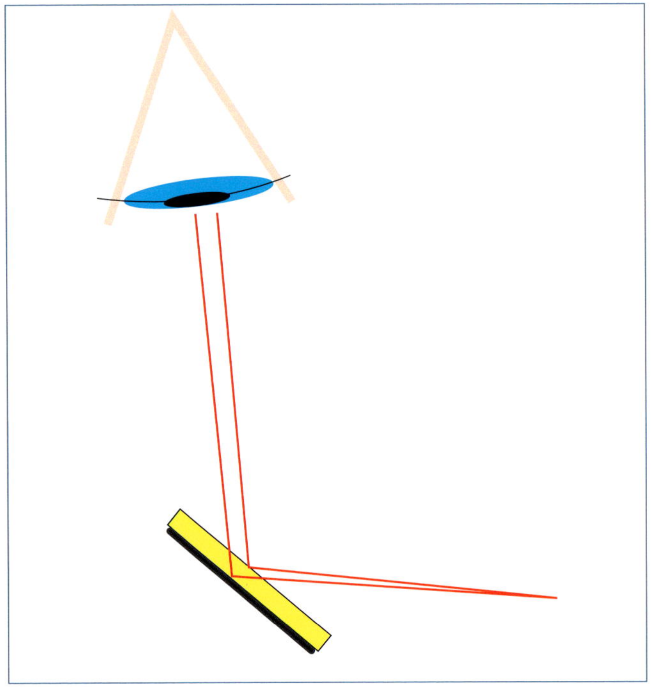

Fig 4–47 "Double" picture created from the front of the glass and the reflective surface behind the glass. Particularly visible (and disturbing) when the angle between direction of vision and mirror is small.

WORKING WITH A MIRROR

When an exterior surface of a tooth and/or interior surface of a cavity on a tooth, or soft tissues cannot be seen directly from a good work posture, then a mirror has to be used.

Different types of mirror

- 15 mm mini-mirror
- 20 mm mirror SE Flex (Hahnenkratt) with stem, which can be bent to a 45-degree angle to shaft
- 20 mm concave enlargement mirror
- 20 mm front surface mirror
- 25 mm large mirror.

Mini mirror 15 mm

If the area where the mirror must be placed is very narrow (due to a small mouth opening or by voluminous soft tissues close to last molars), it is advantageous to have easy access to a smaller mirror of 15 mm diameter (Fig 4–46). This is advantageous to use in around 5 to 10% of treatments. Mirrors for standard use have a diameter of 20 mm.

Flex mirror 20 mm

The stem of the mirror is flexible and can be bent by two fingers. It is bent in a 45-degree angle to the shaft to improve access to the mouth.

Concave mirror for endodontics

A concave mirror is used for enlarging the object being looked at. It has very limited optical properties but placed in right position and distance it enlarges a small visual field. One can only look at an object with one eye, but it is useful for short-term use to search for a point, eg, for localizing very small entrances of root canals. Magnification may be about three times.

Therefore, a concave mirror could be placed in the tray for hand instruments for endodontic treatments. This can be combined with loupes to achieve magnification to a point of the tooth surface, say at 6 to 8×.

Surface coated mirrors

A traditional mirror has a glass surface and a reflective cover on the underside (Fig 4–47).

Under certain circumstances, eg, when the entrance angle of light relating the surface of mirror is small, a disturbing double-reflected picture may result. This is caused by a main reflected image from the reflecting backside of mirror, and a secondary image from the front of the glass.

Mirrors with a reflective front coating do not create double pictures. Rhodium-coated mirrors are often used, but most develop a slightly brownish surface after a few sterilizations in an autoclave. Looking "through" a rhodium-coated mirror is akin to wearing sunglasses, which reduce the precision of vision. New types of coating based on titanium alloys allow almost all light to be reflected, and should therefore be preferred.

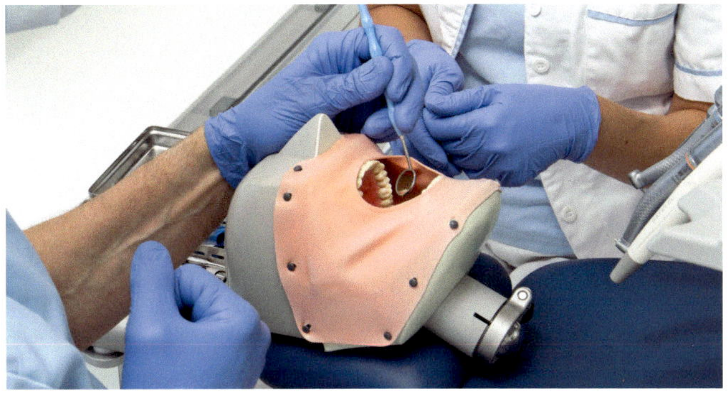

Fig 4–48 Traditional positioning of mirror, close to the tooth being worked on. The dentist is retracting soft tissue. The dentist's left hand is placed at the left side of the patient's head. The dentist's left shoulder may have to be elevated.

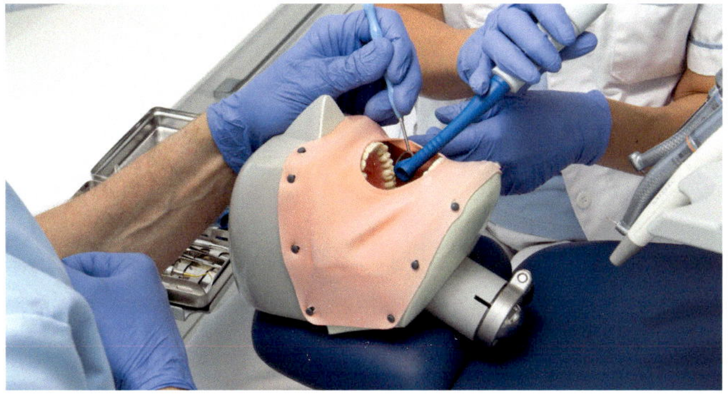

Fig 4–49 The mirror and suction are in conflict if the mirror is placed in the mouth first.

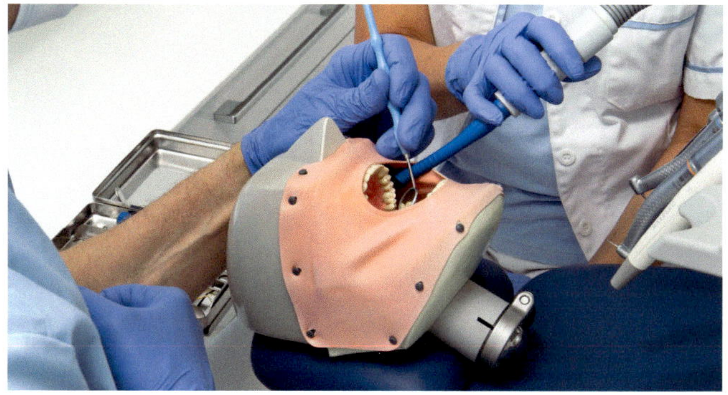

Fig 4–50 No conflict results if the suction is placed in the patient's mouth before the mirror, but the dentist's left hand is still in an inconvenient position at the left side of the patient.

XL mirror 25 mm

For evaluating preparations to bridges, a large mirror with a 25 mm diameter is useful.

The mirror grip

The shaft of the mirror should be long, so it is possible to grip different part of the handle.

The traditional position of the mirror (Fig 4–48) for working in a maxillary left molar, is as follows:

- The mirror is used by the dentist both for retraction of the lips and cheeks, and for looking through to the affected area. The assistant may be inactive.
- The left hand and arm of the dentist have to more or less "embrace" the head of the patient. In this position, the left shoulder is often moved forwards and the left elbow is elevated. The dentist must now use a certain force to retract soft tissues near the field of vision.

Many dentists suffer from muscle tension and pain more on the left side shoulder muscles, than on the right side. Many dentists have a slightly elevated left shoulder. This is probably from a combination of the left hand mirror and retraction position, and a semi-permanent twist towards the left in order to look into the patient's mouth, who is lying inclined.

As described in Chapter 6, one of the assistant's major tasks in four-handed dentistry is to retract the patient's soft tissue on her side, with an aspiration tube shaped for retraction. This saves further work for the dentist.

If the mirror is placed first when working on the left maxillary jaw, the retraction of the cheek is impaired, and the mirror and suction are in conflict (Fig 4–49).

However, if the suction is placed in the patient's mouth before the mirror is placed, then there is no resulting positioning conflict (Fig 4–50). Therefore, the grip of the mirror, can now be changed. The dentist no longer needs to do any retraction, and so therefore holds the mirror close to the end of the grip. A forced grip is not necessary, a relaxed 2- or 3-finger grip is sufficient. The hand of the dentist is carefully supported on the front of the patient. This is a basic condition for a relaxed positioning of the dentist's left arm and shoulder. This is a very important issue for the dentist's posture.

The assistant retracts using the large suction tube with a strong and stable fist grip, by holding her hand (with the suction tube) towards herself.

The angle of the mirror

For general usage, the angle of the mirror to the shaft should be about 45 degrees (standard mirrors, probably made for a half-seated patient, have a mirror-to-shaft angle of say 30 degrees).

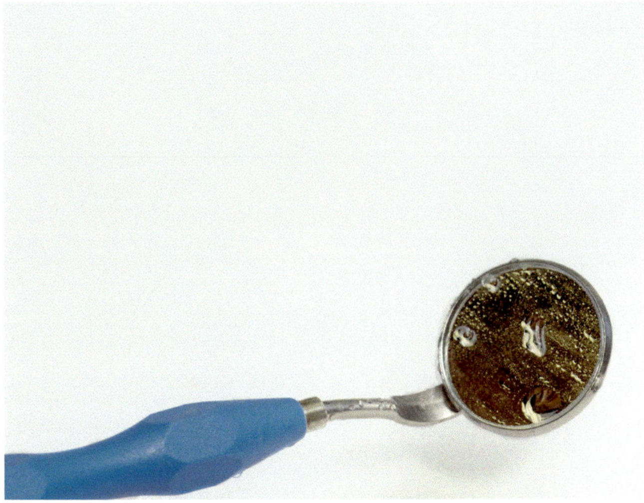

Fig 4–51 Working with mirror and spray.

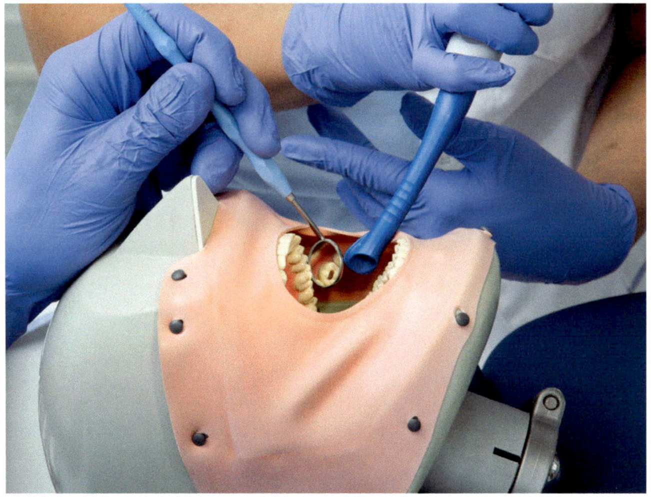

Fig 4–52 Traditional positioning of mirror, close to the tooth being worked on. The mirror is close to the spray as well.

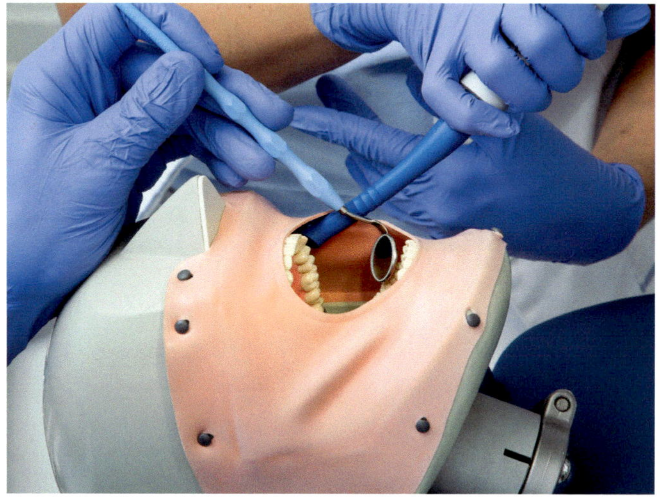

Fig 4–53 The mirror is placed as far as possible from the tooth and the contra-angle. This way, less or no spray touches the mirror.

The frontal-supported grip at the mirror grip has two consequences. The shaft of the mirror must be long, and have a shape made for gripping at the end of the shaft.

How to work with a mirror and spray

When working (for example in the maxillary jaw) with a mirror and spray, the mirror will quickly be covered with spray droplets from the contra-angle (Fig 4–51).

Some 20 to 30 years ago, the spray was composed of water in rather large droplets. These droplets could flow together and form a film of water on the surface of the mirror, so it was more or less possible to see and work with a wet mirror.

The visibility with the water film was improved if the mirror was dampened with a very thin dilution of a detergent. And veterans of four-handed dentistry may remember the original product "Mirrorclair" (or 1 drop of dish wash detergent in ¼ liter water).

These days, ultrasonic scalers produce large droplets, and therefore this technique can be advantageous for use when a mirror is used when using the ultrasonic scaler.

Contra-angles today produce a spray by mixing air and water, producing much smaller droplets that only with difficulty, or not at all, may float together to form a film. The problem of how to work with mirror and spray has to be solved differently (Fig 4–52).

If the distance between the spray and mirror is doubled, then the volume of spray reaching the mirror is quartered (Fig 4–53). When working in the maxillary jaw, the mirror touches or almost touches the teeth in the mandibular jaw. By placing the mirror here the mirror will often stay dry, and reflected visibility is not impaired.

When spray hinders reflected vision, the assistant should keep the mirror dry by using air from the 3-in-1 syringe (Fig 4–54).

For further reading on how to keep the mirror dry, please refer to Chapter 6, page 118.

Geometry of mirror-reflected vision

The geometry of mirror-reflected vision is in some cases quite complex, but in order to be able to train techniques for working with mirror-reflected vision, some examples will be presented here.

Working with a mirror in the maxillary jaw

The geometry of working with a mirror in the maxillary jaw involves the dentist adopting a position of about 11 o'clock (Figs 4–55 and 4–56). A mirror is used for mesial, occlusal and distal cavities in the maxillary molars and premolars, as well as palatal and vestibular cavities, which are not possible to see with direct vision in a good work posture. A mirror is also used at the palatal side of the maxillary incisors and cuspids.

Looking through the mirror:

- A movement to the right side is seen as a movement to the right side.
- A movement to left side is seen as a movement to the left side.
- A movement up is seen as a movement up.
- A movement down is seen as a movement down.

Working with a mirror in the mandibular jaw

The geometry of working with a mirror in the mandibular jaw also involves the dentist using a position of about 11 o'clock (Figs 4–57 and 4–58).

The mirror is used for narrow and deep occlusal cavities in molars, as well as buccal and lingual sides if they cannot be seen with direct vision. The mirror is also useful for distal cavities in molars and premolars, as well as for the lingual sides of the front teeth.

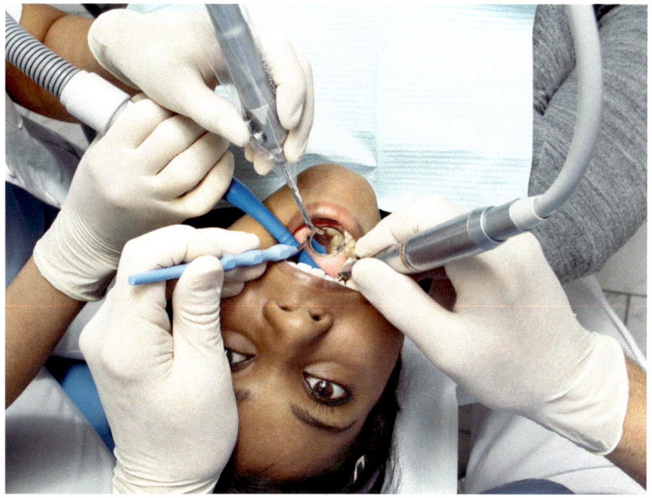

Fig 4–54 The assistant dries the mirror.

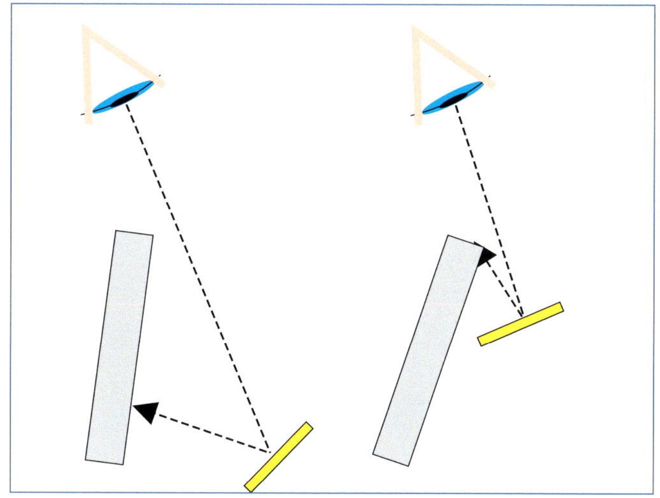

Fig 4–55 Geometry of working with a mirror in the maxillary jaw.

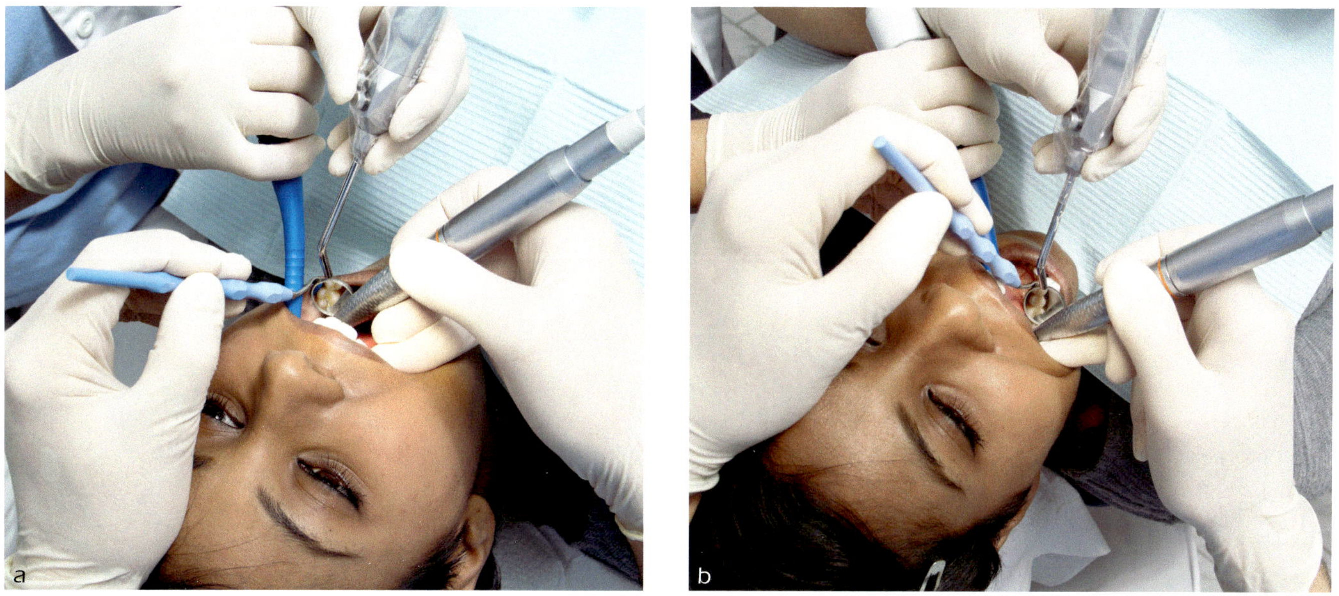

Fig 4–56 (a and b) Working with a mirror in the maxillary.

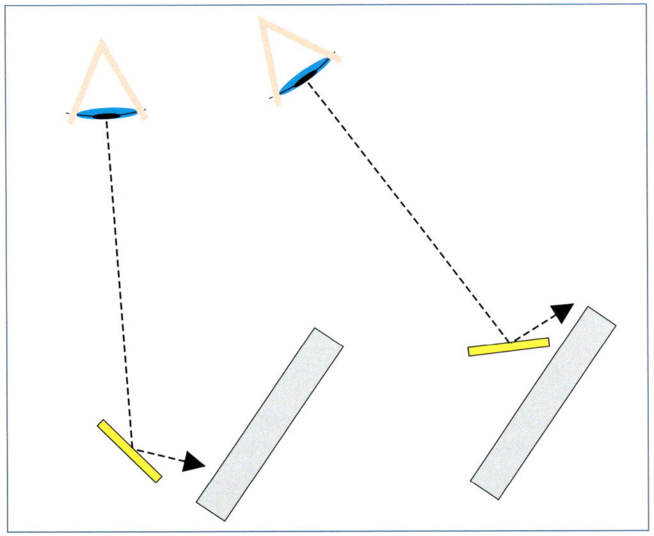

Fig 4–57 The geometry of working with the mirror in the mandibular jaw. The up/down direction of vision is reversed 180 degrees.

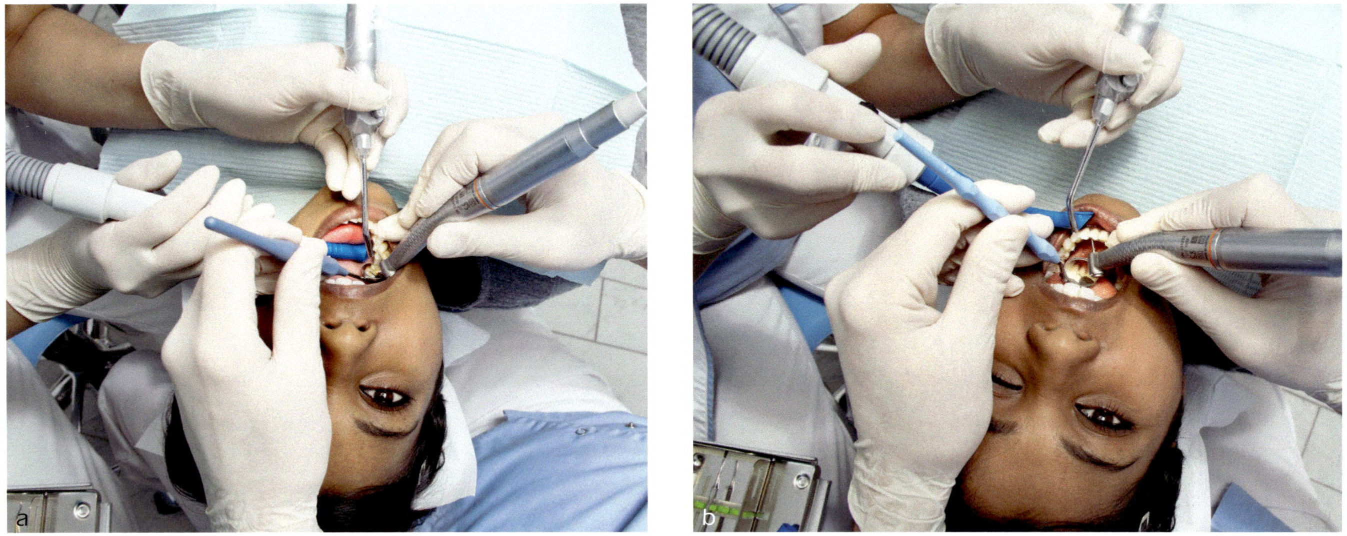

Fig 4–58 Dentist in an 11 o' clock position, while working with a mirror in the mandibular jaw.

Looking through the mirror:

- A movement to right side is seen as a movement to right side.
- A movement to left side is seen as a movement to left side.
- A movement UP (for which the patient is lying for mesial access to a molar) is seen as a movement DOWN.
- A movement DOWN (for which the patient is horizontal for distal access) is seen as a movement UP.
- In the incisal segment, the geometry of vision in mirror on lingual side is following.
- The labial direction is seen as a lingual direction, and the lingual direction is seen as a labial direction.

When seen in a mirror, the image is reversed 180 degrees upside down. This phenomenon strongly influences the technique of scaling with hand instruments. Intensive and deliberate training might be necessary.

A movement following a diagonal line (mesio-occlusal to distogingival buccal) in a mandibular molar is seen as being reversed 90 degrees. However, the 180 degrees upside down turn of the image seen through a mirror in the mandibular jaw is a surprise for most dentists. When the author asked a large number of dentists, not one dentist was found to be aware of this. By testing dentists to perform movements using a mirror in the mandibular jaw with continuous visual guidance, the author discovered that only a very few were able to do it.

This explains one major reason for problems with the sitting posture, caused by working in the mandibular jaw in distal cavities and especially by the use of scalers. Dentists could perform dedicated "eye-to-brain-to-hand training" when necessary, for working with a mirror in the mandibular jaw.

Chapter 5

EQUIPMENT

THE DENTAL UNIT – NEW CONCEPTS FROM THE 1950S AND 1960S

Basic principle:

"The equipment of the treatment room must be adapted to best working methods" and not the reverse.

Dental units and workstations should support the assistant

In 1953, a technical advancement for dentistry was referred by Harold Kilpatrick, who described the so-called "wash field technique," using spray on turbine contra-angles and high velocity suction systems. This technique enabled the patient to lie down in order to improve visibility to the teeth, enabling better work postures and better assistance.

Meanwhile in Paris, France, during the same year Malencon was engaged in the development of the reclining patient chair. In about 1960, Harold Kilpatrick visited Copenhagen, Oslo and Stockholm and some of the other European capitals (the author of this book has met dentists who were with Kilpatrick in Paris, Amsterdam, Madrid and Milan). Kilpatrick presented ideas of four-handed sit-down dentistry with a full-time chairside assistant, and with the patient lying in a Dentaleze patient chair (Fig 5–1). He also worked with a Chayes dental unit, with unit instruments and high velocity aspiration placed above the patient for the use of both assistant and dentist. He presented time and motion analyses, which led to the principles of work simplification.

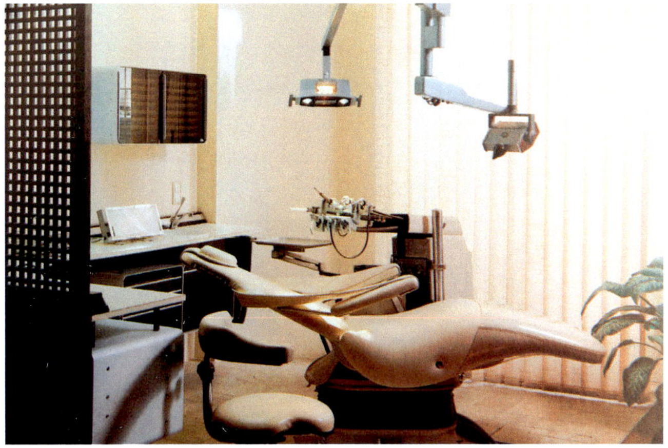

Fig 5–1 Dentaleze chair with a central positioning of instruments in a Chayes dental unit. Both assistant and dentist have access to the unit instruments, supporting high-end assistance. (This was the author's workplace in 1968.)

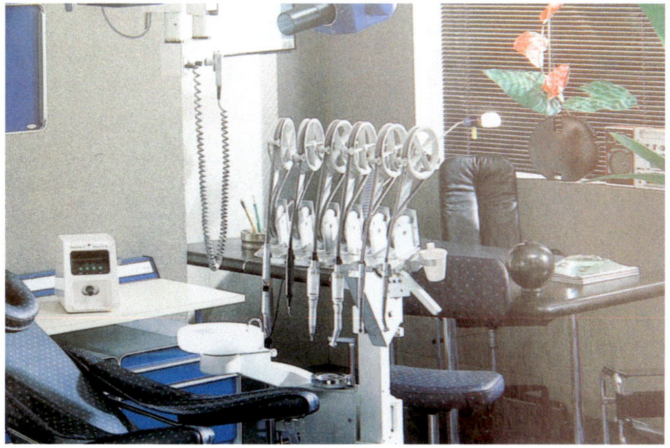

Fig 5–2 Colibri dental unit (Italy), with a central and balanced positioning for instruments. The unit instruments can be reached by both assistant and dentist, also enabling high-end assistance.

This inspired groups of dentists to adapt these principles. In Denmark in 1962, a society of dental ergonomics called "Selskabet for odontologisk praktik" was founded. This society still exists and has yearly meetings with lectures on ergonomics. In Sweden it led to the development of the Anatom dental unit system (1963) by the dentist Dr Lundin, who held courses and demonstrations of four-handed dentistry.

In Italy during 1968, the Colibri dental unit was developed by Carlo Gustamacchia, a dentist who introduced the Strumenti Perdenti Ricuperti Inerte Dobbio Operabilita (SPRIDO) system (Fig 5–2). This nomenclature translated to "hanging retractable instruments with double use" (for dentist and assistant). The dental unit holding the instruments was balanced so the dentist did not need to carry the weight of the unit instrument in his or her hand.

In 1969 in Denmark, the Alternativ dental unit was developed and produced by the author of this book (Fig 5–3). This author made the ergonomic design, mechanics, engineering, pneumatics and electronics personally. The Alternativ also had balanced instruments. The unit was developed to support the principles of "best ergonomical practice."

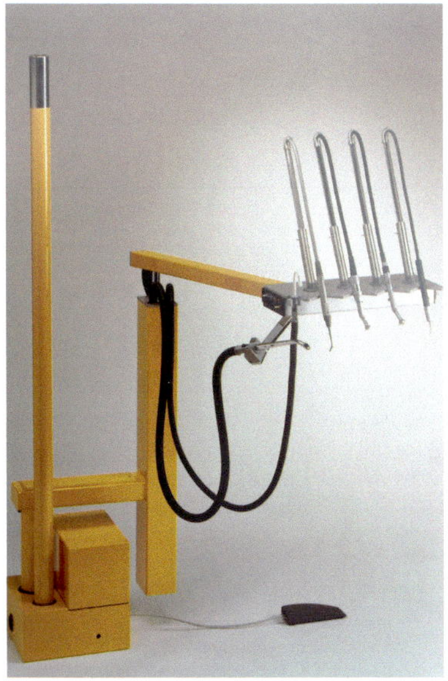

Fig 5–3 An Alternativ dental unit, made between 1968–69. There is a central positioning of instruments, and again both assistant and dentist can reach the instruments. There is an integrated suction holder so they are always at the correct and accessible position. The unit arm is placed in the "parking" position on the assistant's side. The height adjustment is accomplished by an electrically controlled spindle motor.

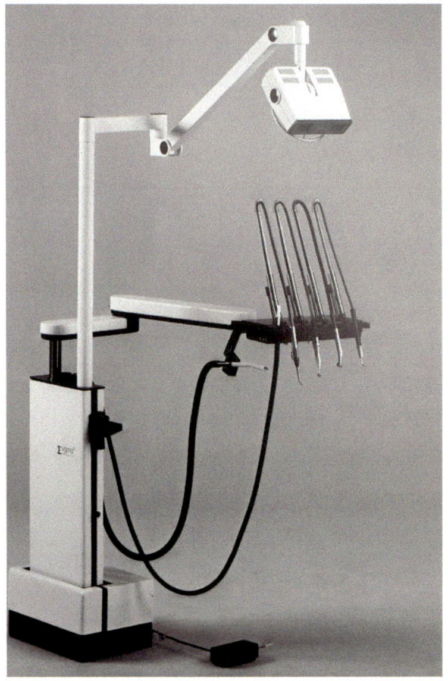

Fig 5–4 Alternativ dental unit from about 1980. The automatic speed regulation is controlled by the pressure on the diamond/bur, with a programmable variety of speeds. The height regulation is telescopic and contraweight balanced to perfect balance. The valves and controlling system is built in the arm system. The small foot controller reacts on vertical or sideways touch, and its cover controls spray selection.

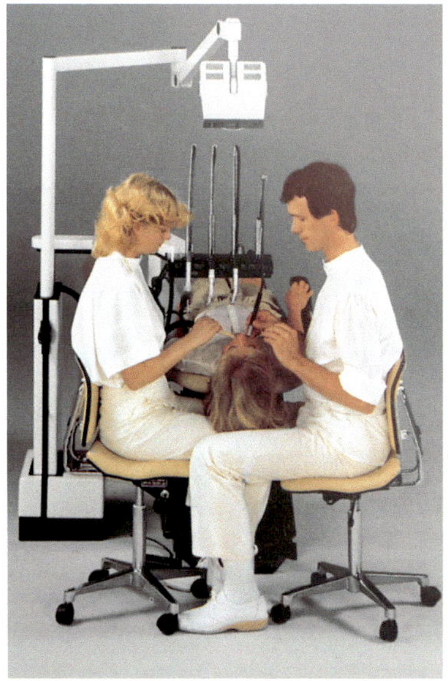

Fig 5–5 Alternativ dental unit – the perfect place for teamwork.

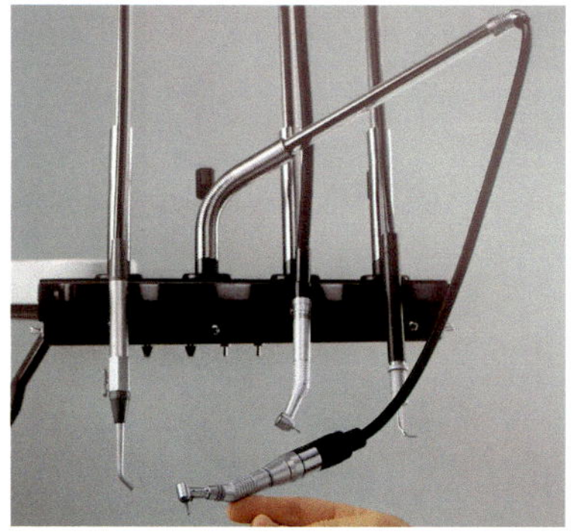

Fig 5–6 Even when in a side position, the unit instruments are perfectly balanced.

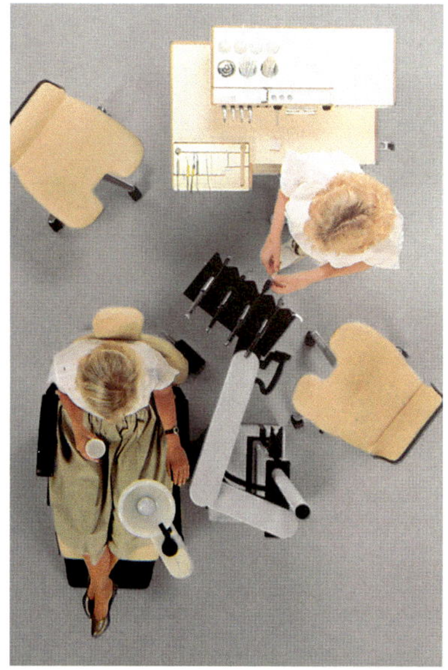

Fig 5–7 The dental unit is placed in the "parking position" on the assistant's side when the patients come and go, so the assistant doesn't need to walk far in order to dismount, disinfect and prepare unit instruments. The assistant has a concentrated workplace. The cuspidor is motorized and moves in front of the sitting patient.

The features of this dental unit included:

- Unit instruments placed in a central position over the patient in between the dentist and assistant. The unit instruments are perfectly balanced, so the dentist does not need to carry the weight of the unit instruments by hand. The balancing of unit instruments enables important side movements.
- Aspiration tube holders with inclined mounting on the dental unit close to the multifunction syringe for easy and simultaneous grasp of both for the assistant (with automatic suction valves).
- A small foot controller, with on-off function and programmable speed selection. For each speed selection it also has an automatic load generated speed control of up to 40% of the increased speed (hyper compensation).
- A water spray in two levels (two solenoid valves).
- A parking position at the assistant's side. An automatic chipblow dries the cavity when the unit instrument stops.

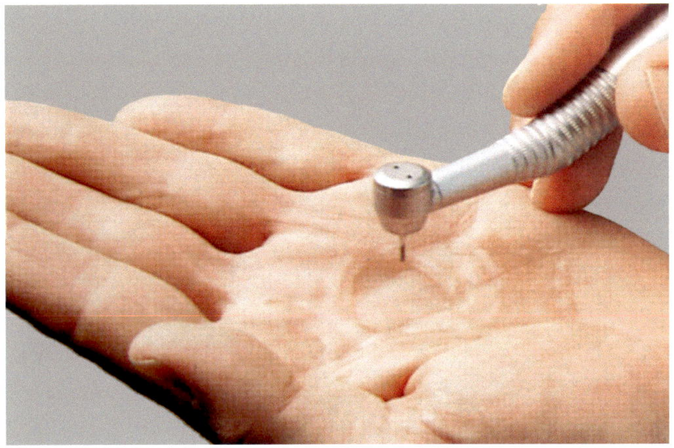

Fig 5–8 An automatic chipblow dries the cavity when the unit instrument stops. Hundreds of changes to the 3-in-1 syringe for drying the cavity are avoided. An important simplification of the visual control of the cavity/surface in/on tooth.

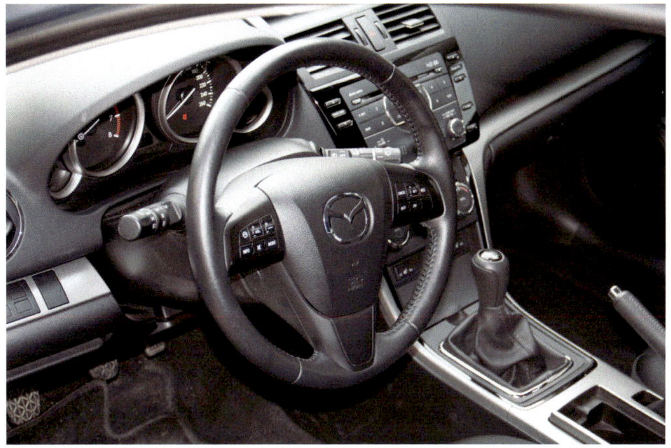

Fig 5–9 An analogy for an ideal workplace. The "driver" can have full and undisturbed concentration on "traffic" and almost all functions within reach, without having to lose eye contact or move hands away from the steering wheel. This is a good standard of practice for a dentist, and for any other workplace.

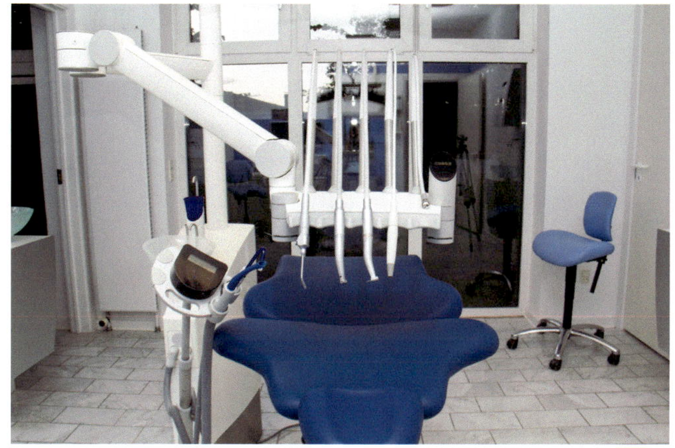

Fig 5–10 The dental unit as seen from the 12 o'clock position. The suction holder is close to a 3-in-1 syringe.

The author produced 300 of these dental units in three "generations" during some 12 years (Figs 5–3 to 5–8). About 150 to 200 units are still in use 25 to 30 years later because of their unsurpassed ergonomics and function. A wide number of units using the same principles as for four-handed dentistry were constructed in the year that followed. These construction principles are universal and are as applicable today as they were when the unit was constructed.

Then 50 years later – what now?

One could expect that principles of fine functionality were generally accepted and well known. But that is unfortunately not the case.

New generations of dentists still are copying old unpractical habits, and dental units are still made as though nothing has changed in the past 50 years. It is therefore time to remember that there is a lot of knowledge, know-how and skills that many dentists could profit from.

Dental unit for maximal teamwork

The basic principle of a dental unit is that the dental unit of the treatment room must be adapted to best working methods and not the reverse. A good dental unit supports assistance and undisturbed concentration for the dentist (Figs 5–9 and 5–10), whereas some units obstruct assistance and concentration.

Taking advantage of teamwork

When working with the assistant (who is chairside), the ability for her to reach the unit instruments adds a new dimension to her work.

The central position of the dental unit, placed over the horizontal patient and in between the dentist and assistant, was recognized 50 years ago as being a basic requirement for assistance, and still is today.

The immediate reaction from dentists in some countries may be that they do not find this an acceptable arrangement for the patients. It is essential to deal with this reaction however.

Unit instruments placed at the right side of the patient are very visible just in front of the waiting patient sitting in the chair. The argument that unit

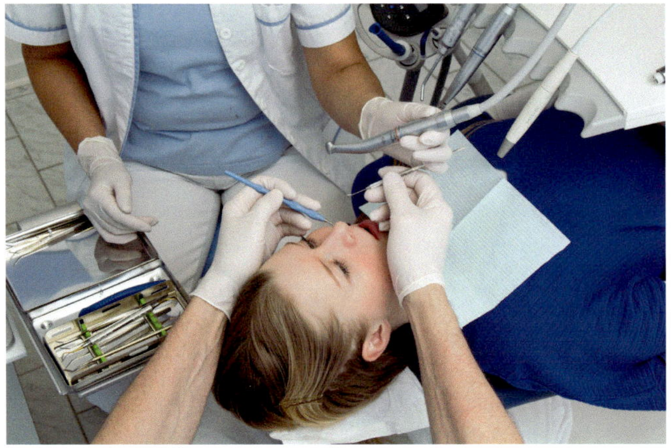

Fig 5–11 The assistant transfers the micromotor.

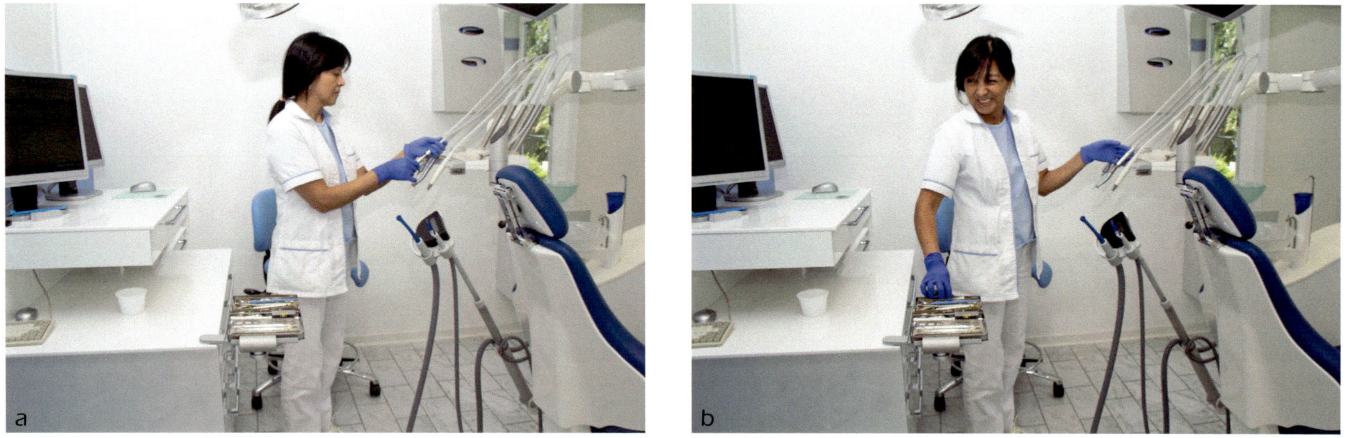

Fig 5–12 Dental unit parked at left (a) and behind (b) of patient. The assistant prepares the unit instruments.

instruments are visible to the patient originates from the time when patients were treated semi-reclined. The unit instruments are placed about 6 cm over the patient's chest area, out of their sight. The top of the balanced instrument support may however be seen.

What is very visible just over the patient's head is something different – the dentist's face. But how does the patient experience this? If the dentist's attention has to be in different directions (eg, in order to grasp and later return the unit instruments or hand instruments far away from the patient) this will be disturbing for the patient, because the dentist's concentration is distracted. The patient easily notices this.

If the dentist maintains a relaxed concentration while working in the mouth, the patient's experience will be very different. The dentist can maintain their eye level and be very calm, thus relaxing the patient.

The central position of the dental unit supports assistance

The central position of the dental unit enables the assistant to use the multifunction syringe in front of her. She can change contra-angles and mount diamonds, burs, ultrasonic inserts and so on, so the dentist's work is not interrupted by having to do it themself (Fig 5–11).

The assistant can also transfer unit instruments into the dentist's hands, therefore the dentist can be relaxed, without needing to do anything outside the patient's mouth.

The parking position of the dental unit

Traditionally centrally positioned units can be moved to the dentist's side for the "parking position." The dentist does this when the treatment is finished.

The assistant's "jogging program"

The parking position for the unit instruments is far away from the assistant's working area. To dismount used contra-angles, tips of multi-functional syringes and insertion of ultrasonic scalers, the assistant has to walk about 4 to 5 m around the base of the dental unit and to the unit instruments, and than 4 to 5 m back to place them on the tray with the used instruments. Then she has to walk all the way back a second time for the disinfection procedure with a wipe. And then again, when gloves are changed, for a third time for mounting new contra-angles, and for mounting new burs and diamonds.

Unit instruments at the assistant side

If the geometry of the dental unit is created for this position, the work of the assistant is much more easy (Fig 5–12). When the unit is parked close to the assistant's workstation with the hand instrument tray, the dismounting of used items at the unit instruments is very easy, and they are immediately placed on the hand instrument tray to be carried to the sterilization room afterwards.

Balanced unit instruments

An important feature of a centrally placed dental unit with suspended unit instruments, is balancing the instruments in the dentist's hand (Fig 5–13). The unit instruments are supported while they are in use, so the dentist does not need to bear the weight of them. The balanced instruments are supported in different positions, and side movements are especially important.

The balanced instrument reduces fatigue in the dentist's hands and improves tactility, an important precondition for precision work. The first two dental units with balanced instruments were both developed by dentists, and independently of each other:

- the 1968 Colibri, by Gustamacchia, Italy
- the 1969 Alternativ, by the author, Denmark.

Take care – not all dental units with central positioning have balanced unit instruments.

The vertical position of unit instruments in relation to the floor

Important: The unit instruments must be placed so high above the floor that there is room for the dentist above the horizontal patient.

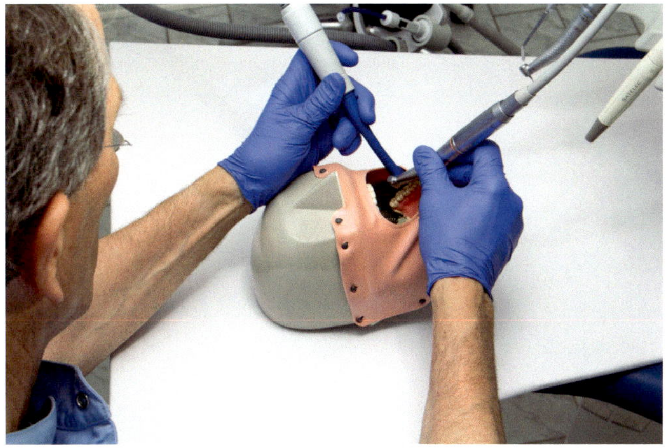

Fig 5–13 Balanced instruments.

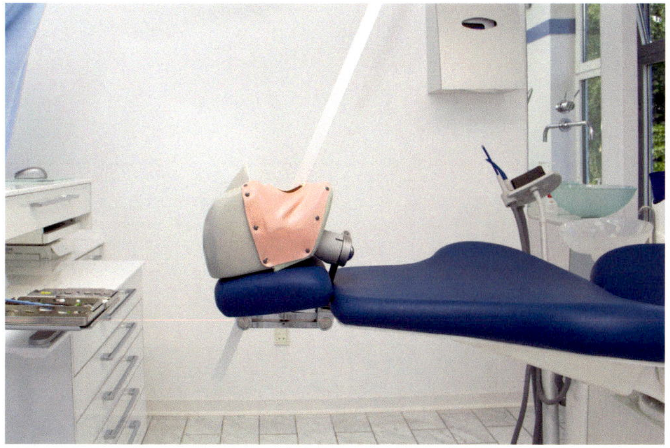

Fig 5–14 Horizontal patient chair.

For a dentist of average height working with a horizontal patient, the horizontal backrest of the patient chair should have a maximum positioning of 80 cm above the floor. For dentists taller than 175 to 180 cm, this should be 90 cm above the floor (Fig 5–14).

The unit instruments should be placed 25 to 30 cm higher than the horizontal backrest of the patient chair. For the dentist of average height, the maximum position for the unit instruments must be 105 to 110 cm. For taller dentists, this should be 115 to 120 cm above the floor. Some dental units do not have enough vertical mobility of the arm system for carrying the unit instruments. These units will have to be delivered in two versions, one of which is suitable for a dentist of maximum 175 cm in height, with unit instruments a maximum of 105 cm from the floor. The arms that carry the unit instruments are mounted 15 cm higher in the version for the taller dentist. (In most European countries, more than 50% of males are taller than 175 cm.)

Measurements of the dental unit

The supporting arms of the dental unit must be so long that the unit instruments in the working position are placed 25 to 30 cm from the top of the headrest, with the back of the chair in a horizontal position.

Taking care of construction

Many dental units with centrally placed unit instruments do not fulfill this important requirement. To construct a dental unit with the instruments placed centrally is more complicated than the manufacturers expect. The functionalities and measurements have to be precise, as there are many things that can go wrong.

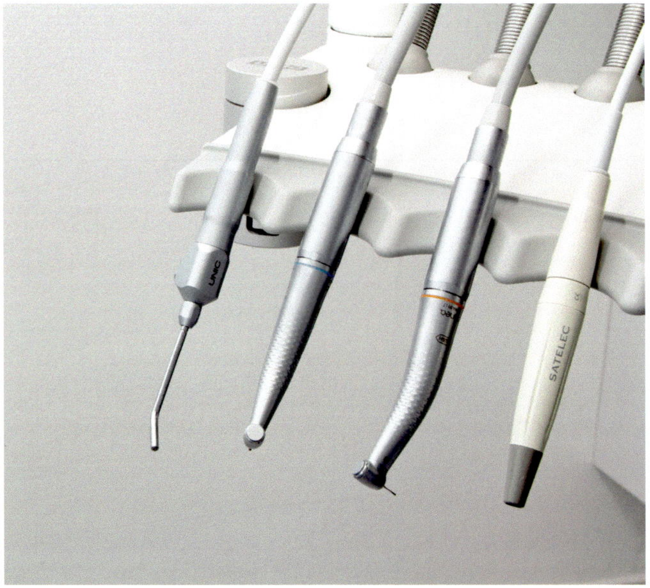

Fig 5–15 Four unit instruments (including the 3-in-1 syringe) supplemented by cordless rechargeable instruments.

UNIT INSTRUMENTS

The 3-in-1 syringe

The 3-in-1 syringe used with suspended (balanced) unit instruments must be straight, and the tip easy to dismount for sterilization. It is very important that the dosage of air, water or combination spray is easy to regulate in delicate levels, so you can create sprays of different force: soft spray, medium spray and strong spray. On this point, there are big differences on the syringes. One of the most used syringes on the market (in 2012) is difficult to regulate to other levels, than no spray or maximum spray.

The syringe handpiece can be covered by a special disposable plastic bag, retained with an orthodontic elastic (Fig 5–15). The plastic cover is disposed of and replaced when changing patients.

Micromotor with red 5x-multiplication contra-angle compared with a turbine

The advantages of replacing a turbine with a second micromotor used with red 1:5 multiplication high-speed contra-angle (using turbine burs and diamonds) is described in detail in Chapter 4.

Two micromotors and no turbine

One micromotor is normally mounted with a blue contra-angle, and occasionally with other contra-angles. This micromotor is the one closest to the assistant, so she can easily change the burs and diamond. The micromotor in the next position towards the dentist is mounted with a high-speed multiplication contra-angle.

Ultrasonic scaler

Composite polymerization lamps with a rechargeable battery and very high power output are now on the market. They may well replace the use of dental unit-based polymerization lamps. They are used like hand instruments and transferred by the assistant to the dentist.

The intraoral camera is an excellent tool for patient information. It may be mounted on a dental unit, but can also be connected directly to the computer and the praxis-software by USB connection or even wirelessly.

Hose with multicoupling

Some patients have such sensitive teeth that the use of an ultrasonic scaler causes a lot of pain. An airscaler is both effective and is tolerated by the "sensitive" patient. The airscaler can be mounted on the multi-coupling, as well as a prophy jet air polisher (be attentive to risk assessment regarding the inhalation of abrasive articles by dentist, assistant and patient).

Four unit instruments are enough:

- a 3-in-1 syringe
- two micromotors
- an ultrasonic scaler.

A battery powered polymerization lamp and battery-powered endomotor (both separated from the dental unit) are useful.

Contra-angles for the micromotor

The micromotor replacing the turbine is mounted with a red 1:5 multiplication contra-angle. This contra-angle uses same size diamond (CVC) turbines (Fig 5–16).

The second micromotor is mounted with a blue 1:1 contra-angle for general use (Fig 5–17).

A green 2,7:1 contra-angle (or similar reduction of speed) runs with 2,7 reduced speed and about 2,7 of increased torque.

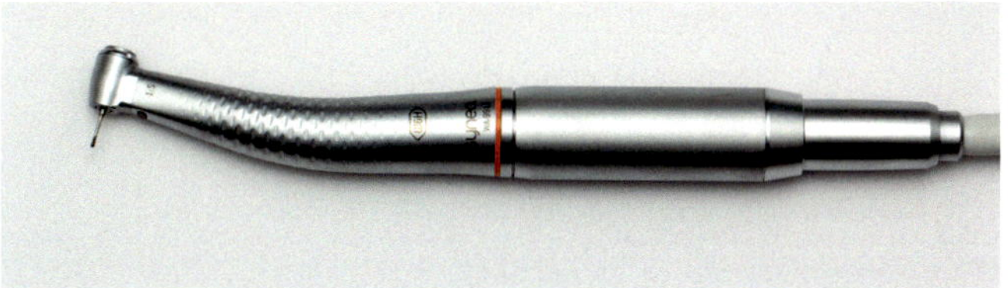

Fig 5–16 A high-speed contra-angle.

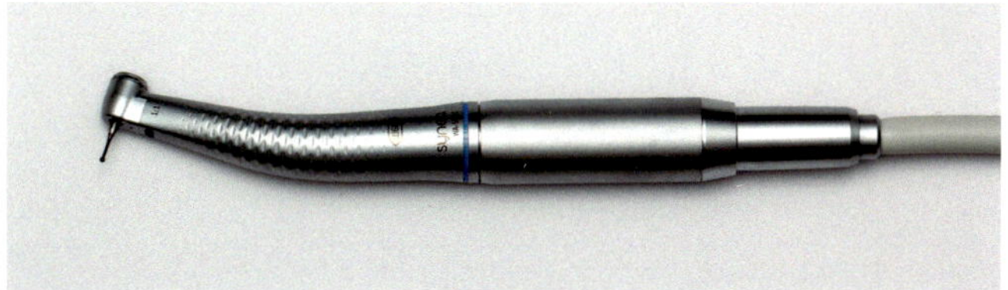

Fig 5–17 A blue 1:1 contra-angle for general use.

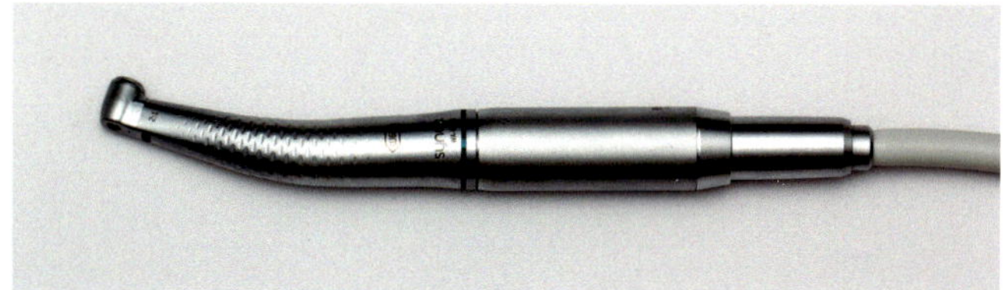

Fig 5–18 A green 2,7:1 contra-angle (or similar reduction of speed).

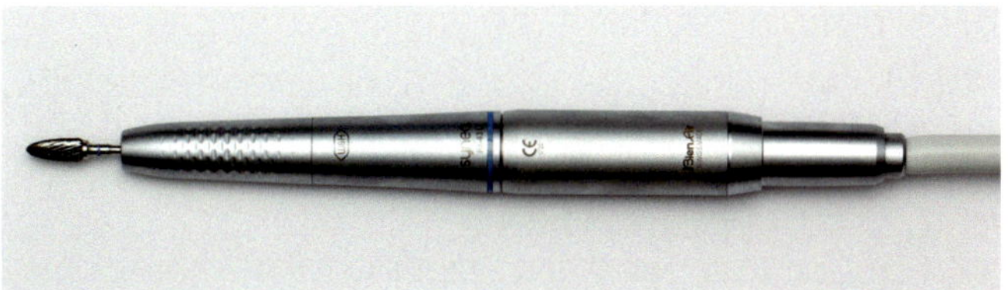

Fig 5–19 A 1:1 handpiece for technical procedures.

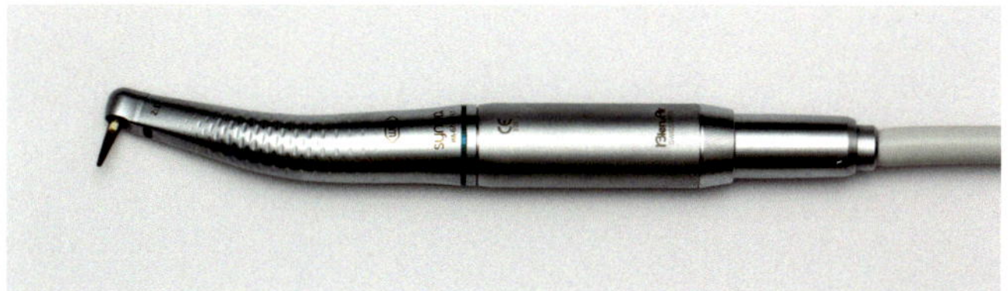

Fig 5–20 Prophin contra-angle with different tips.

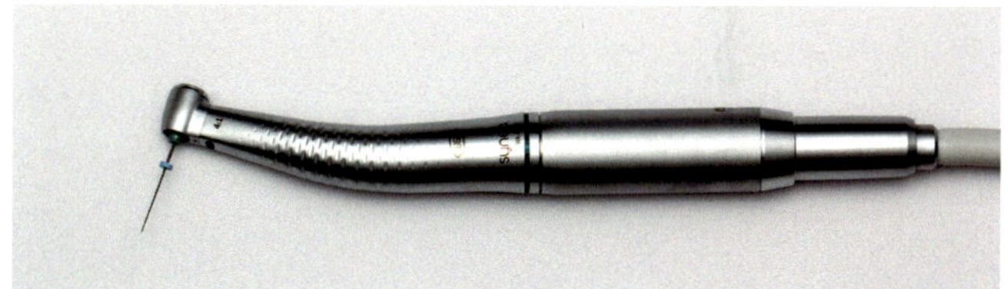

Fig 5–21 Endo contra-angle oscillating movements for hand files.

This is useful for preparing for root-posts, and the low speed might also be used for preparing parapulpal posts (Fig 5–18).

A prophycontra-angle, for use with a screw-on rubber cup to polish teeth as a part of a general scaling, is mandatory. The head is very small and enables good access. The head is specially sealed against the polishing paste. For details and use, see Chapter 10.

A 1:1 handpiece for technical procedures, eg, corrections of dentures, outside the mouth of patient. Some surgeons may use handpieces for certain surgical procedures (Fig 5–19).

A less well-known but excellent tool, a Profin contra-angle is used with different small diamond coated polishing tips (inserts), and is mostly flat or slightly curved (Fig 5–20). The tips can be fixed in any angle and work with reciprocating movements. It is very suitable for polishing approximant margins for example, where a pointed diamond is very difficult to use.

The endo contra-angle can be mounted with standard files and moves with 60 degree reciprocating movements (Figs 5–21 and 5–22). The possible uses will be explained in Chapter 10.

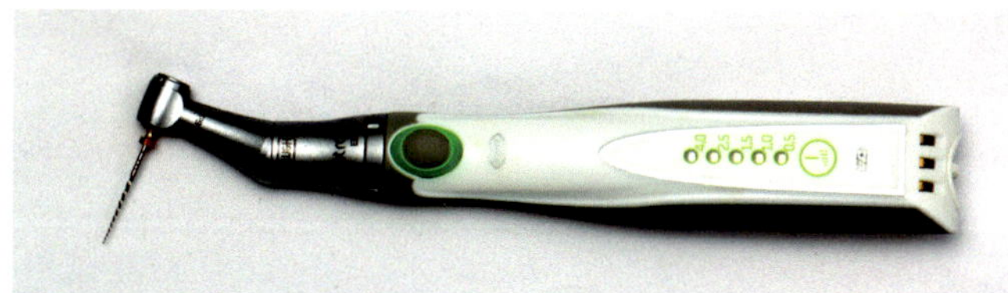

Fig 5–22 Endomotor for rotary files, with fixed speed and torque limitations.

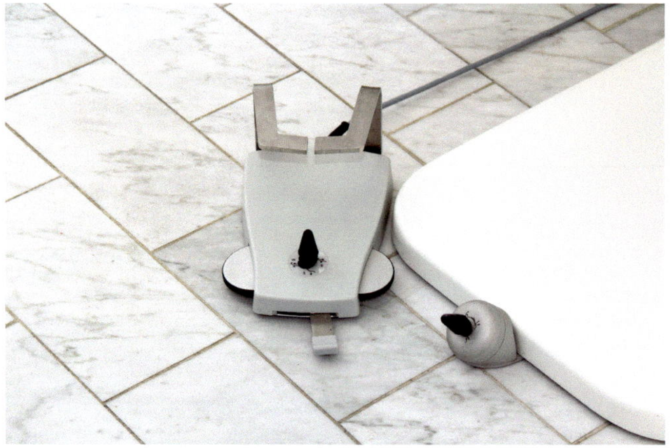

Fig 5–23 Foot controller and chair base.

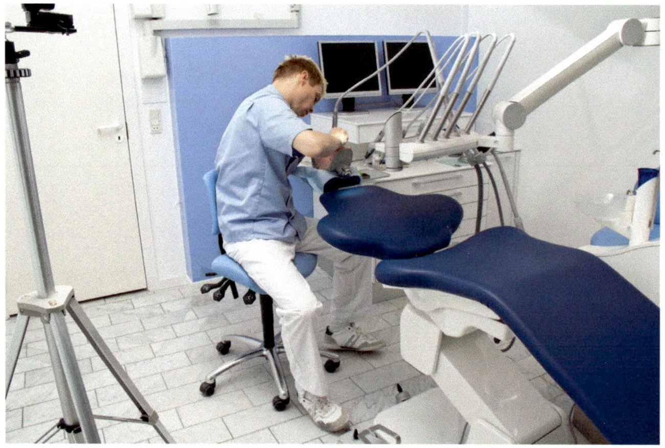

Fig 5–24 Foot controller on the right side of the chair base.

THE FOOT CONTROL

The dentist needs space for free seating in clock positions from 9 to 12. The foot control must be placed under the patient chair at left backside of the base of the patient chair. Therefore it is very important that the base of the chair is small (Fig 5–23).

If the chair base is too big, the foot controller has to be placed at the right side of the patient chair base (Fig 5–24). This makes it very inconvenient for the dentist to work in a 9 to 10 o'clock position, when these positions are indicated (working on surfaces at the right side of the teeth).

If the foot controller is placed at the left side of the chair midline, the dentist can activate the foot controller independently of whether he or she is working in a 9, 10, 11 or 12 o'clock position. (For more on speed regulation and selection of the automatic chip blow, see page 56.)

SUCTION TUBE HOLDER

The suction tube holder positions the large and small suction tubes so they can be easily reached by the sitting assistant. The large suction tube has a double function: aspiration and soft tissue retraction. It is lifted off the holder and used by the assistant's right hand, so the left hand is free to perform other functions, such as using the multifunction syringe, or transferring hand or unit instruments to the dentist.

In order to enable the assistant to take the large suction tube with the right hand, the suction tube holder must be precisely positioned in between the multifunction syringe of the dental unit (the unit instrument closest to the assistant) and the left shoulder of the assistant.

This space is quite narrow, so the suction tube holder must be small, and placed so that the tip of the large suction tube is about 12 cm from the tip of the multifunction syringe. And the tube must be inclined forward, so that it is easy for the assistant to grasp (Figs 5–25 and 5–26).

Other positions have been tried, but have been found to have a negative impact on the work of the dentist and assistant. If the suction holder is behind the assistant sitting in a work position, she has to move back in order to take it.

A large aspiration tube behind the patient will hinder the dentist sitting in a 12 o'clock position. Furthermore, this positioning of the suction holder may disturb the position and use of the hand instrument tray (and the dentist's solo left-to-right hand instrument transfer). The small suction tube sits close to or above the large tube.

With regard to an open or closed holder for the suction tube, it is easier to take and return the suction tube if the holder is closed, however the holder must be very smooth inside.

Through the years, there have been two different types of flexible suction tubing. The first version is light and very flexible, yet rough outside and inside. Depending on the air velocity, it may produce a whistling sound. If the adapter between the suction tube and the flexible tubing has a sliding closure valve, the volume of passing air can be regulated to avoid the whistling sound. If these valves are used, they should be dismounted at least once a day for cleaning.

The other kind of flexible suction tubing has a smooth inner and outer surface. It is a bit heavier and less flexible and is unfortunately quite "sticky," and so is difficult to slide into a closed suction holder. If the closed suction holder has rolls (usually three pulley-like rolls), even this aspiration tube will be very easy to pick up and replace.

Working solo

If the dentist needs to take the suction tube, the holder for it should be moved closer to the dentist (Fig 5–27).

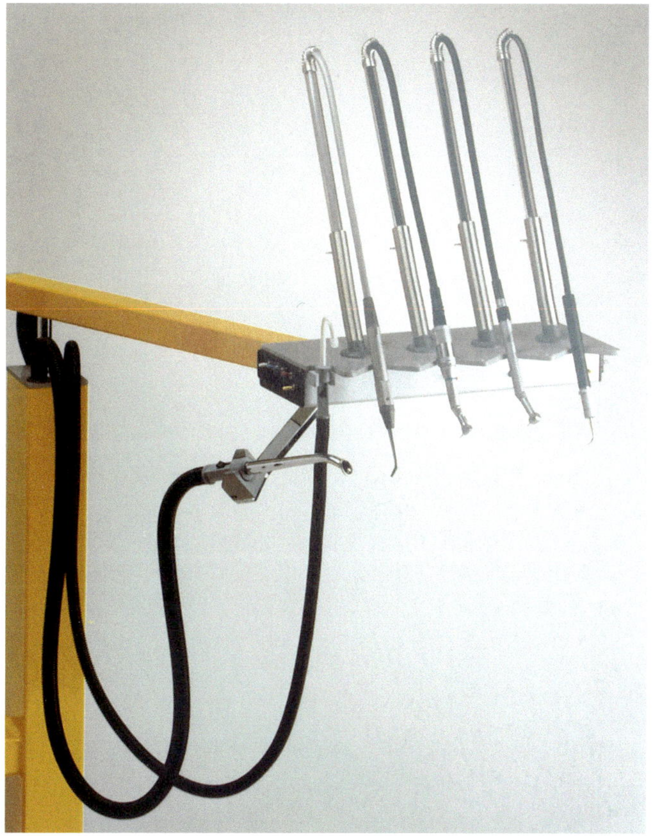

Fig 5–25 This is the ideal position for an aspiration tube holder on this 1972 Alternativ dental unit. The suction tube holder is fixed to the unit instruments support, so it is well positioned for the assistant to simultaneously pick up the aspiration tube and 3-in-1 syringe. This has the implication that the parking position of the unit is on the assistant side of the patient chair.

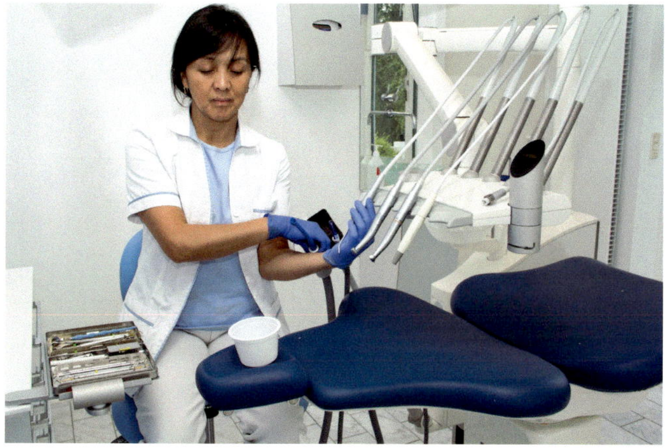

Fig 5–26 Here the unit instruments and suction holder are separated, but in the same position. The short distance between the suction tube holder and the 3-in-1 syringe makes simultaneous pick up possible for the assistant. The patient's acceptance of a horizontal position is very important for rinsing the mouth.

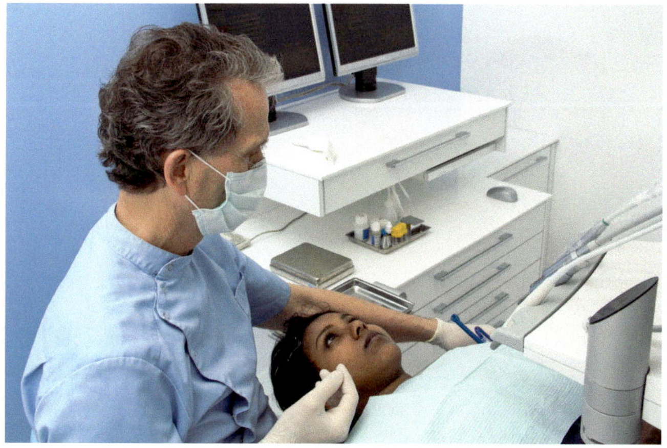

Fig 5–27 The dentist takes a suction tube with the left hand.

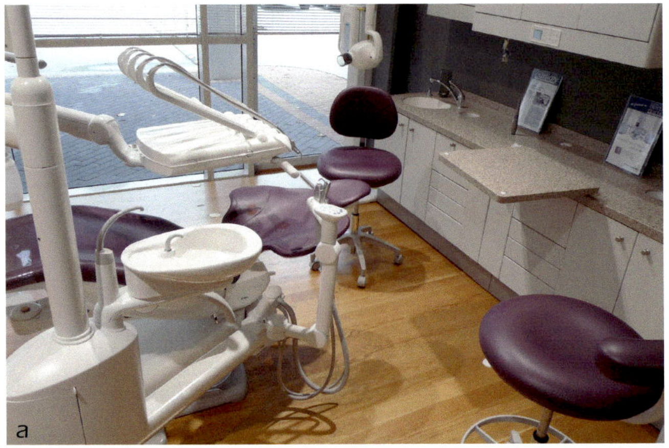

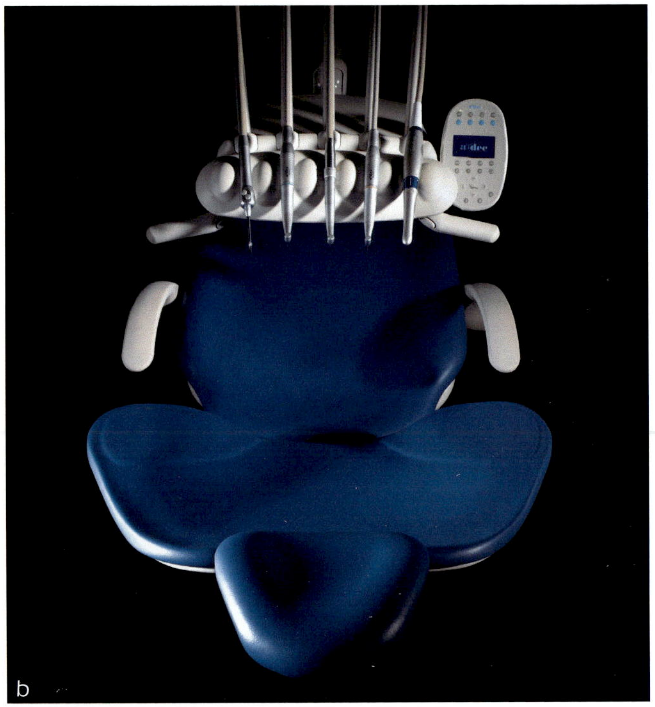

Fig 5–28 (a and b) An A-dec dental unit with central unit instruments and suction holder. The horizontal patient chair supports optimal assistance if combined with a good workstation.

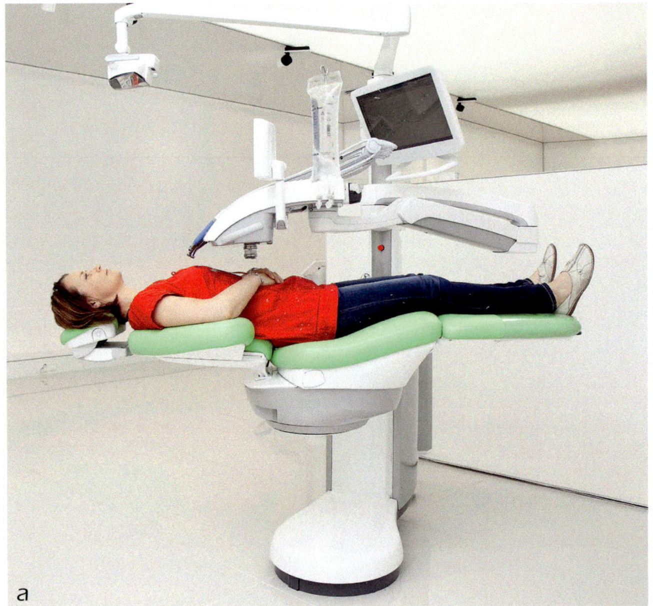

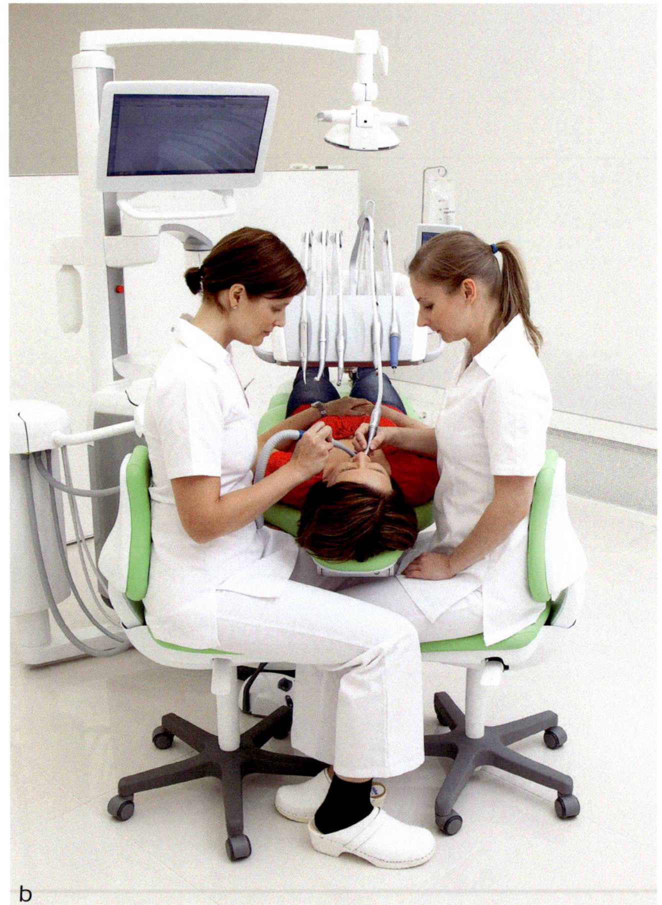

Fig 5–29 (a and b) A Planmeca dental unit with central unit instruments and suction holder. The horizontal patient chair supports optimal assistance, if combined with a good workstation.

Dental unit positioning

There are dental units on the market with patient chairs that seem to fulfill these principles, eg, horizontal patient + access of both dentist and assistant to dental unit = centrally placed unit.

But when the back of the patient chair is horizontal, the dental unit cannot be placed in properly because the arm system is too short and/or does not move up enough to leave place for the patient.

There are many dental units with centrally positioned unit instruments on the market (Figs 5–28 to 5–30). Please test them according to the principles described in this book.

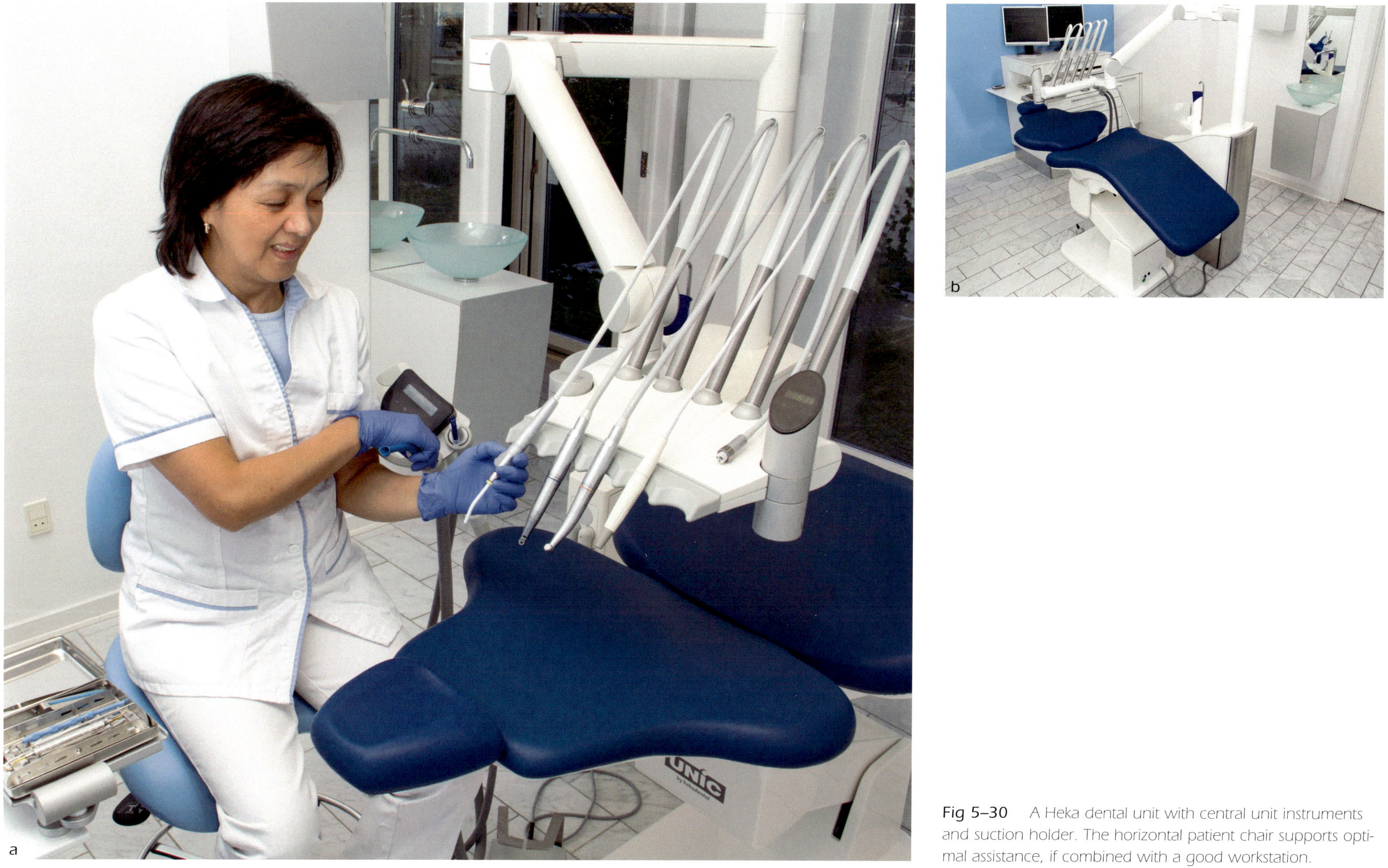

Fig 5–30 A Heka dental unit with central unit instruments and suction holder. The horizontal patient chair supports optimal assistance, if combined with a good workstation.

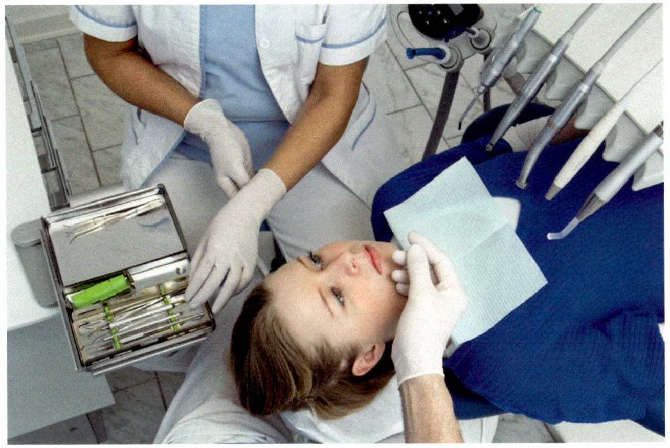

Fig 5–31 The assistant picks up a hand instrument.

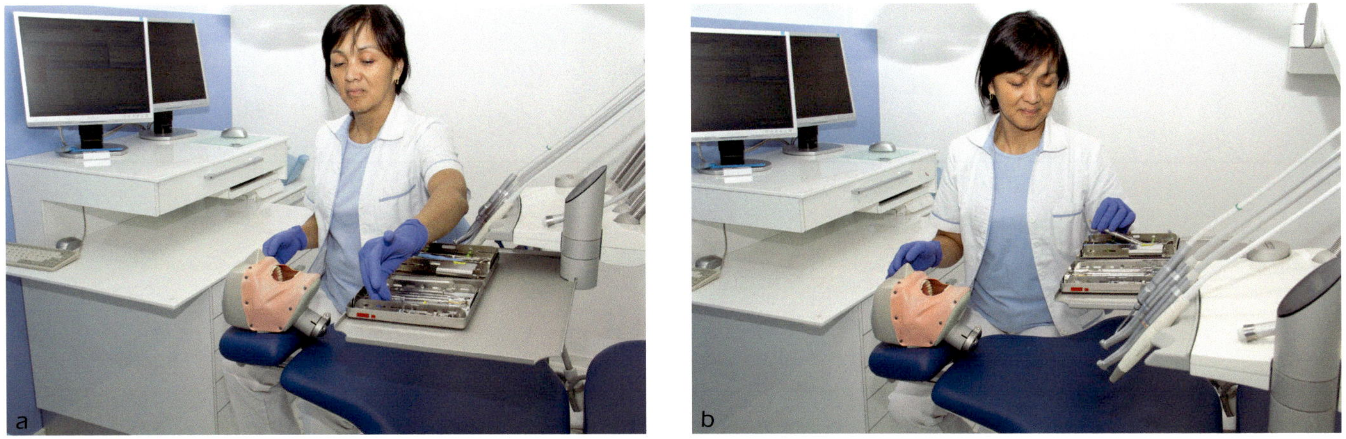

Fig 5–32 (a) The dental unit with a hand instrument table at the right hand side. (b) The hand instrument table placed over the patient.

HAND INSTRUMENT TRAY TABLE POSITION

Position of hand instruments – analysis and conclusions

The position of the hand instrument tray for four-handed dentistry has been a matter of discussion since early the 1960s. The hand instrument transfer from assistant to dentist is made in front of the mouth of the horizontal patient.

The hand instrument table is placed as shown about 15 cm left and back from the patient's head (sometimes called the "cervical tray position") (Fig 5–31). The assistant can take instruments from the instrument table and materials from the worktable, and give them to the dentist.

If the table is positioned at the right side of the dental unit, it cannot be used by the assistant, but can be used by dentists who do not want assistance for the transfer of hand instruments.

Meanwhile, if the hand instrument table is positioned at the left side of the dental unit, it comes into conflict with the aspiration tubes. If the patient is lying, the instruments are placed uncomfortably high for the assistant (Fig 5–32).

A hand instrument table over the patient's side hinders the unit use, so the unit then must be placed on the right side of the patient (for the disadvantages this position leads to, please see Chapter 6).

The hand instrument table should carry a full instrument tray/cassette as per European standards, measuring 28.0 × 18.5 cm, or two half trays/cassette as per European standards, measuring 14.0 × 18.5 cm for using with overseas trays (Fig 5–33).

The hand instrument table must have a certain mobility, so it can be moved a little to the assistant's side when the dentist must sometimes sit in a 12 o'clock position (Fig 5–34). It may need to be moved closer to the patient's head, if the patient is short.

The arm carrying the hand instrument table could be about 15 cm long, and the adapter for it could furthermore allow a sliding movement of about 25 cm. The vertical position above the floor could be about same height as the height of the headrest for the horizontal patient chair. This height will depend on the size of the dentist and

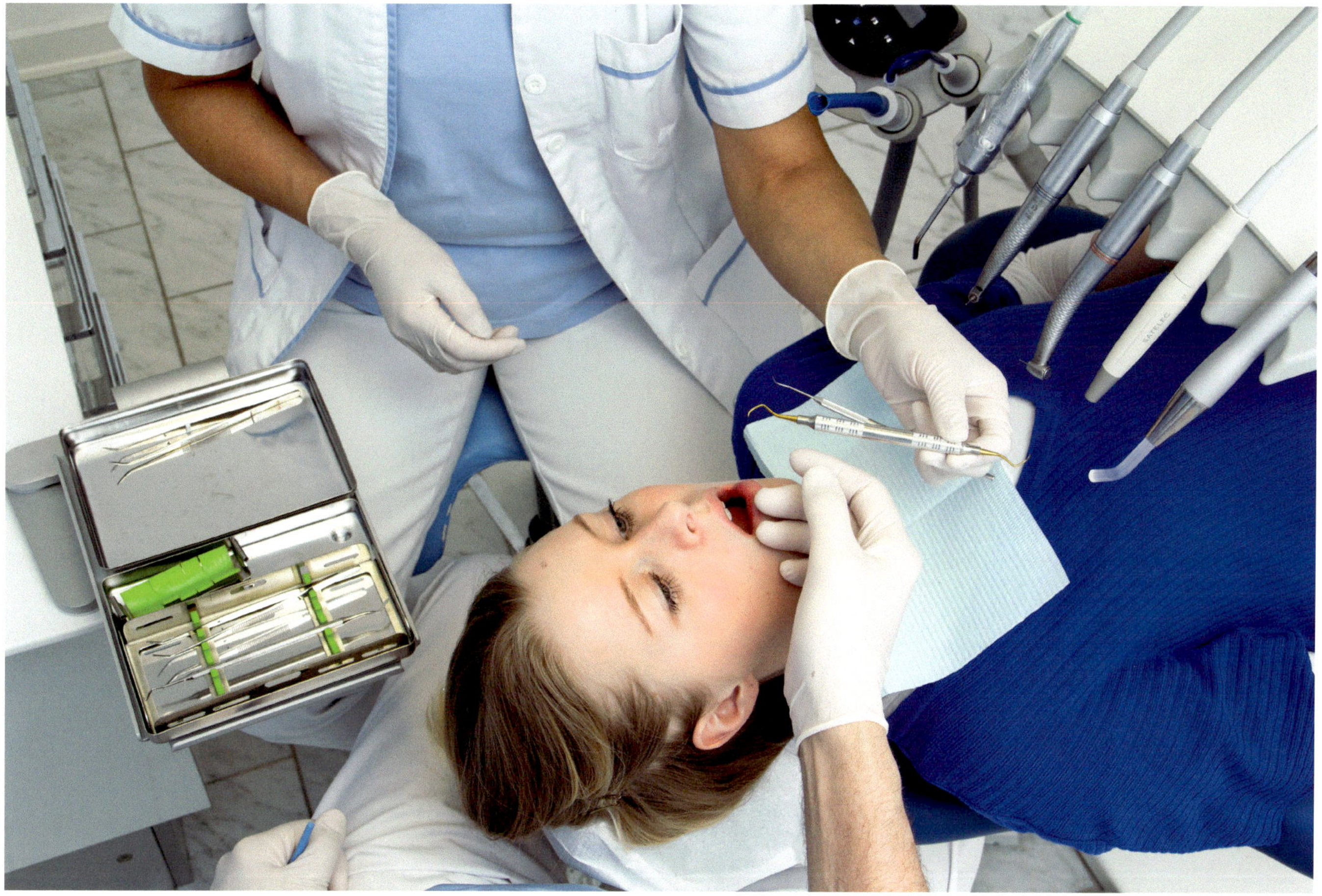

Fig 5–33 The hand instrument table should carry a full instrument tray/cassette, as per European standards.

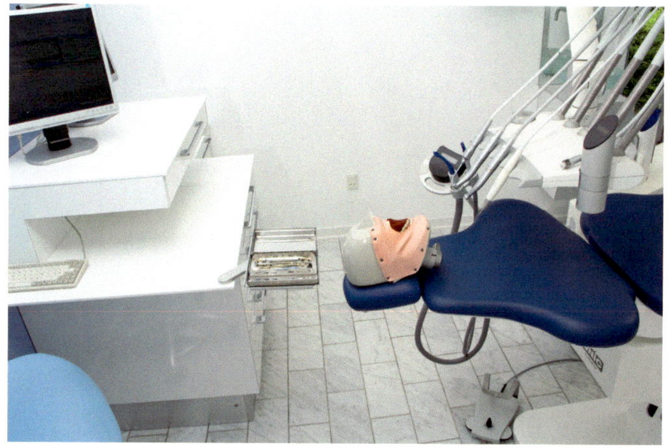

Fig 5–34 The hand instrument table in a standard position.

how inclined her/his thighs are while sitting in balanced sitting position.

A height for an average dentist could be about 75 to 80 cm. If the dentist is taller than about 180 m, the height could be 8 cm higher (and an 8 cm-higher socket from the workstation). The hand instrument table is placed between the assistant and dentist, so it serves them both. The assistant can take hand instruments from the table and transfer them to the dentist (eg, four-handed dentistry) (Fig 5–35). The dentist can also use special techniques, shown and described on page 135. The methods can be trained and ready to use after 50 to 100 repetitions of about 15 minutes each.

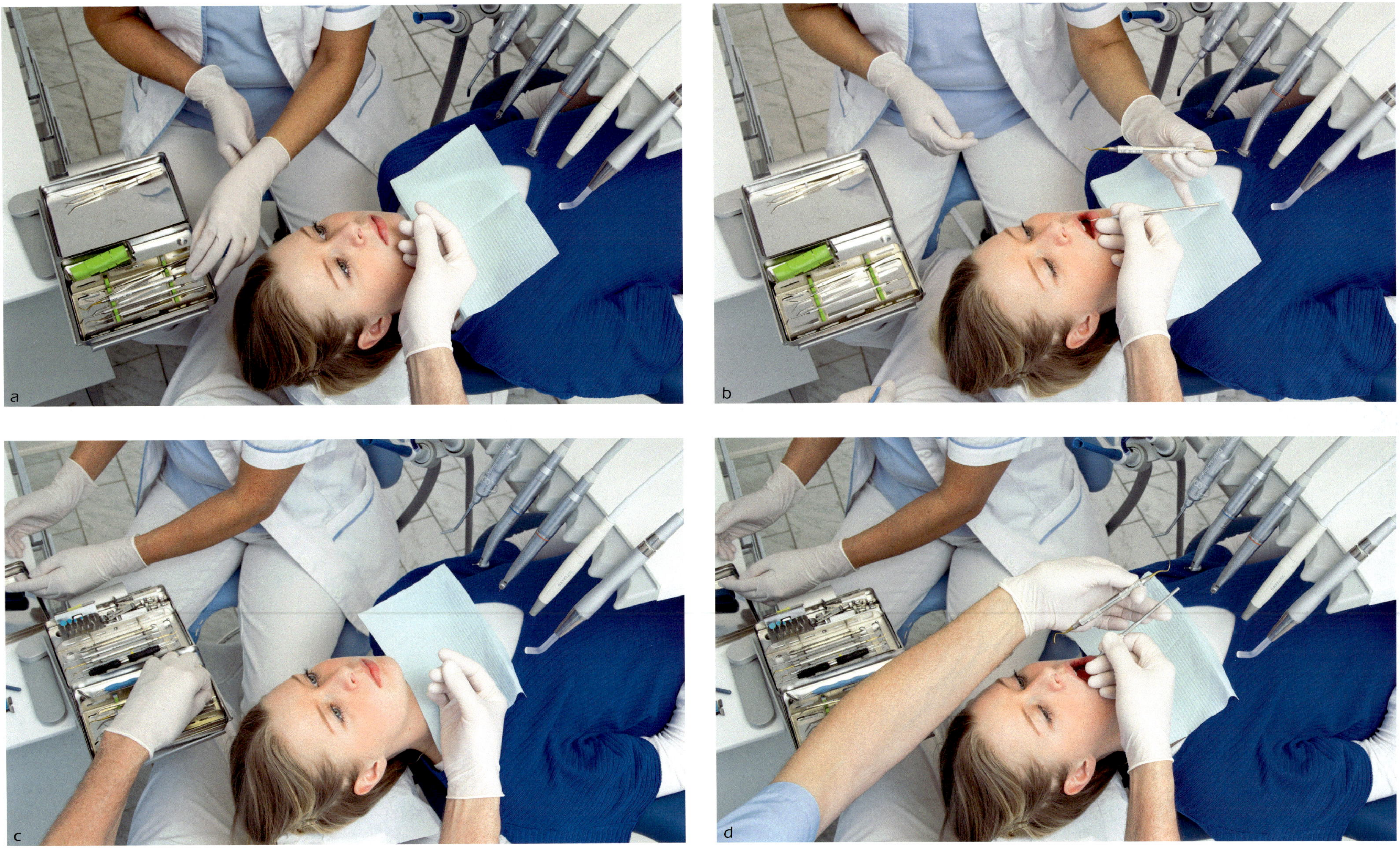

Fig 5–35 The hand instrument table: (a and b) the assistant takes an instrument, then (c and d) the dentist takes an instrument.

Chapter 6

WORK RELAXED – SAVE TIME AND ENERGY

Management of practical work by protocols

PROTOCOLS

Protocol-guided work is also a quality safety system

When a specified treatment or other action is to be performed with the dentist and assistant working in a team, both need to agree about what each of them should do.

This agreement is the protocol.

The protocol is the standard step-by-step procedure for a treatment, including the preparation as well the treatment itself. The protocol is the procedure that should usually be followed.

A protocol may have different options where a choice has to be made.

For each treatment, the dentist has to decide the step-by-step content of the protocol. In most cases this is easy to do, because it is the accepted, most-used standard procedure. When creating the protocol, the dentist needs to consider the relevance and objective of every detail, in order to create a sequence of actions based on reason.

If the protocol includes high-end assistance, the assistant transfers all hand instruments, unit instruments and materials to the dentist.

A protocol is made for every treatment or procedure, which describes everything used for a procedure, including the materials, instruments, unit instruments, burs, and contra-angles. The protocol reflects the materials selected and the rules for handling them. The protocol is the "rule of the game," and both dentist and assistant need to follow it, or inform the other in advance if deviations are needed.

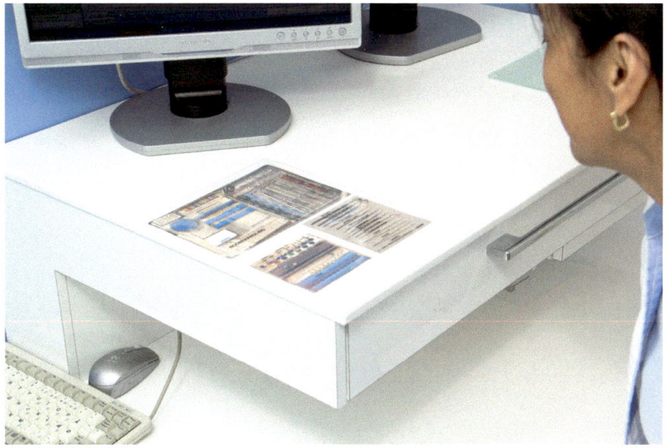

Fig 6–1 A photo can be used for showing everything that should be prepared for each treatment.

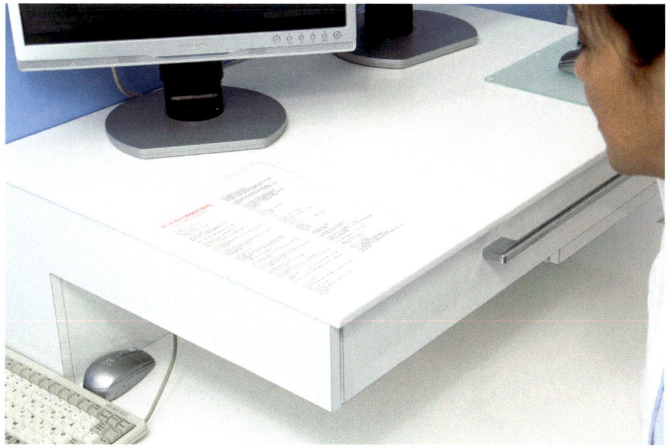

Fig 6–2 Abbreviated protocol text may be placed a visible place fort he assistant.

The protocol will include a lot of manual procedures and skills for both dentist and for assistant, which will have to be taught and learned. If a dentist does not have well-defined procedures, then the assistant will not be able to give proper support.

Protocol-guided working makes the dentist predictable. This means that the assistant can plan their next step without needing to ask, and provides a mental and practical simplification.

Documentation of the protocols

1. Learned by heart
   Procedures performed often will naturally be quickly learned by heart.
2. List of keywords for sequential procedures
   The protocol keywords can, after printing, be laminated in plastic and placed in sight at the workplace. It can be used until the actual protocol is learned by heart. If something is difficult to remember, it may be underlined or emphasized.
3. Digital photo prints
   This is an excellent solution for the preparation of materials and instruments. The names of the different items may be overwritten in hand.
4. Photos can be shown on a computer screen or may be a "digital photo frame" in the sterilization area or in the treatment room (Figs 6–1 and 6–2).
5. Short videos
   These are especially useful for training new assistants.

When the protocol is developed, the dentist and assistant make an agreement, then protocol is agreed upon. And from now on there is no doubt about what to do. This means that the dentist and assistant follow the protocol exactly, if there is no reason for deviations and if no other information is given.

Working with protocols does not mean that you cannot perform the treatment differently. You may choose between different protocols for a specific treatment – or of course you inform the assistant of what should be done. When the protocol is followed, the dentist has no need to say or ask for anything, as the assistant transfers all hand instruments, materials, and in most cases unit instruments too, automatically to the hand of the dentist.

Let's say that protocols can be used 80–90% of the time for a given treatment. This means that for 80 to 90% of the time, the dentist does not need to tell the assistant what to do. This is quite a relief, because the dentist does not need to think about it any more. Only 10 to 20% of the time will you need to ask for something different from the protocol. It is also a relief for the assistant who no longer has an endless number of instructions from the dentist.

Rare or unforeseeable branching or deviations are not "built in" to the protocol. But frequent "branching" is integrated into the protocol, such as perhaps questions from the assistant, eg, "What kind of matrix system do you need?"

Also, in this case the dentist can remain concentrated on his immediate task and relax because the assistant takes care of the planning and pose her question in due time before the matrix system is needed.

Metaprotocol 1

A protocol is made. It can be summarized as the following: "When we have made a protocol we use it from now on and it cannot be changed unless we have a reason to do so and a mutual agreement about it."

We are all different. The assistant or dentist may forget the smaller or larger details of the protocols.

Metaprotocol 2

This is needed if the assistant or dentist forgets elements in the protocol, the other party commits her/himself to helping the other by remembering the forgotten details, and maintaining a friendly ambience.

The advantages of protocol-guided teamwork

The assistant can prepare materials and instruments prior to being needed. The assistant can anticipate what is going to be done even before the dentist has realized it. This enables the dentist to maintain concentration on the task she/he is performing.

In Chapter 3, we have seen that visual perception and cognitive activity has a tendency to dominate over "sensations for body movements." However, what is sensible for fine motor body movement is exactly what is needed during precision work. So the less you have to think and to perceive visually, the more can you be aware of your own physical motor movements.

Using a protocol that both dentist and assistant can follow liberates a lot of energy and time. Most of the teamwork is performed "automatically," and the practical work will be relaxed and highly effective at the same time.

Every practice has to make its own protocols

Over the years, the author has met dentists from different countries with almost identical protocols. The reason for this is that there is very little variation in the solutions when optimal work is combined with optimal work postures.

Further comments

All of our protocols are based on four-handed teamwork, where the assistant – with perfect timing – passes all instruments, unit instruments materials etc, to the dentist. The dental unit, workstation, hand instruments, contra-angles, organizational systems, skills, working methods etc, are all described in this book.

(By mailing your request to dancinghands@mail.dk, the author will be happy to send you an example of recommended protocols.)

HIGH-END TEAMWORK

A dentist can work:

- DUO, with assistance
  The dentist is working with a full-time chairside assistant – see below.
- DUO-SOLO working
  Dentist is working some of the time with the assistant, the other without – see page 156.
- All SOLO
  The dentist is working alone – see page 162.

DUO, high-end teamwork

Four-handed working methods are demonstrated in the following pages with a centrally-positioned dental unit ("over the patient delivery system"). This enables the four-handed teamwork to include unit instruments.

At page 166, you will see the modifications necessary for four-handed working with a unit at the right side.

At page 175, you will see the modifications necessary for four-handed working with a unit in a 12 o' clock position.

Responsibilities of the chairside assistant

The assistant is seated close to the patient, as described in Chapter 9.

1. She has easy access to unit instruments with the 3-in-1 syringe on her side (Fig 6–3a).
2. The suction tube holder is placed close to the 3-in-1 syringe (Fig 6–3b).

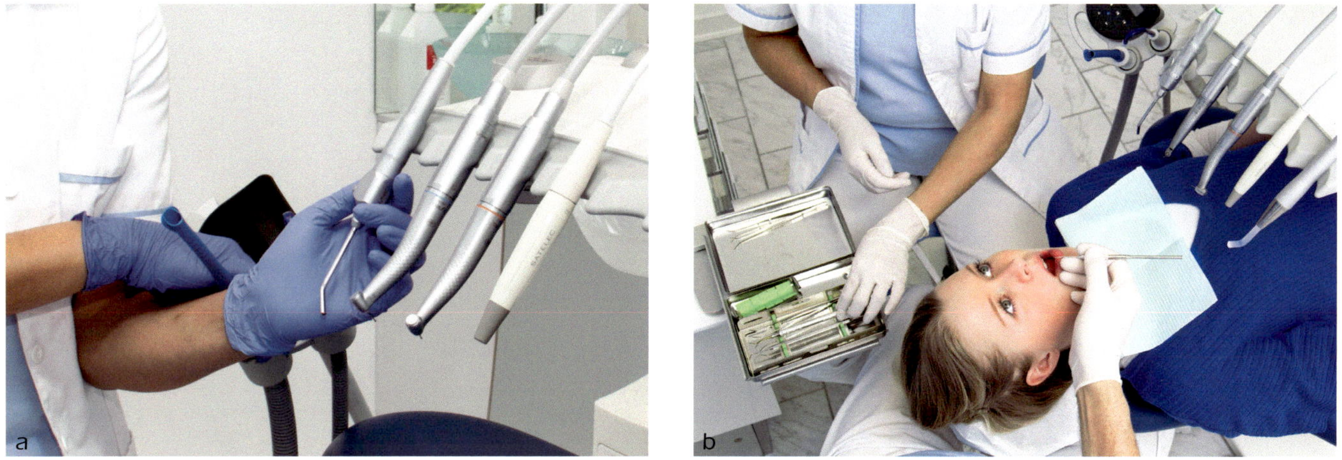

Fig 6–3 (a) The assistant takes a large suction tube at the same time as the syringe. (b) The assistant takes a hand instrument.

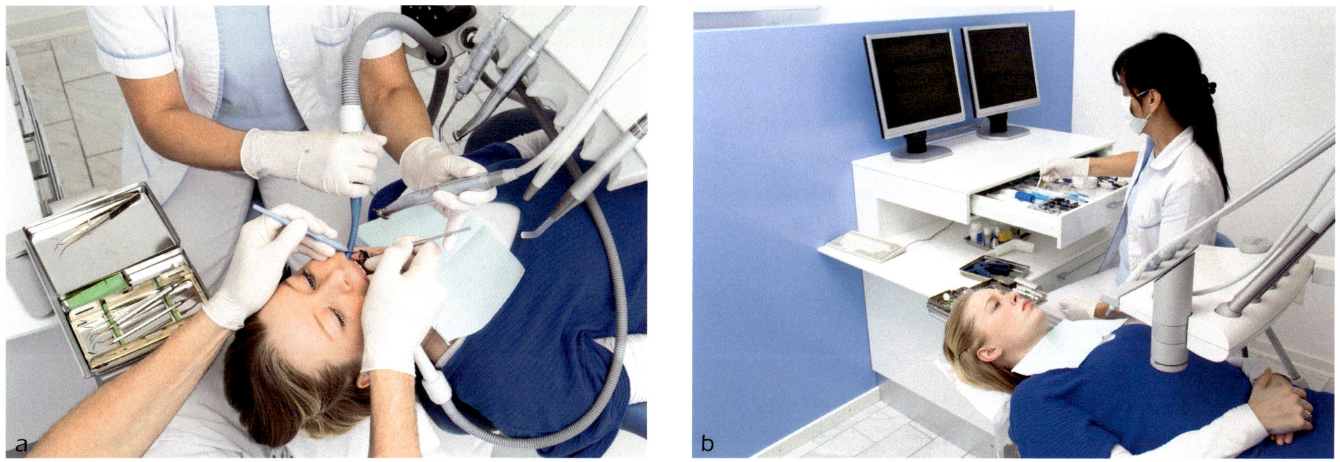

Fig 6–4 (a) The assistant takes a unit instrument. (b) The assistant prepares material on the worktop.

3. To her right side (left and behind the patient's head), she has the hand instrument table (Fig 6–4a).
4. She is also beside a worktop surface for preparing materials (Fig 6–4b).

Later on in this chapter, the last three elements of the workplace for the assistant will be described.

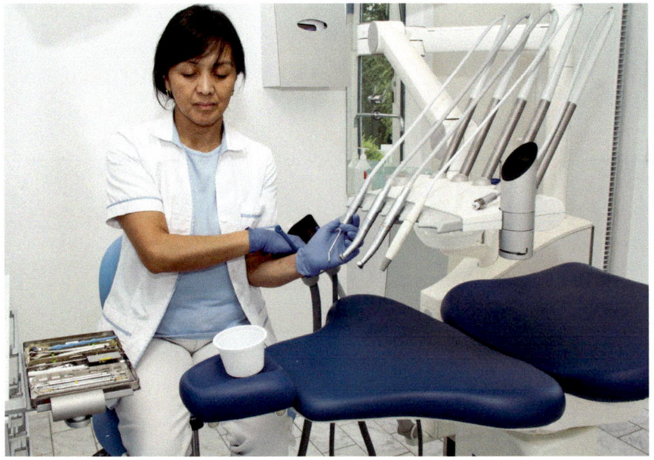

Fig 6–5 Picking up a large suction tube and a 3-in-1 syringe, at the same time.

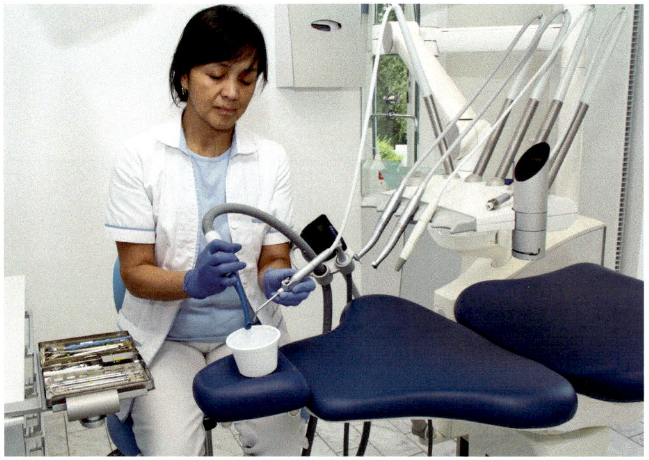

Fig 6–6 Holding a large suction tube and a 3-in-1 syringe at the same time.

Training the simultaneous pick up of large aspiration tube and 3-in-1 syringe

Here is the basic training program for the assistant:

A water cup is placed on the patient's headrest. The right hand grasps the large suction tube at the same time as the left hand takes the syringe (Fig 6–5). The large suction tube is always taken with by the assistant's right hand in order to free the left hand, which at the same time is using a syringe (Fig 6–6). Later on, the other functions of the assistant's left hand will be presented. Examples are the transfer of hand instruments and transfer of unit instruments to the dentist's right hand.

Here both hands are ready to act. Now the assistant activates the 3-in-1 syringe for first for air, then soft spray, then hard spray, then soft spray, then air and stop (Fig 6–7).

In most 3-in-1 syringes, it is easiest to activate the buttons for air and water with the left hand thumb.

This training protocol is repeated 25–40 times a day over 3 days (it takes 5 minutes).

Retraction and aspiration using the large suction tube

The large suction tube has a dual function. It is used for aspiration and also for holding soft tissue away from the working area. This is called retraction. So the large suction tube is used for aspiration and retraction. In order to be able to do this, the large suction tube must have an extended part suitable for this retraction. This is the suction tube most often used for retraction (Figs 6–8 and 6–9).

The suction tube holders are placed in the rather narrow space between the 3-in-1 syringe on the dental unit and the left upper arm of the assistant. Because the space is narrow, the position of the suction tube holder must be precise.

The large suction tube is grasped with the assistant's right hand, so the left hand is free for the simultaneous use of the 3-in-1 syringe, or for the transfer to the dentist of hand instruments or unit instruments (Fig 6–10). The large tube is normally taken and held in a fist grip (Fig 6–11), which is a forceful grip in order to protect the assistant against overstraining the muscles of the hand and arm.

The "fist grip" is used because this grip is so strong that only a small part of the total force is used to hold the suction tube in a stable position. If less than about 10% of muscle force is used for the isometric retraction position, then the risk for symptoms of over-arching muscles or tendons is low.

The suction tube is slightly bent, so the part held by the assistant's right hand does not hinder her in seeing the tip, and keeps the hand away from the dentist's field of vision.

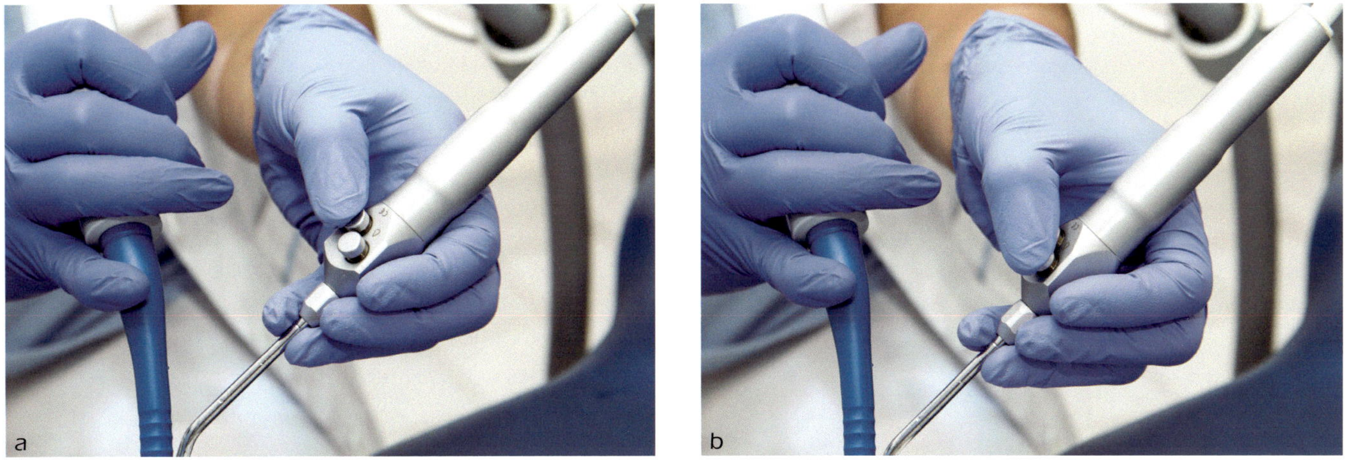

Fig 6–7 (a) Pressing air button. (b) Pressing air and water button.

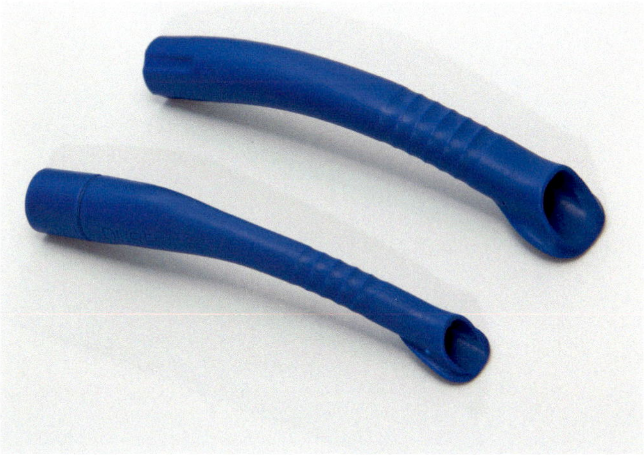

Fig 6–8 Small and large version of large suction tube.

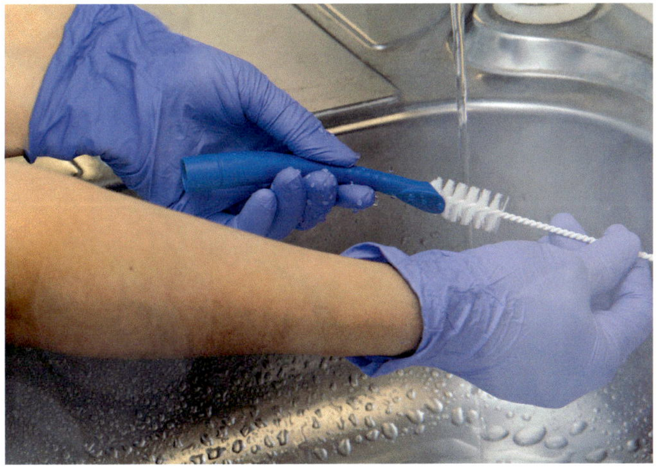

Fig 6–9 The suction tube is cleaned manually before placed in instrument washing machine and later autoclave.

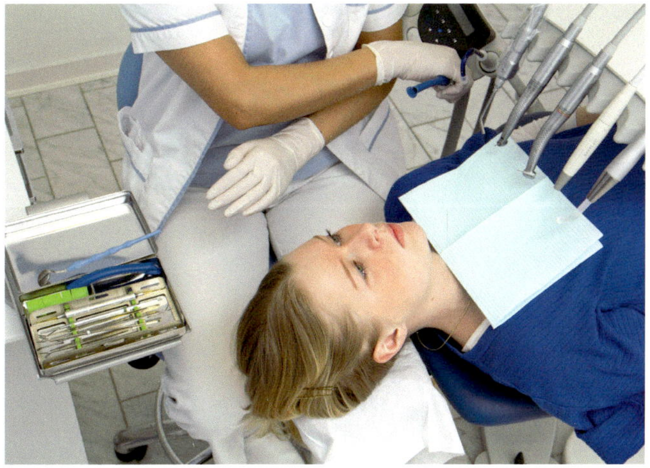

Fig 6–10 Assistant's left shoulder near the unit instrument. The suction holder is in between, grasped with the right hand.

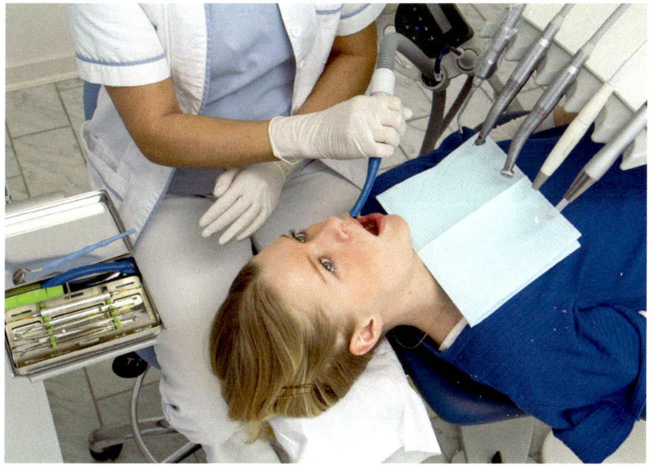

Fig 6–11 Large suction tube in the mouth held by a fist grip, for secure retraction and aspiration.

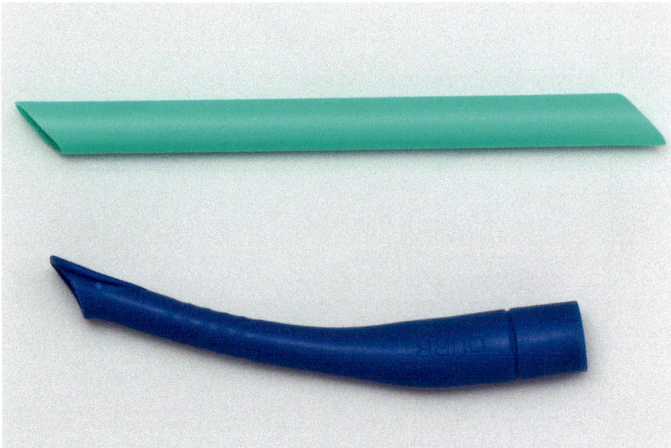

Fig 6–12 Disposable suction tubes (green), compared with the proposed sterilizable tube (blue).

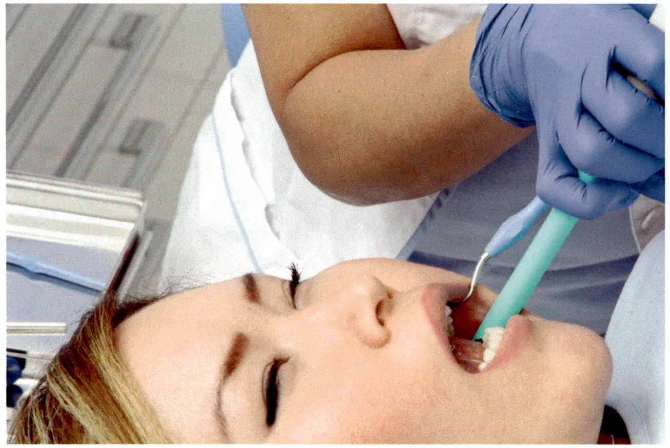

Fig 6–13 The assistant uses a straight tube and mirror for retraction, held with both hands. In this case the many functions of assistant's left hand are lost. The left hand is occupied for retraction instead of using the right hand for combined aspiration and retraction.

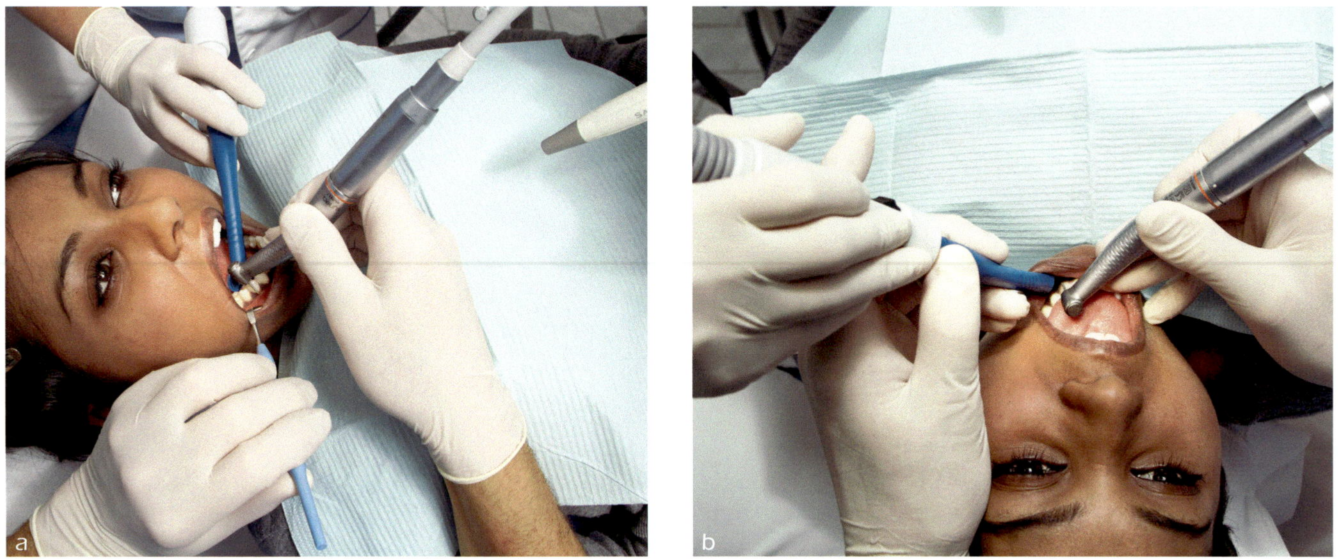

Fig 6–14 (a) Opening of the aspiration tube parallel to the buccal side of the teeth on the mandibular right side. (b) The mandibular left side.

Disposable straight suction tubes

Disposable suction tubes are too soft, lack extension for retraction, and the assistant has to angle her hand so that it does not obstruct her working field of vision (Fig 6–12).

Straight aspiration tubes cannot retract soft tissues properly, and in a "safe" way. Then the assistant needs to use a mirror for retraction, and she has "lost" a hand for other tasks. The disposable type of large aspiration tube should not be used because it is obstructive for fine assistance (Fig 6–13).

The large suction tube is used for aspiration and at the same time – from the assistant's side – for retracting the patient's cheek, lips or tongue, so the working field is visible and free to work in for the dentist.

The "tip" of the suction tube is placed at a distance of 5–7 mm from the tooth, where the dentist is working. The retraction shield is directed towards the tooth root, except for last molars where it is inclined in relation to the tooth. The suction tube is held so the opening is parallel to the assistant side of the actual tooth. The middle of the opening of the suction tube is level with the occlusal plane of the molar or premolar (Fig 6–14).

Sometimes it is difficult to retract the tongue or cheeks enough with the small version of the suction tube, which is used most often. The cheek or tongue may "fold around" this suction tube indicating that a larger version will be needed. This may be the case in say 5 to 10% of the cases, so large suction tubes must be stored in a position that is easy to access.

The dentist uses the mirror from the right side to retract the mouth of the patient. The angle of grip of mirror depends on the clock position of the dentist. The angled grip ensures that the dentist can keep the wrist straight and prevents bending of the wrist particularly in say 11 or 12 o'clock positions where the grip is almost reversed.

The assistant should be attentive to the double function of the large aspiration tube (Fig 6–15); it should not be left from a retraction position while the dentist is working. This is in contrast to common working methods, which can be described as follows:

- When working with spray and a large aspiration tube for aspiration and retraction, the large aspiration tube evacuates the majority of spray, but some spray and saliva can accumulate in the bottom of the mouth. In order to remove this, the assistant leaves the large suction tube from a retraction position to aspire spray and saliva in both sides of the bottom of the mouth, in order to maintain the patient's comfort.
- In the meantime, the dentist must wait. Then the assistant moves the large suction tube back to the retraction and aspiration position.
- Sometimes these interruptions may happen very frequently during the use of spray from the unit instrument.

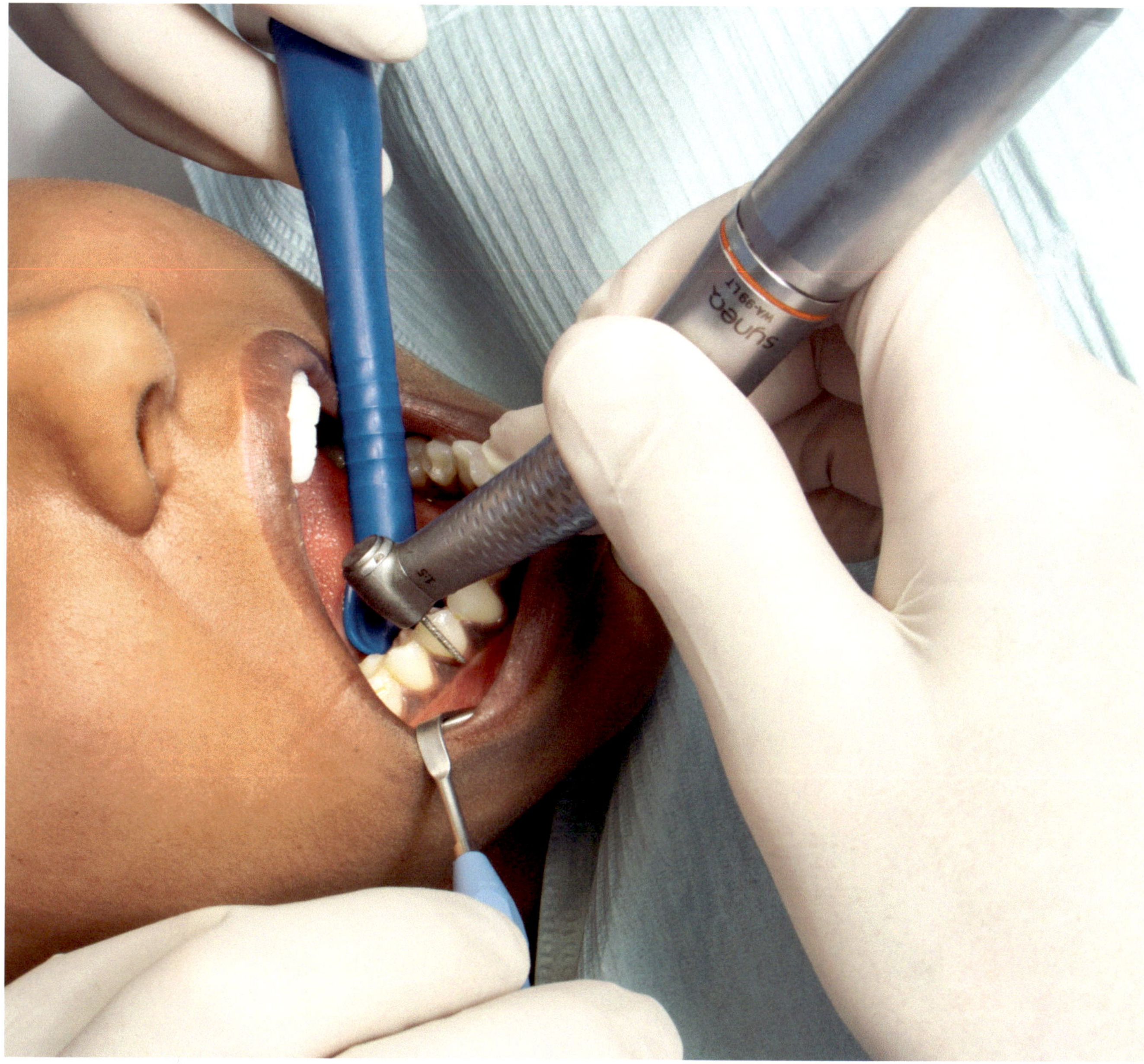

Fig 6–15 Dentist is retracting using a mirror.

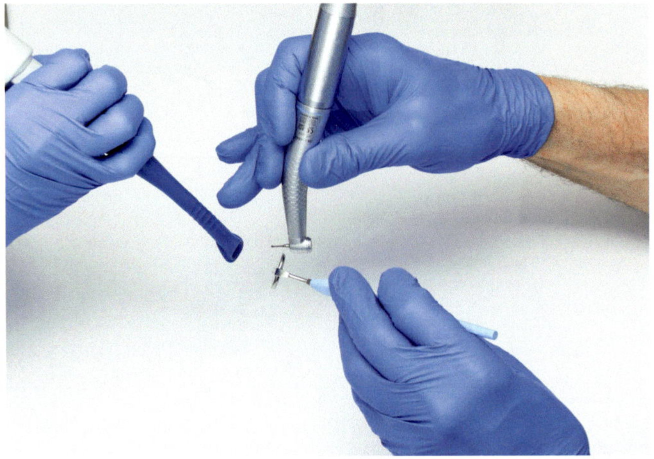

Fig 6–16 Mandibular left – the assistant supports the retraction of the chin with the aspiration tube. The dentist performs the lingual retraction with a mirror.

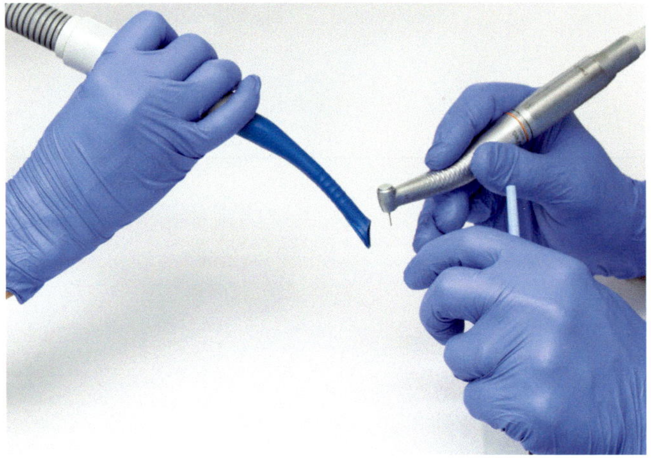

Fig 6–17 Mandibular right – the assistant retracts (depresses) the tongue with the aspiration tube. Meanwhile, the dentist performs the retraction of the chin with the left hand index finger.

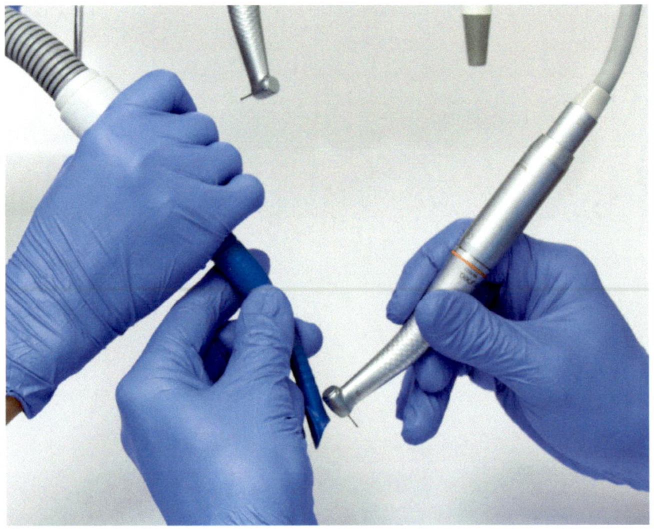

Fig 6–18 Mandibular right, lingual surface – the assistant retracts the patient's tongue with the aspiration tube. The dentist also assists if necessary by holding the aspiration tube if the tongue is forceful.

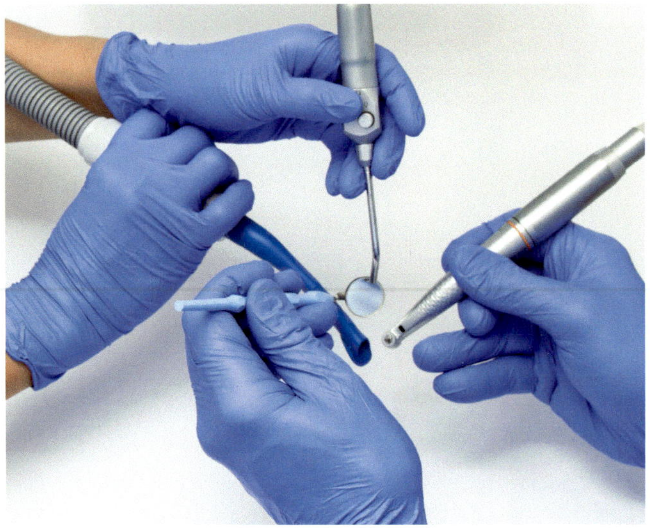

Fig 6–19 Maxillary right, using mirror – the assistant retracts (depresses) the tongue with the aspiration tube. The dentist supports the right ring finger on a cotton roll in the upper vestibulum, and retracts tissue at the same time.

However, it is often the case that the assistant keeps the large suction tube down at the bottom of the mouth in order to remove saliva and spray here. Then the retraction is lost and there is no aspiration by the work field and, if spray and mirror is used, no way of keeping the mirror dry for a good reflected vision.

But fortunately there is a simple solution: the small aspiration tube is used. Its bent tip is placed behind the last mandibular molar in order to evacuate the "bottom of the mouth." The result of this is that the large aspiration tube can be held permanently in the retraction and aspiration position, as long as the unit instrument is in use.

Some examples of retraction are detailed, in Figs 6–16 to 6–26:

Dentist's retraction of soft tissue while working DUO

Generally while working DUO, the assistant retracts from the left side and the dentist retracts from the right side. The dentist may retract with a mirror, if that is not being used for vision. Alternatively, the retraction can be made by a finger.

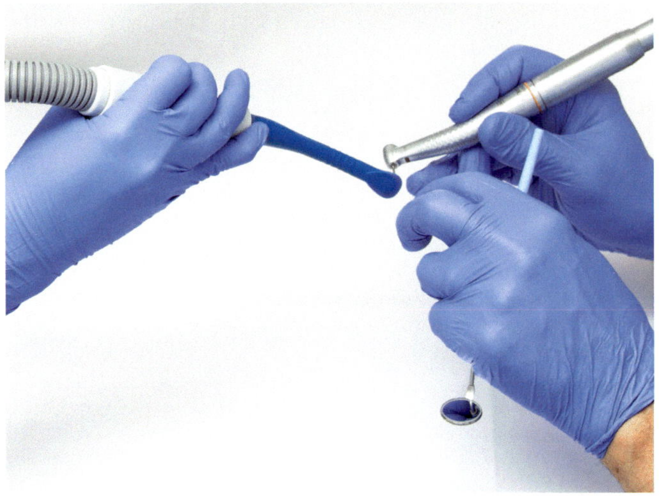

Fig 6–20 Maxillary right, direct vision – working parallel to the buccal surface. The assistant retracts as per Fig 6–19. The dentist retracts at the right side with his finger.

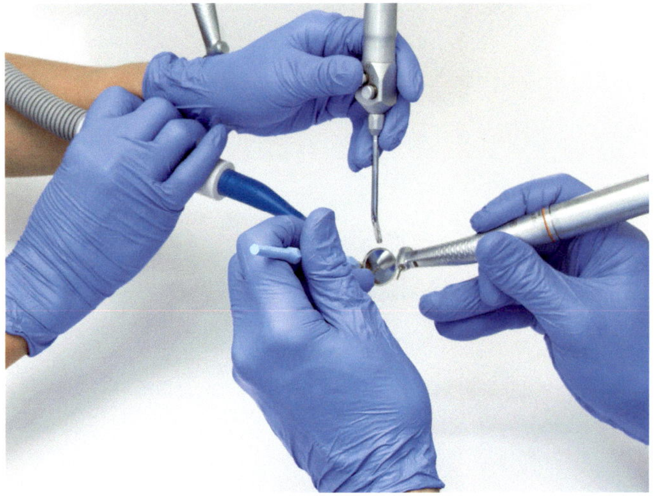

Fig 6–21 Maxillary left – the assistant retracts the chin with the aspiration tube – there is no retraction from the dentist. If the mirror is used, the assistant dries it.

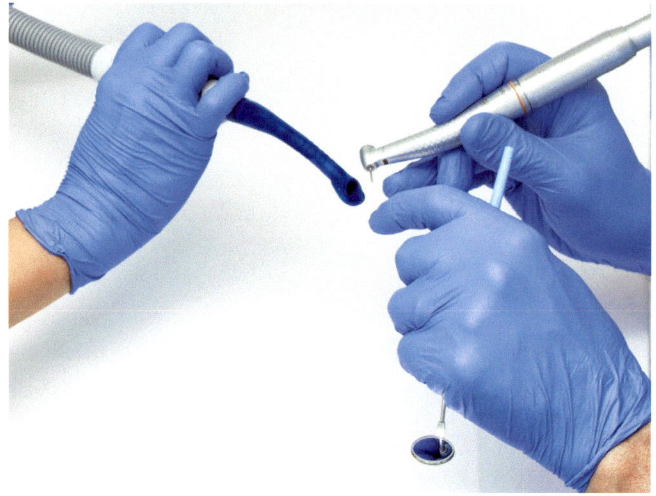

Fig 6–22 Maxillary front – retraction by aspiration – labial or patina or with a finger (either the assistant or dentist can do this).

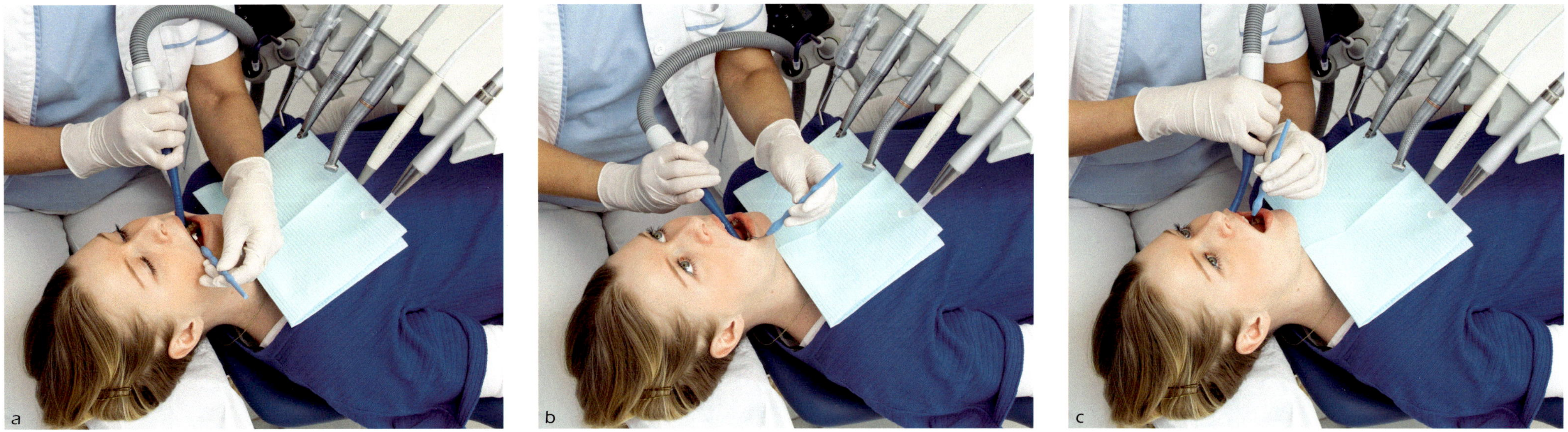

Fig 6–23 (a to c) Retraction from the left side is done by the assistant using the suction tube. The lip, chin and tongue are retracted to create free access and vision to the working field. Retraction from the dentist's side may sometimes be done with mirror (or aspiration tube).

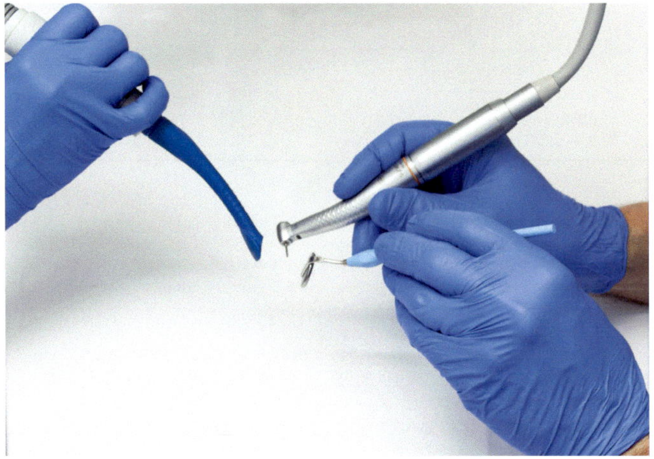

Fig 6–24 Retraction position 26 – with the suction tube, the assistant retracts the patient's lip, cheek and tongue from the left side.

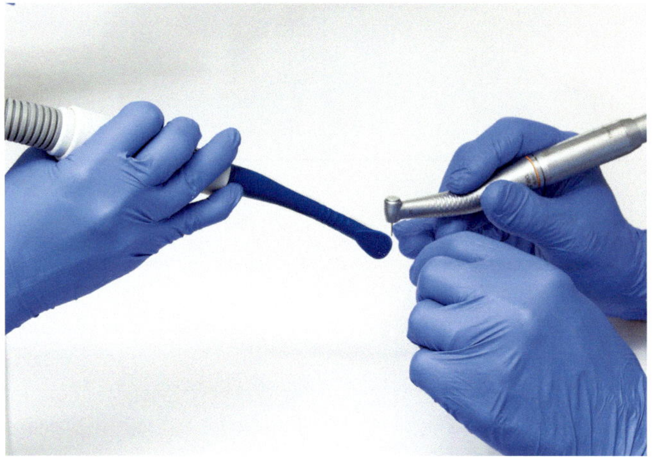

Fig 6–25 In the front region, a finger may be used for retraction.

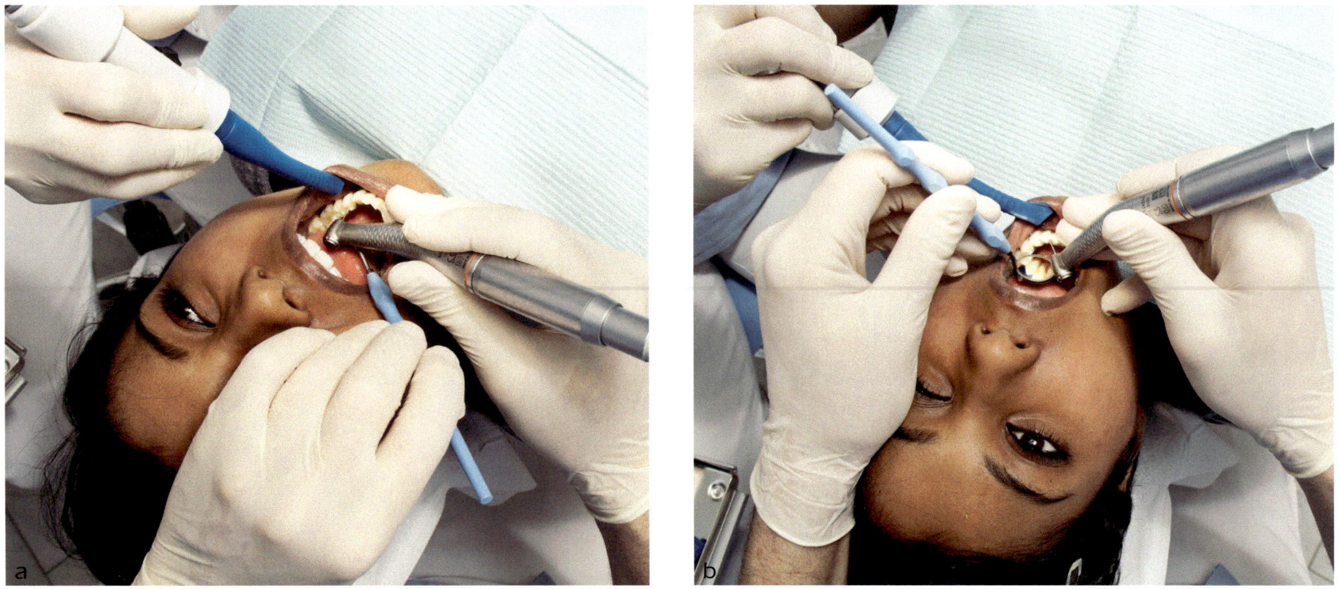

Fig 6–26 Dentist performing retraction position 36, with the mirror at a 9 o'clock position (a), and 12 o'clock position (b). In some cases, a finger is best for retraction.

USE OF THE SMALL SUCTION TUBE

Chose a type of small suction tube which can easily bend, and where the tip can be removed.

The small suction tube is always in use. It is used to aspirate water and saliva in the "bottom of the mouth of the lying patient" in the lowest position convenient for the patient (Figs 6–27 and 6–28). This position of the point of the small suction tube is at the trigonum retromolare, behind the last mandibular molar. With this position, continued aspiration removes spray and saliva, while the tip does not touch the tongue and cause inconvenience to the patient.

The small aspiration tube is bent so it remains in this position. If the patient's mouth is large, then the distance from the angle of the mouth to the position of the tip of the small suction tube is short. In this scenario, the suction tube is bent close to the tip. If the patient's mouth is small, the distance from angle of mouth is larger and the bending is a little further away from the tip. The assistant could also hold the small aspiration tube (Fig 6–29).

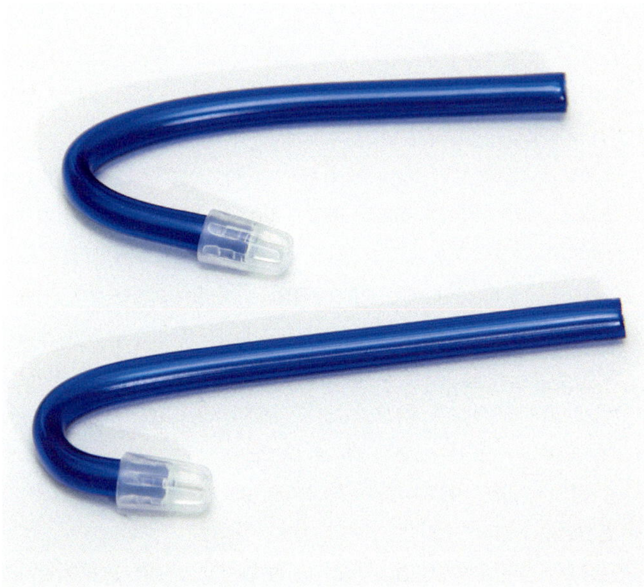

Fig 6–27 Small aspiration tubes: the lower tube is bent in a short distance from the tip for a large mouth, where the distance from angle of mouth to the retromolar area in the mandibular jaw is short. The upper tube is bent in a longer distance from the tip for a small mouth, where the distance from the angle of the mouth to the retromolar area in the mandibular jaw is longer.

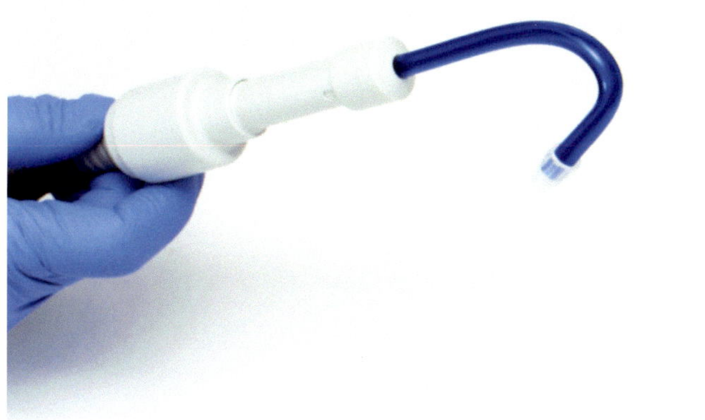

a

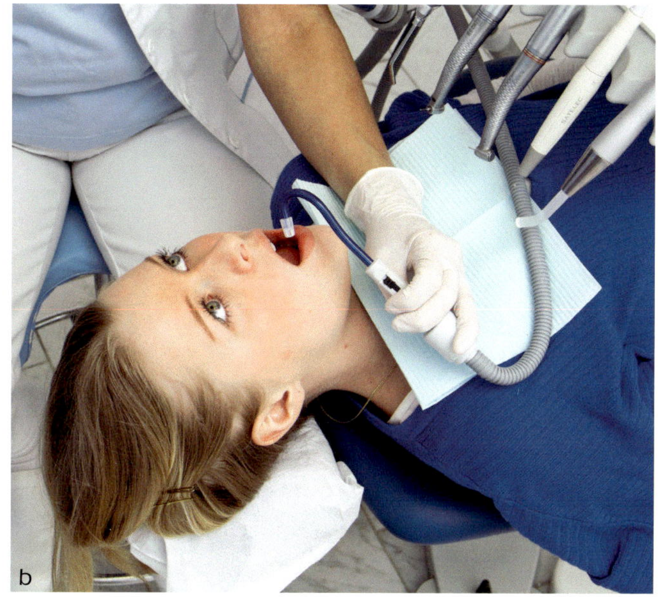

b

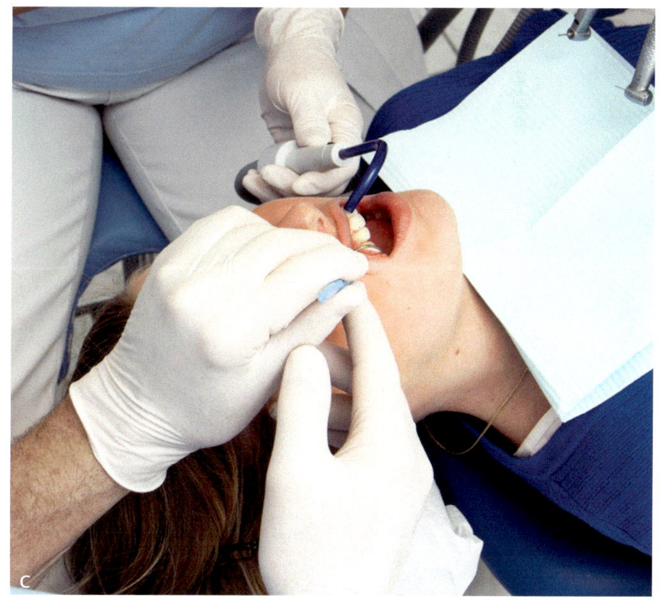

c

Fig 6–28 Small aspiration tube mounted (a) right side, tube arranged on serviette (b). On the left side, the tube is hanging down (c).

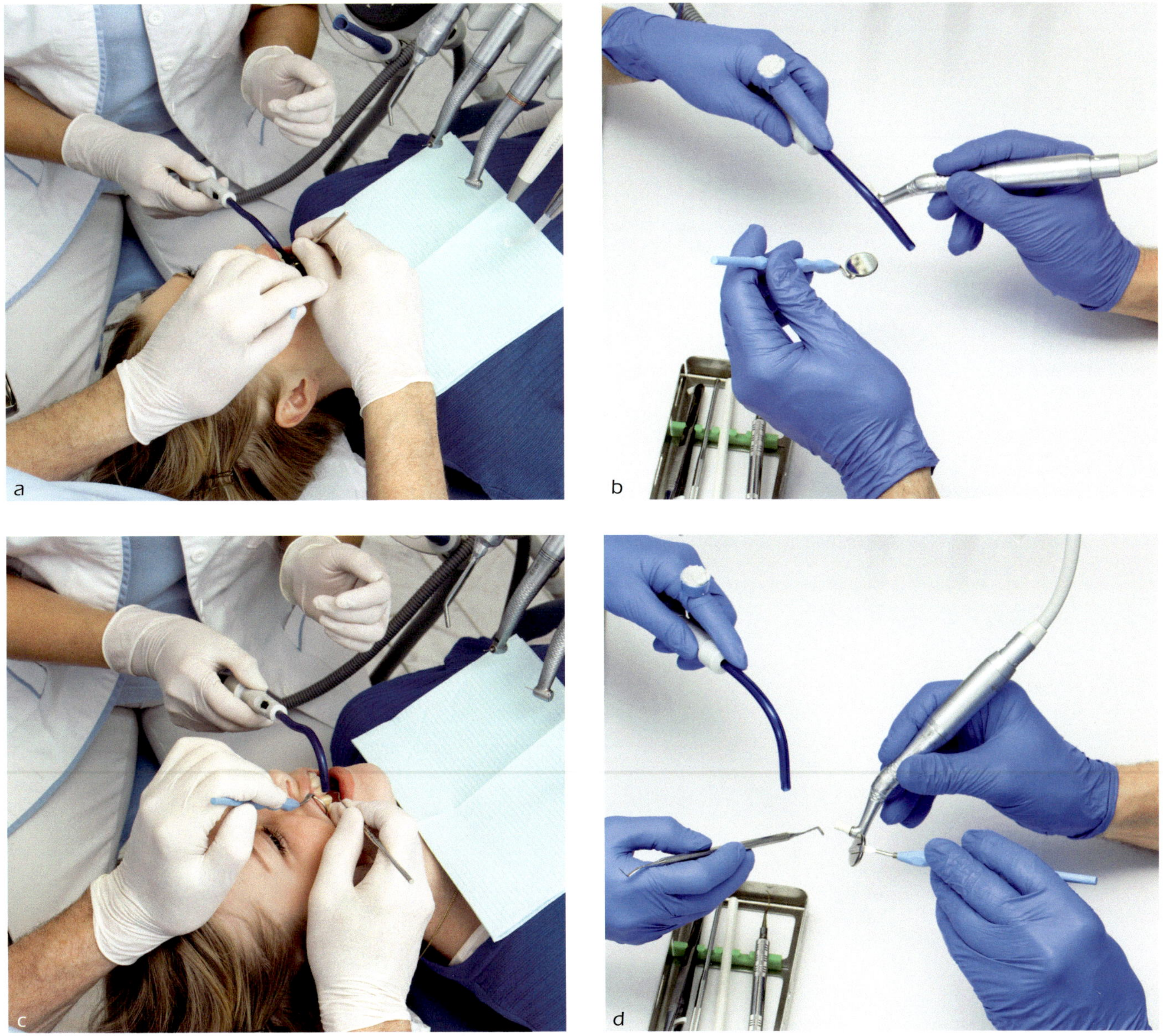

Fig 6–29 "Spot aspiration" at the gingival maxillary left (a and b) and mandibular right (c and d). The assistant can hold the small aspiration tube by hand.

Here is a useful little protocol to use if a dentist sees a particle (eg, of an old amalgam filling) in the patient's mouth (Figs 6–30 and 6–31):

1. The dentist lifts up the small aspiration tube and the assistant removes the tip. Dentist removes particle on tongue and the assistant replaces the tip of the small aspiration tube. The dentist places it in the patient's mouth again.
2. A small aspiration tube is used for picking up amalgam particles (if making an amalgam filling see section on Amalgam, page 202).
3. A small aspiration tube is used by four-handed polishing with a rubber cup (see section on Scaling and polishing, page 215).

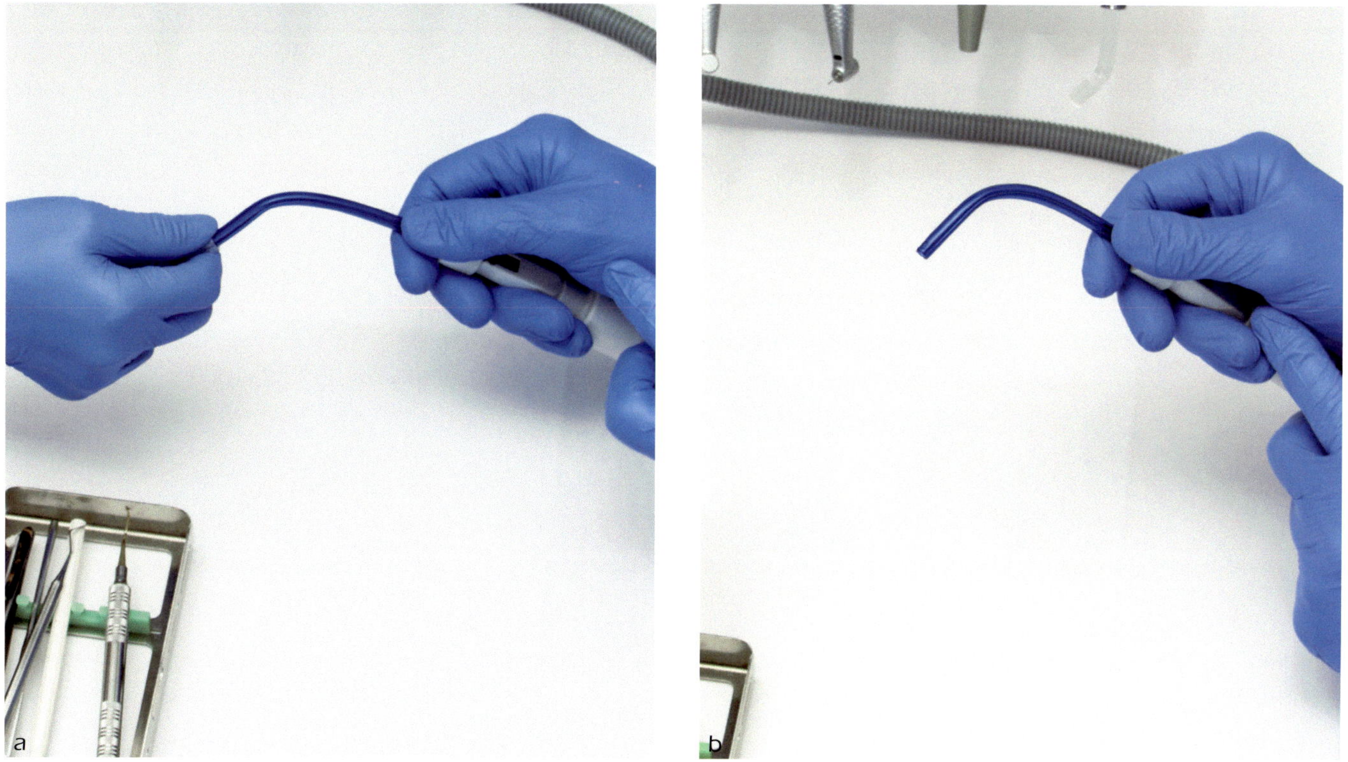

Fig 6–30 Here is a protocol to use if the dentist spots a particle (eg, from an old amalgam filling) in the patient's mouth. Aspiration on the right side (a). The dentist lifts the tube and the assistant removes it (b).

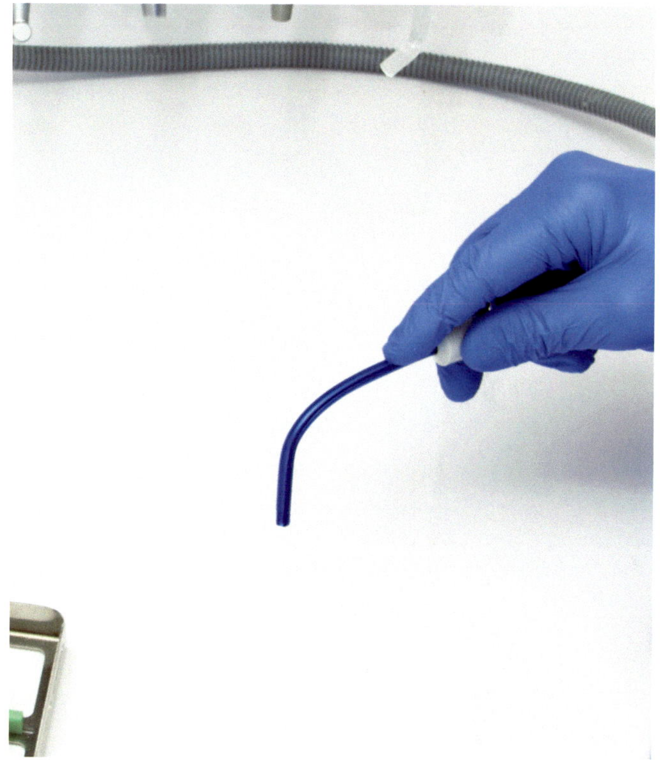

Fig 6–31 The dentist removes the particle on the tongue.

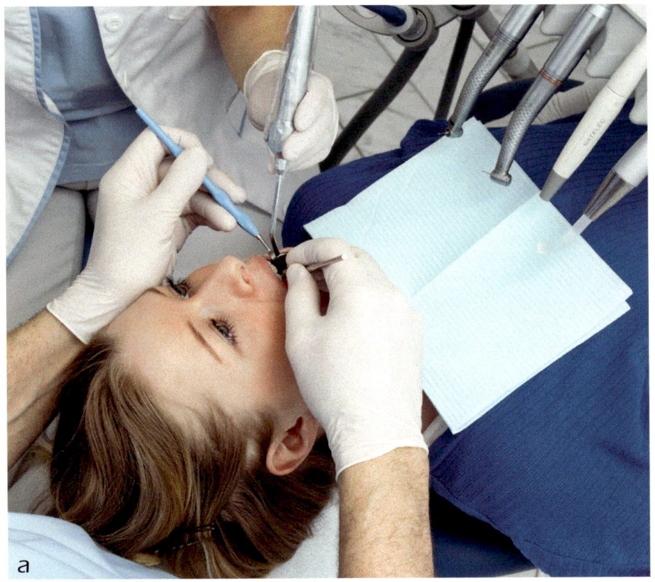

Fig 6–32 (a and b) Use of air for drying.

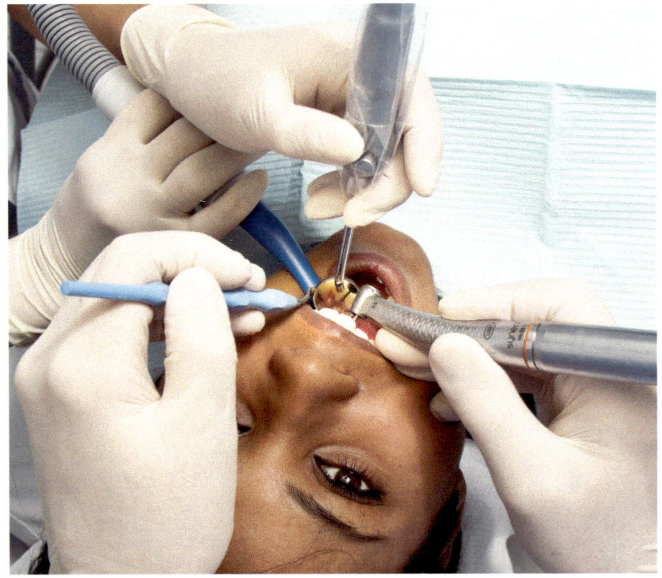

Fig 6–33 The mirror at the maxillary left almost touches the mandibular teeth.

THE ASSISTANT'S GENERAL USE OF 3-IN-1 SYRINGE AND SUCTION TUBES

3-in-1 syringe used with air

The assistant can use the 3-in-1 syringe for drying the teeth with air during examination. The drying is done with "shaking" movements to create air turbulence, so surfaces and possible cavities are dried even if the direction of the air is not precise (which may be difficult to see for the assistant) (Fig 6–32).

The assistant has to imagine the direction of air coming from the angled tip of the 3-in-1 syringe. This three-dimensional animation is sometimes a bit difficult and may need specific training. A careful soft blow of air may be used in order to dry gingival tissues (from saliva or blood) for measuring periodontal pockets. When stopping work with the contra-angle and spray in a cavity, the assistant uses air for visual inspection of the cavity (with small shaking movements) to dry the cavity.

Keeping the mirror dry when working with spray and mirror

How to see through the mirror

The protocol for how to see through the mirror is very important:

- The mirror is placed as far away from any spray as possible.
- If the distance between the spray and the mirror is doubled, the volume of spray reaching the mirror is quartered.
- When working in the maxillary jaw, the mirror touches or almost touches the teeth in the mandibular jaw (Fig 6–33). Placing the mirror here will, for about 30 to 40% of the time, keep it dry and visibility through will not be disturbed. In this position, the mirror surface is easy for the assistant to see.

What to do when spray hinders reflected vision in mirror

When working with mirror and spray, droplets from the spray will rapidly cover the mirror. The assistant keeps the mirror dry by using air from the 3-in-1 syringe.

The force of the continuous air blow must be rather high. The volume of air from some disposable tips to the 3-in-1 syringe is not sufficient. It may be better to buy the tips in a metal that can be sterilized (Fig 6–34).

The tip of the 3-in-1 syringe should be 1½ to 2 cm from the mirror (if it is too close, then vision is disturbed). It should also be directed about 45 degrees towards the surface of the mirror (if the angle is too large then vision is disturbed, if too small the mirror will not dry).

Directed towards the middle of the mirror, the syringe tip is moved from side to side, with 1 cm long movements to keep the major part of the mirror dry. Three movements per second should be used (two is not enough and four is too difficult).

The movements are made by "oscillations" of the assistant's arm. If movements are made from the wrist, they are very tiring and therefore difficult to continue. The mirror will not always remain completely dry, but when the dentist stops using the contra-angle (and therefore stops the spray), then the assistant continues to dry the mirror, which is completely dry almost in a fraction of second. If debris is stuck to the mirror, it will need to be cleaned with a serviette (Kleenex type).

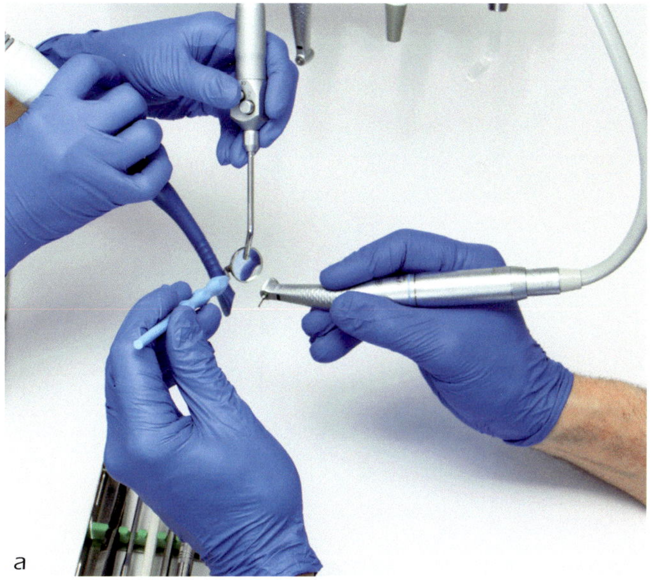

a

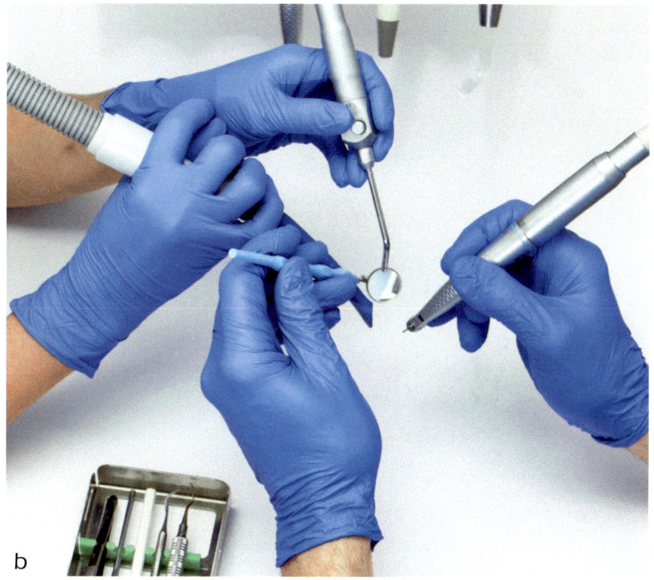

b

Fig 6–34 Airblow positions (a and b).

Automatic chip blow

The drying of the mirror combined with an automatic chip blow after stopping the spray, dries the cavity with air for 1 second. The dentist can then (without doing anything but stopping the contra-angle) inspect and control the working surface (Fig 6–35a).

If the dental unit does not have an automatic chip blow, then the protocol is as follows.

After the dentist stops the contra-angle and spray (and the mirror is now dry), the assistant now leaves the mirror with the tip of the 3-in-1 syringe and dries the cavity with a strong air blow and hand movements. The short shaking movements create a turbulence of the air, therefore drying the cavity, even if the direction of the air is not perfect (Fig 6–35b).

3-in-1 syringe used with spray

The syringe should regulate the spray in three levels: soft, medium and hard. Unfortunately, the most commonly used 3-in1 syringes are very difficult to regulate. The movement of the activation button is so short that it is very difficult to activate soft or medium spray. The function is either almost no spray or full spray.

This syringe (Fig 6–36) is easy to regulate. The thumb is able to roll over the two buttons, first activating the airblow and with a continuous "roll," gradually activating the spray, to soft spray – medium spray – strong spray.

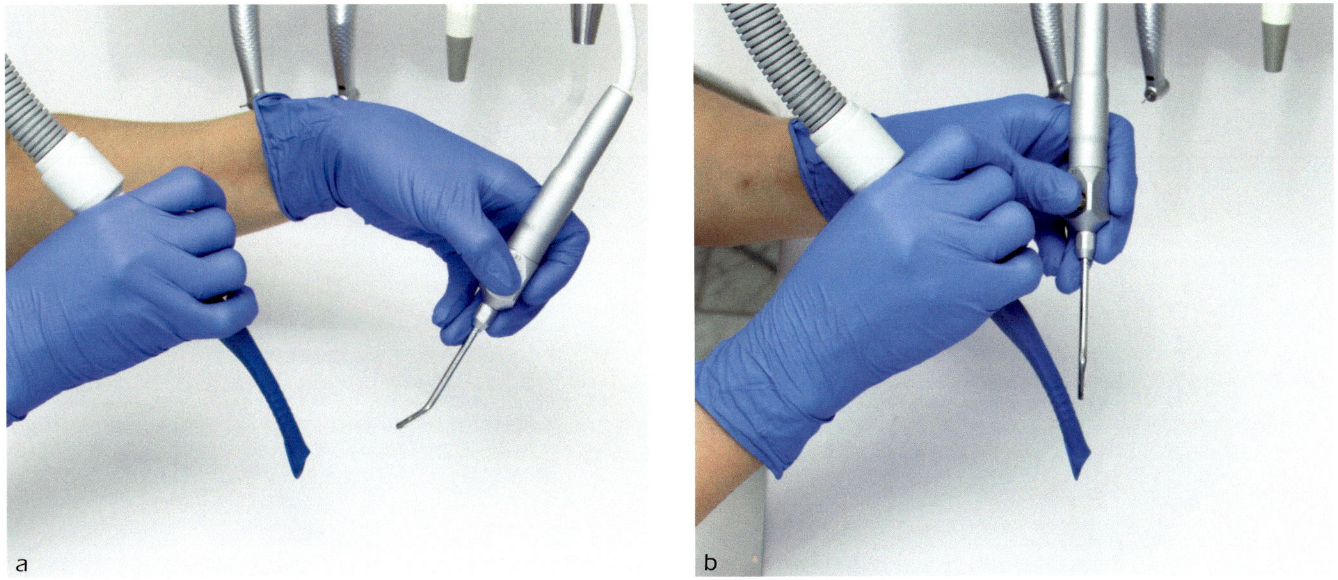

Fig 6–35 Airblow position on a mirror (a), and on a cavity (b).

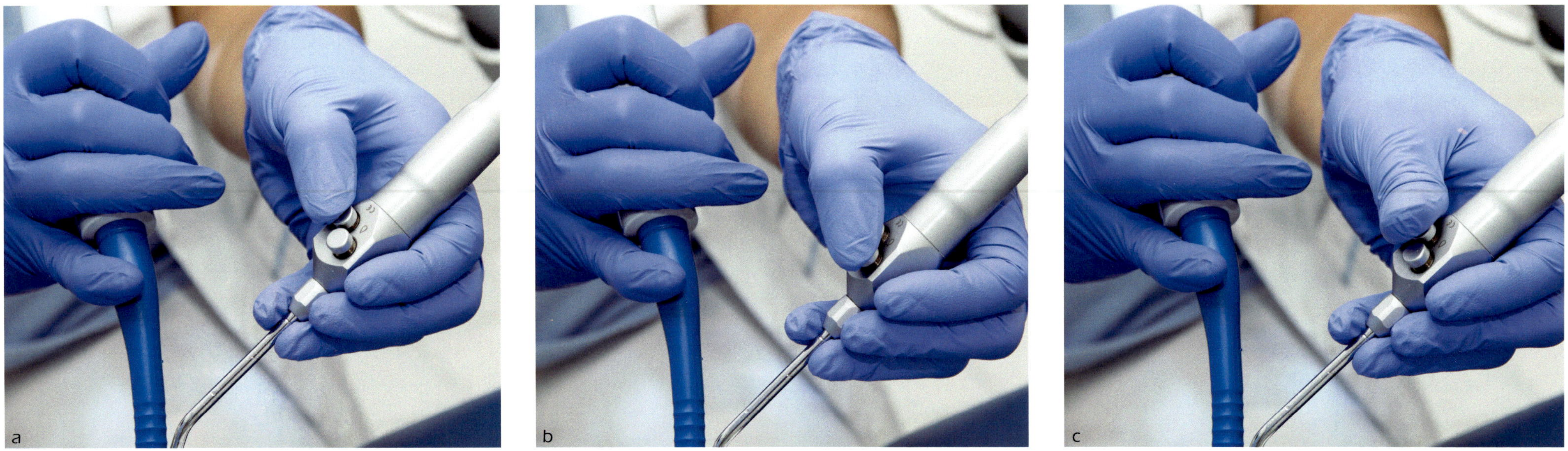

Fig 6–36 (a) Activating air. (b) Activating soft spray. (c) Activating hard spray.

RINSING THE PATIENT'S MOUTH

If performed carefully, the patient will accept a horizontal treatment position. position and refrain from rinsing her/himself at the cuspidor. By using this technique, about 1 hour a day can be saved.

Spray is used for rinsing the mouth of the patient during an examination (in case of high viscosity saliva). It is used for cleaning the patient's mouth when preparations have left debris and particles or when polishing paste has been used. The large suction tube is not used in the middle of the mouth (uvula aspiration is no fun for the patient!) but is placed often at the assistant's side of the patient's mouth. Then the 3-in-1 syringe is used from the other side for rinsing the back of the mouth towards the aspiration tube. See Fig 6–37 (a to f) for the various rinsing positions that can be used. Whole mouth rinsing (including the vestibulum) is done with coordinated movements of the large suction tube in the right hand, and a medium spray from the syringe in the left, where a careful retraction is made by the syringe or by large suction tube. The incisors are rinsed with a soft spray, in order to avoid an extaoral douche.

A careful and attentive rinsing of the mouth is made to secure the comfort of the patient in a horizontal position. The patient is informed that she/he can ask for (or give a signal to) careful rinsing when it feels right. Careful mouth rinsing when the patient needs it is very important for their comfort, and the acceptance of treatments in horizontal position. If mouth rinsing is not offered, the patient will usually like to rinse her/himself, which causes quite an interruption to the treatment and a total estimated loss of 1 hour a day. Spray from the 3-in-1 syringe may also be used during periodontal examinations in case of bleeding.

The small aspiration tube

As described above, the small aspiration tube is placed behind the last molar in order to evacuate the bottom of the mouth on a lying patient. The rinsing of the patient's mouth should be trained intensely by the assistant alone and in also when in a team. This training can be done repeatedly on a friend, family member or a paid teenager.

The dentist and assistant rinsing techniques can be seen in Figs 6–38a to 6–38f.

The rinsing is performed with coordinated movements from both dentist and assistant.

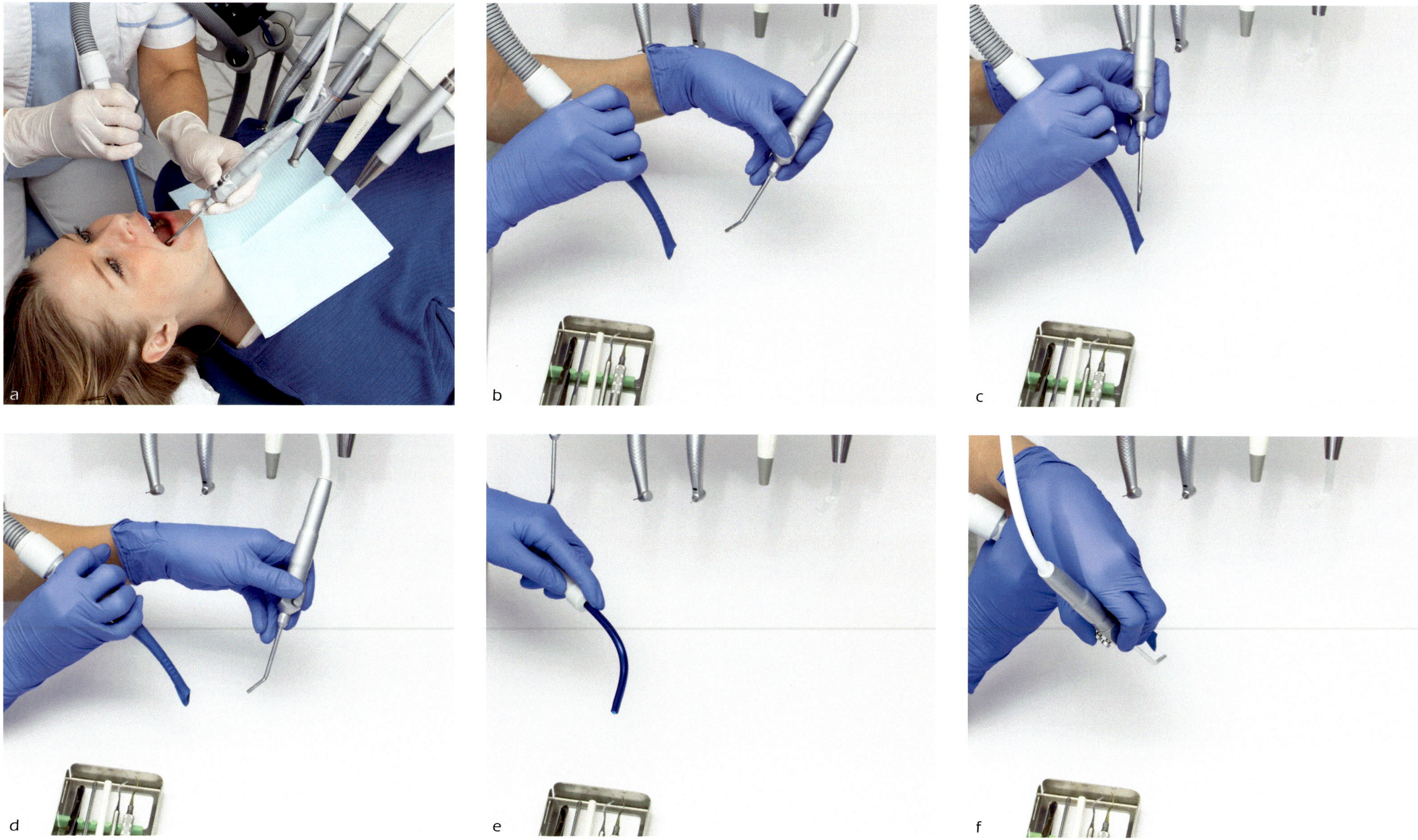

Fig 6–37 Various rinsing positions. (a) Upper left. (b) Sideways rinsing towards the upper left. (c) Inside the maxillary incisors. (d) Labially by the maxillary incisors. (e) Aspiration with small aspiration tube without tip. (f) Drying a cavity.

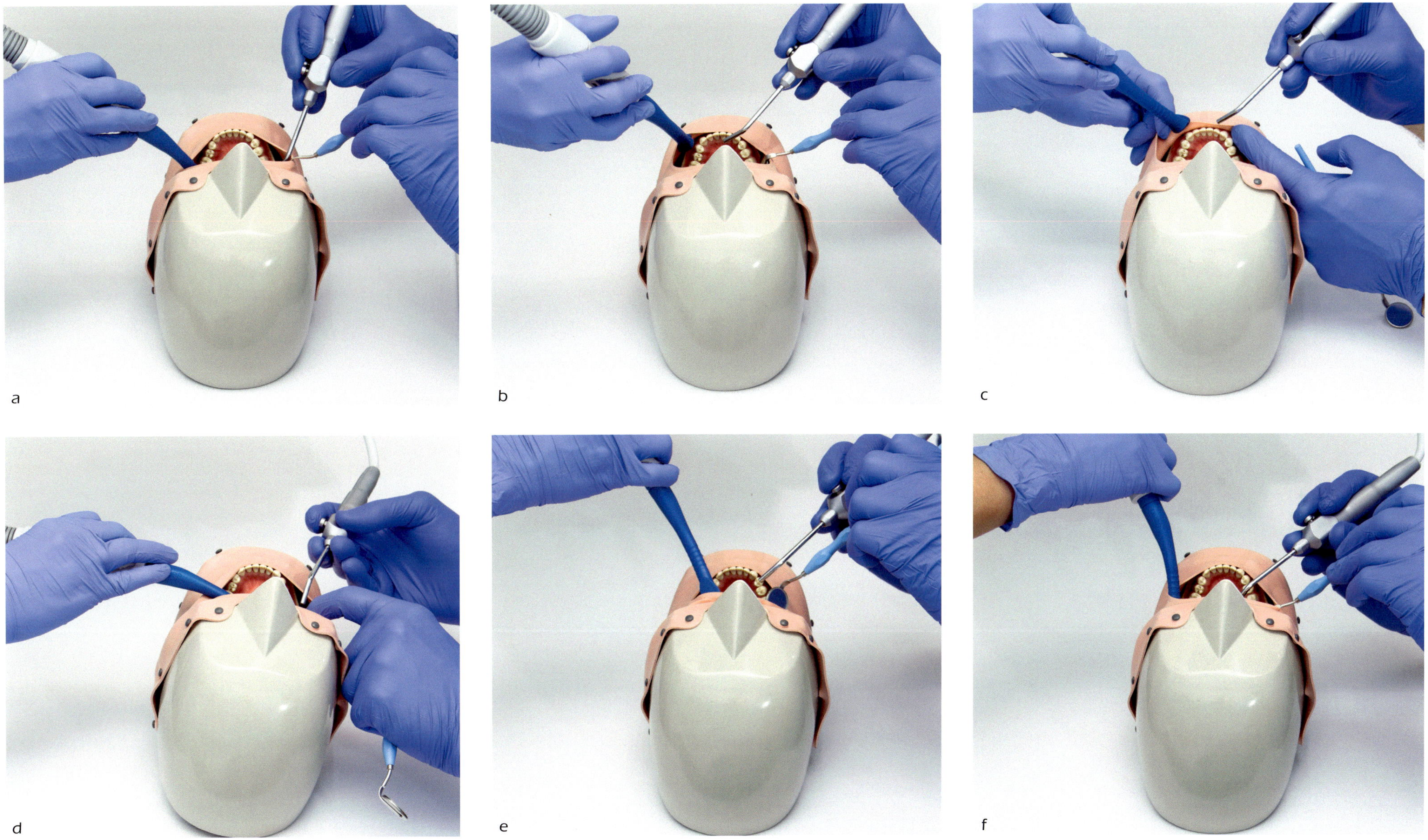

Fig 6–38 (a to f) Rinsing the mouth of the patient in different positions. The assistant retracts and aspires with a large suction tube, while the dentist rinses with a 3-in-1 syringe and retracts with a mirror for access and vision.

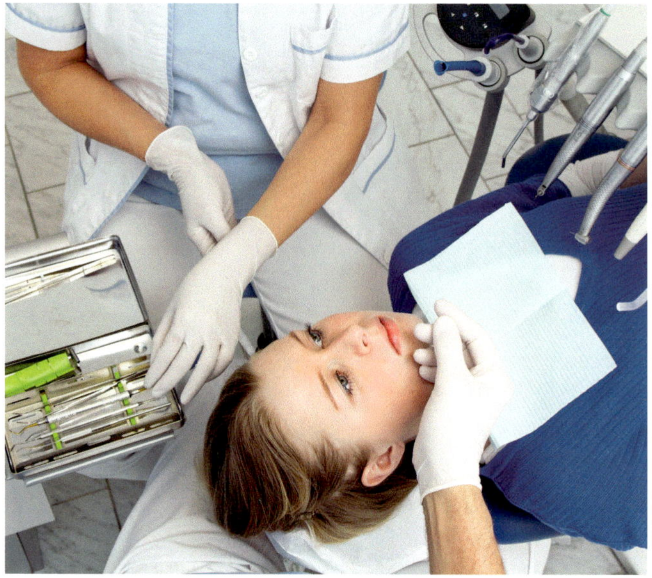

Fig 6–39 The assistant picks up a hand instrument.

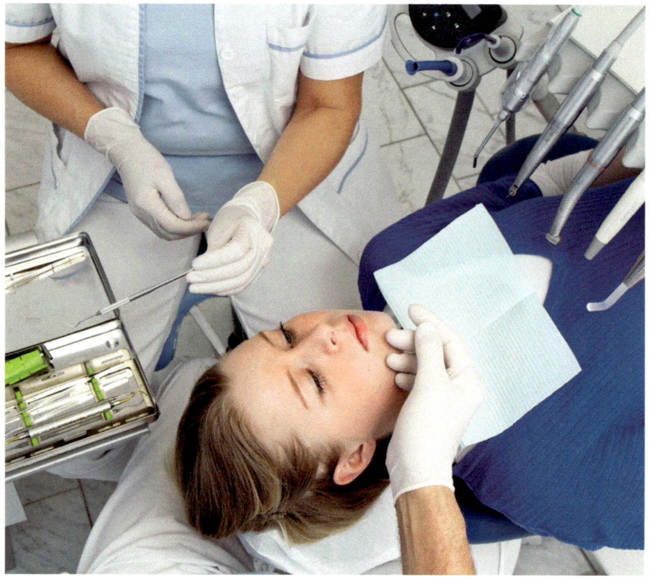

Fig 6–40 Hand instrument transfer position 1.

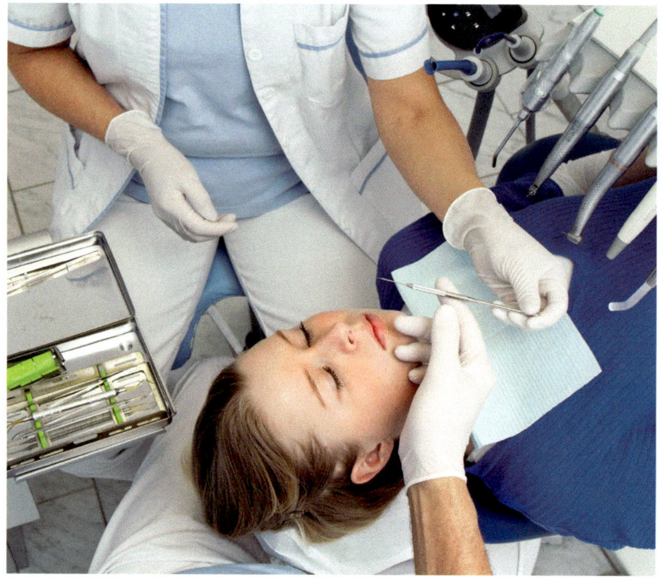

Fig 6–41 Hand instrument transfer position 2. The prepositioned instrument is now ready.

HAND INSTRUMENT TRANSFER TRAY

When transferring hand instruments (and other items) to the dentist, the assistant uses the left hand, and for the large suction tube, the right. The hand instrument transfer is done close to and in front of the patient's mouth, which only can be reached with the assistant's left hand. The assistant's right hand may be occupied with the large aspiration tube.

The hand instrument tray cannot be placed over the patient, as this is where the unit instruments are placed so they can be used both by the dentist and assistant. In addition, a hand instrument tray over the lying patient has an inconveniently high position for the assistant, unless the dentist is of shorter stature.

The conclusion (page 270) is that the hand instrument tray is placed to the upper left side of the patient. From here, the assistant picks up the hand instruments with her left hand.

Hand instrument pickup by assistant

The tray with hand instruments is placed on the hand instrument table, so the hand instruments have the same direction as the axis of the patient (Fig 6–39).

The assistant's left hand is moved to her right side with the palm of the hand downwards, and picks up the hand instrument at the closest part of the grip. The instrument must not be taken in middle of the grip, because this will hinder the transfer to the dentist's hand, and disturb their grip.

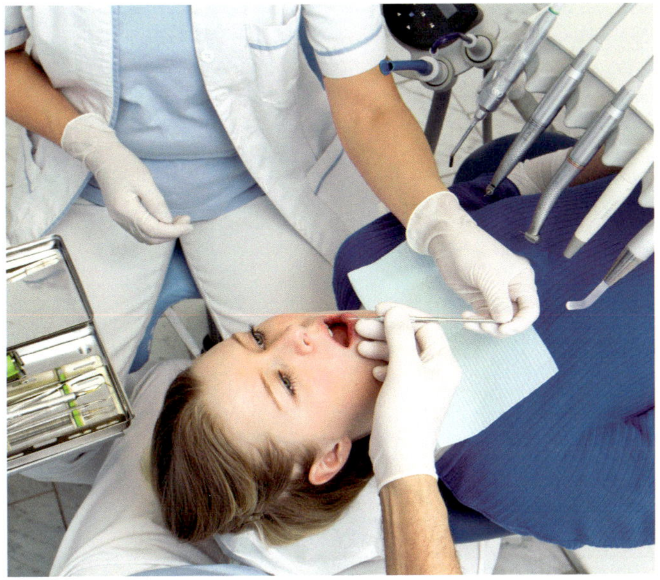

Fig 6–42 The instrument transfer is made with a little firm contact to the dentist's hand, which is now closed while applying a right positioned instrument grip.

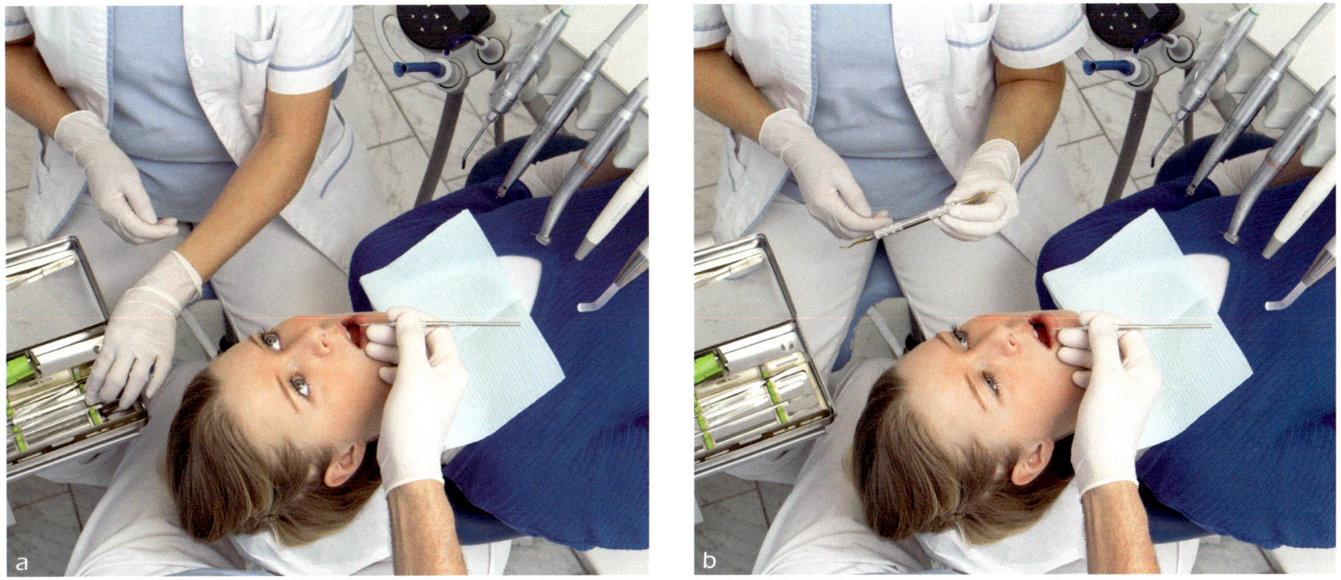

Fig 6–43 (a) The next hand instrument is grasped in the instrument tray, and (b) is carried towards the mouth of the patient.

The hand with the hand instrument is now moved to the left, and so low to the left side of the patient's head that the instrument is not visible to the patient. At the same time as this movement is being performed, the left hand of the assistant is twisted anticlockwise until the palm is directed upwards. The instrument remains almost horizontal (Fig 6–40).

During the side-movement and twisting of the left hand, the finger grip on the instrument is slightly loosened, until the instrument stays almost horizontal while the hand is twisting. It is a little difficult to follow from a textbook, but is quite easy to do after a bit of practical training.

The assistant is now ready with her prepositioned instrument (Fig 6–41). This means that the new instrument is delivered parallel to the used one, and even with the working tip in the same direction (up or down, forwards or backwards). The transfer is made so close to the patient's mouth that the dentist does not need to move the hand away from the mouth, and in many cases can maintain the finger support (Fig 6–42).

Prepositioning

Everything the assistant passes to the dentist should be prepositioned, which means it is precisely in place for the direction and position in which it is going to be used (Fig 6–43). When the dentist receives it, it is not necessarily to change the grip. This principle is used by the transfer of hand instruments, unit instrument, eg, a contra-angle on a micromotor, pellets on a pair of pliers (pincette), paper points, gutta-percha points or root files, wedges presented with pliers, mounted matrix-holders, or composite "pistols."

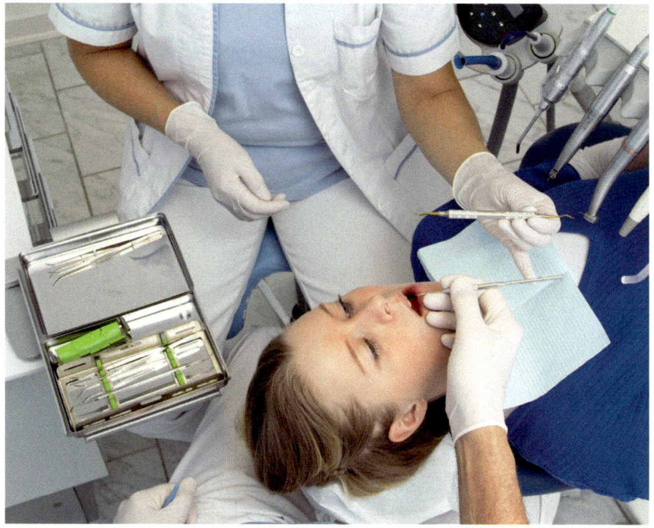

Fig 6–44 The prepositioned hand instrument ready for transfer, as the dentist makes the "shift signal."

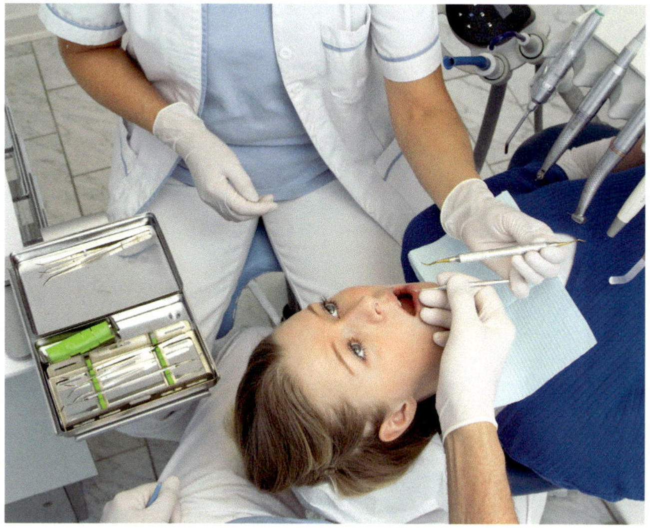

Fig 6–45 The assistant closes to the left-hand little finger around the instrument in the dentist's hand.

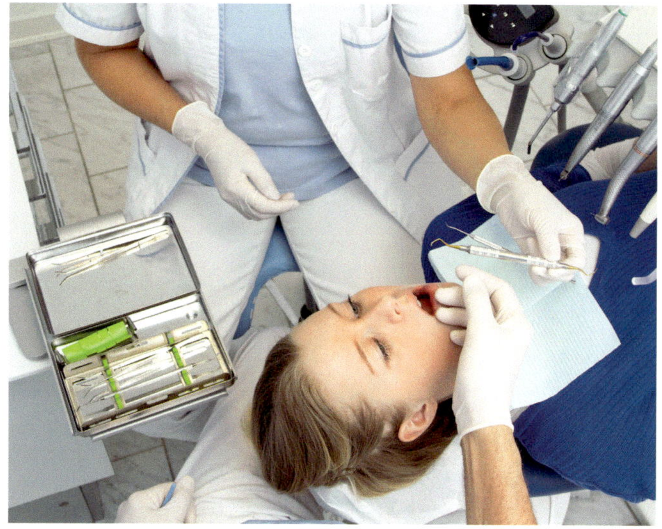

Fig 6–46 The assistant places a new instrument in the dentist's hand.

When the dentist is ready for next hand instrument, he/she moves the used instrument out so the working part is free of the mouth. This movement is done with a little marked tilt, which at the same time is the shift signal to the assistant to change to the next instrument (Fig 6–44). The support of the finger/hand of the dentist is in most cases maintained.

The assistant now takes the used instrument with her little finger (Fig 6–45).

In the same movement, she places the new instrument into the dentist's hand, ready to use (Fig 6–46). The assistant looks at where the dentist's fingers are placed on the instrument grip, and places the new instrument in the same grip position.

Now the assistant "closes" her little finger, so that the hand instrument is placed in the "security position" close to her wrist, so it does not "hang down" and touch or harm the patient (Fig 6–47). The hand instrument is now moved to the instrument tray and is placed there without being turned around.

This tray delivery needs training. For a more advanced technique, placing the thumb underneath can support the instrument, just before placing it in the tray (Figs 6–48 to 6–51).

The sequence of instruments

Protocol

To be of support to the dentist, the assistant must know what will be the next hand instrument for the dentist to use. This is noted in the protocol for the actual treatment. From frequent repetition, the protocol is learned by the assistant.

Timing = no lost time. The assistant is ready with the next instrument – according to protocol – before the moment of transfer. If the assistant cannot anticipate which instrument is going to be the next, the dentist must in due time tell which instrument is the next to be used, about 4 to 5 seconds before needing it. If the dentist forgets this, then the assistant may remind the dentist until he remembers to do so. The details in the instrument transfer must be well studied, and are proposed to be repeated under supervision 100 to 125 times the first day, and 50 times a day for the ongoing 3 to 4 days (for 5 to 10 minutes a time).

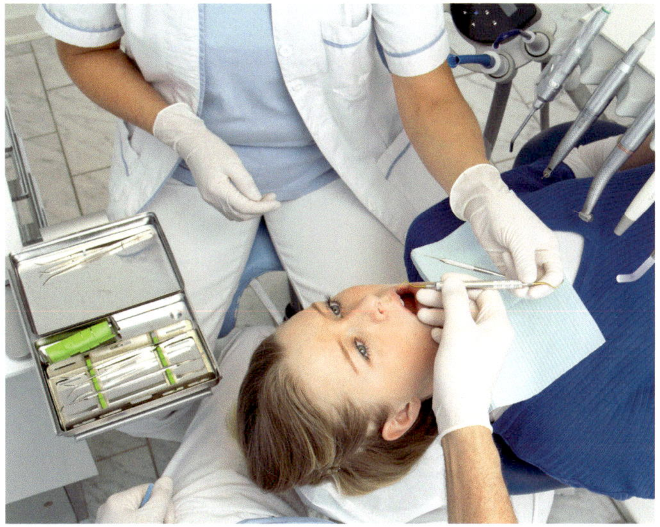

Fig 6–47 The assistant receives the hand instrument and moves it into the "security position."

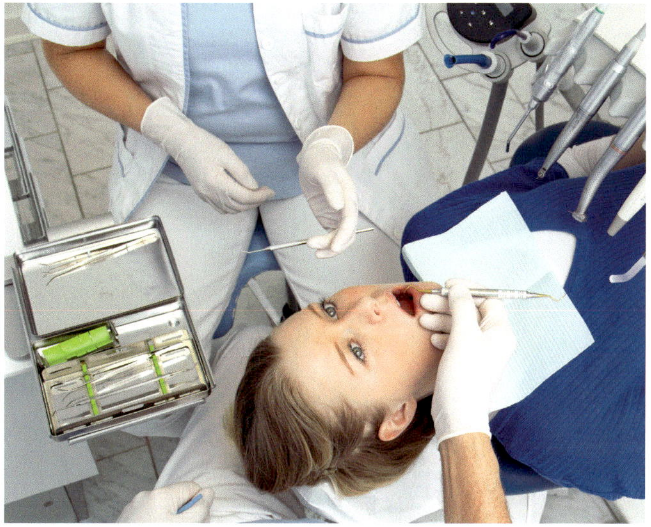

Fig 6–48 The instrument on its return, below the assistant's line of vision.

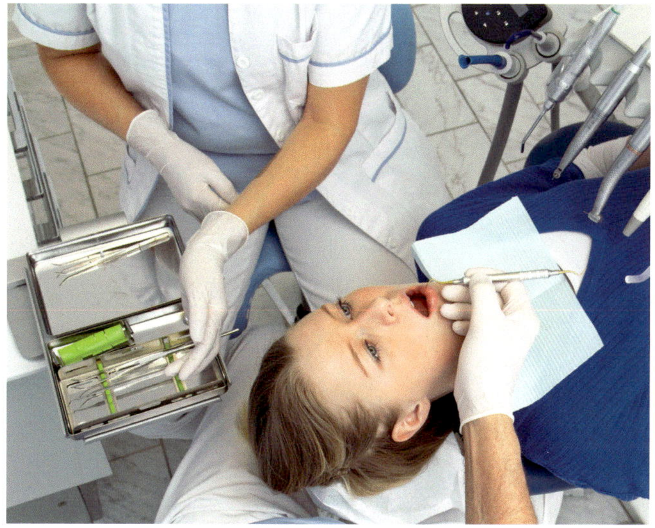

Fig 6–49 Delivery in the tray.

Instrument transfer between two hand instruments

When two hand instruments are used alternately, they are not placed back in the tray, but instead are kept in the hand with a modified transfer, which is quite easy to learn (see Figs 6–52 to 6–56).

Instrument transfer between hand instrument and unit instrument

When hand and unit instruments are used alternately, they are not placed back in the tray (as above), but are kept in hand with a modified transfer, which is quite easy to learn (Figs 6–57 to 6–60).

This protocol is valuable and used very frequently, eg, for excavating caries using a round bur for exca-

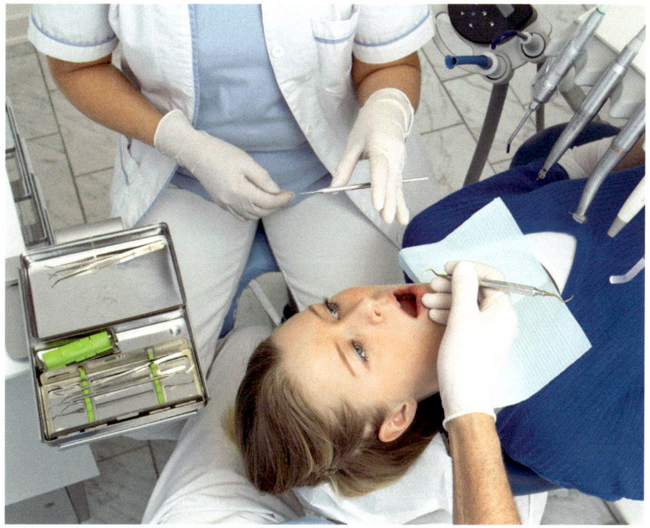

Fig 6–50 When trained, the assistant can place the thumb so it supports the instrument grip from underneath, while carrying the hand instrument towards the tray.

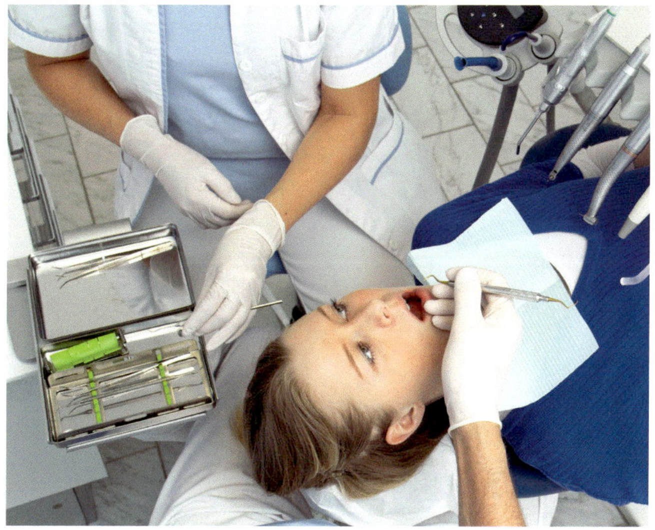

Fig 6–51 This grip faciliates a precise placement of the instrument in the tray.

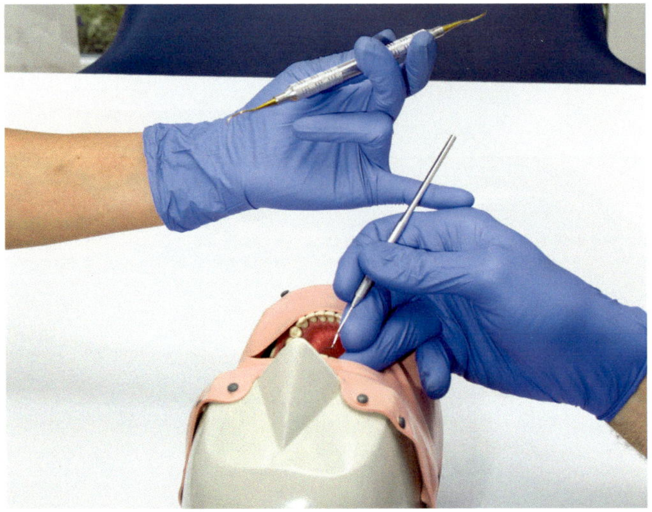

Fig 6–52 The assistant is ready for the next instrument; the little finger is open.

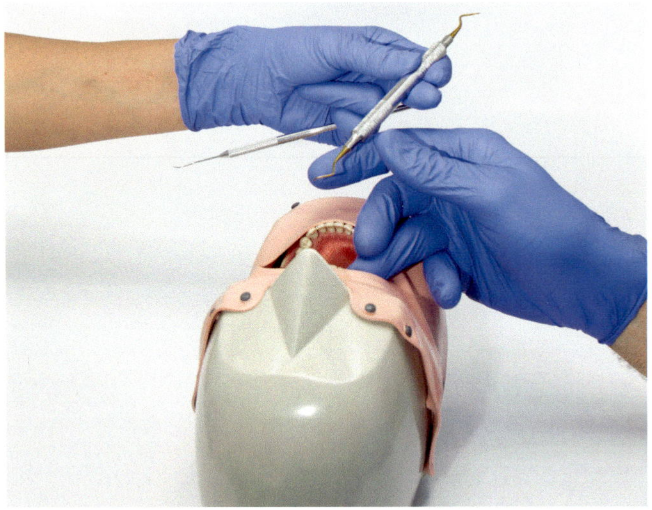

Fig 6–53 The assistant takes the used instrument.

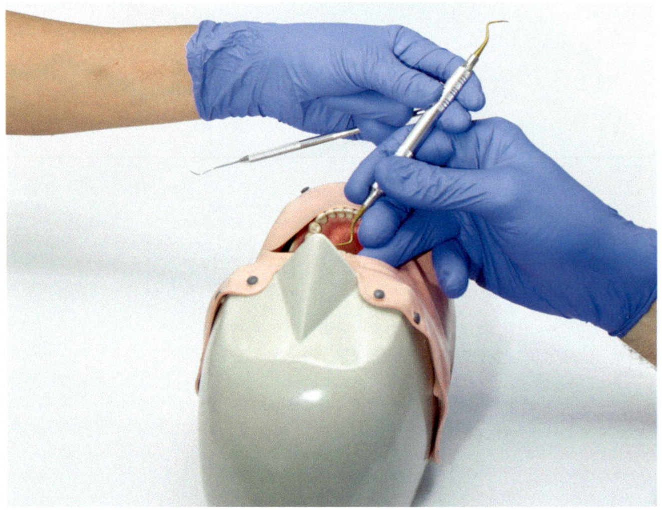

Fig 6–54 The assistant transfers the new instrument, and places the used instrument in the "security position."

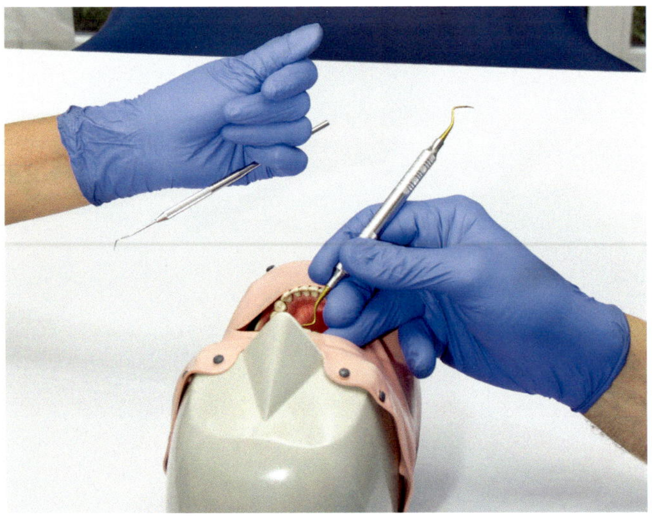

Fig 6–55 The already-used instruments are held by the assistant's little finger; the dentist uses the hand instrument.

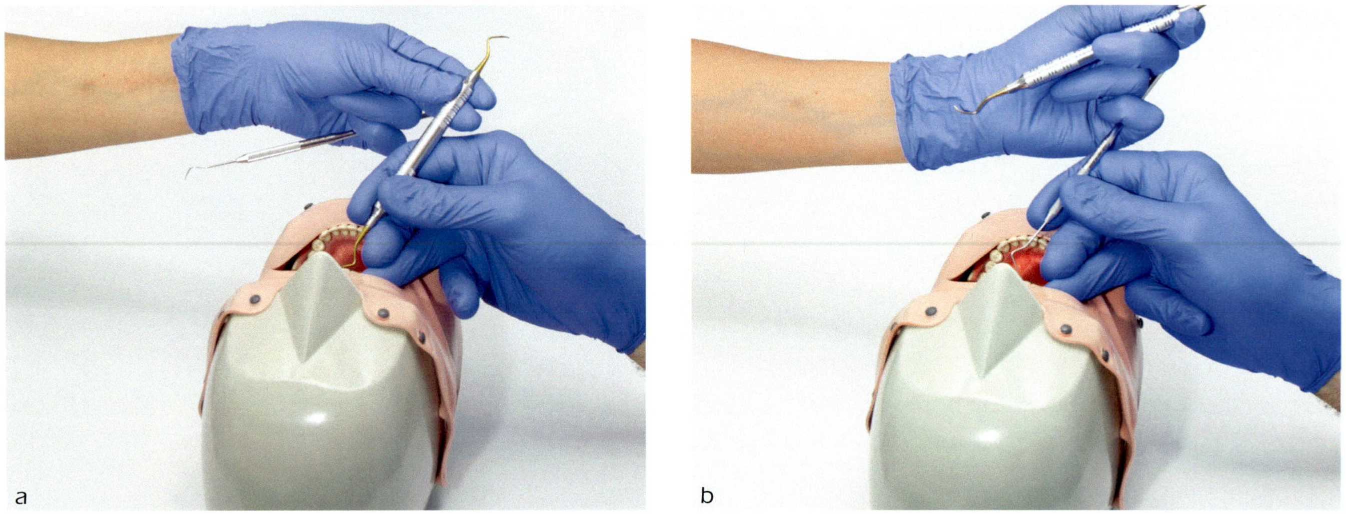

a b

Fig 6–56 (a) The assistant takes the used instrument between the index finger and thumb. (b) The assistant transfers the new instrument supported by her little finger to the dentist.

vation and a probe for control – or for a contra-angle with a flame-shaped diamond for correcting approximal margins, with a probe for control.

Instrument transfer between hand instruments and 3-in-1 syringe

When a 3-in-1 syringe and hand instruments are used alternately, the hand or unit instruments are not placed back in the tray, but are kept in the hand with a modified transfer, which is quite easy to learn (Figs 6–61 to 6–63).

Instrument transfer between two unit instruments

When two unit instruments are used alternately, again the hand instruments are not returned to the tray, but are kept in the hand with a modified transfer, which is quite easy to learn (Figs 6–64 to 6–66).

Working with a unit instrument with spray, drying mirror, drying cavity, transferring to probe and back to unit instrument

This is high-end assistance, but it is not as difficult as it looks. This protocol provides perfect efficiency in a procedure with the alternating excavation of caries and examination of the cavity with a probe. The dentist is working in the maxillary jaw with mirror and spray. The mirror must therefore be kept dry by the 3-in-1 syringe. The assistant holds the probe at the same time, with the left hand little finger.

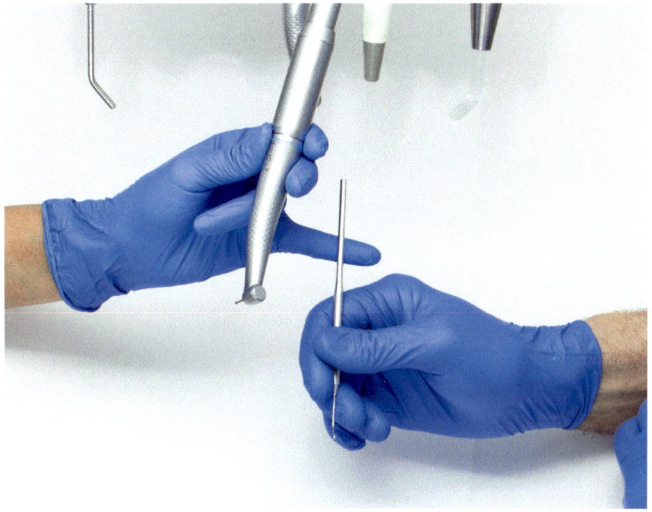

Fig 6–57 The assistant is ready with the unit instruments; the little finger is open.

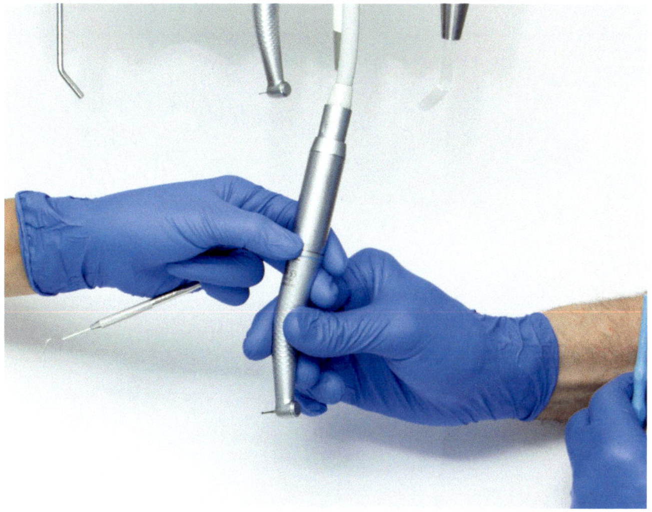

Fig 6–58 The assistant takes the used instrument, which is kept in the security position to avoid touching the patient, and transfers the new unit instrument to the dentist.

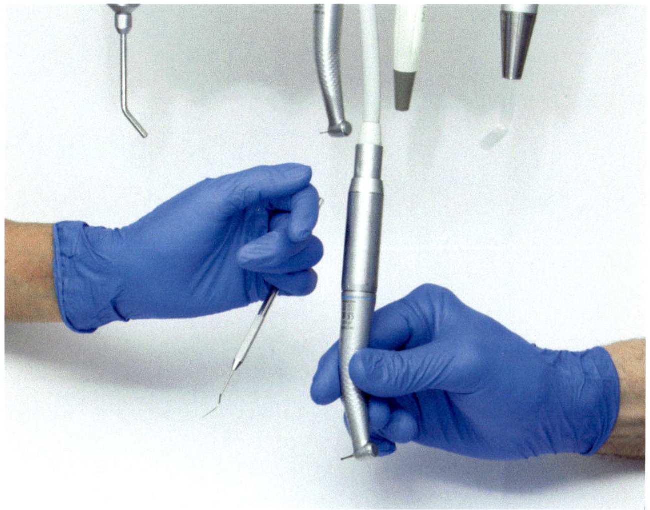

Fig 6–59 The already-used instruments are held on the assistant's little finger; the dentist is using the unit instrument.

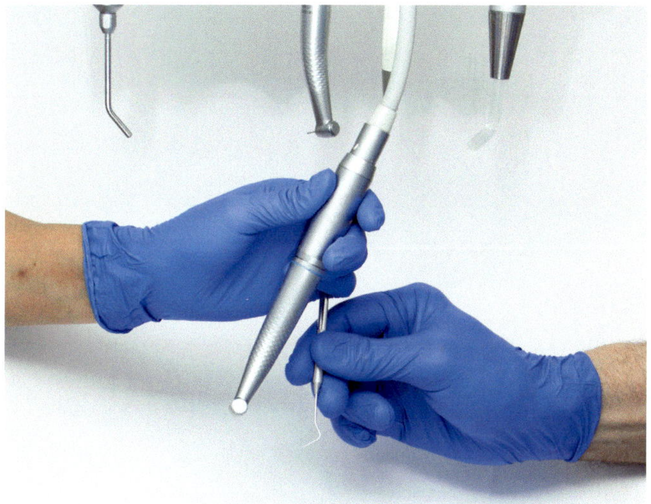

Fig 6–60 The assistant takes the unit instrument with the index finger and thumb, transferring the hand instrument with the "little finger position" to the dentist.

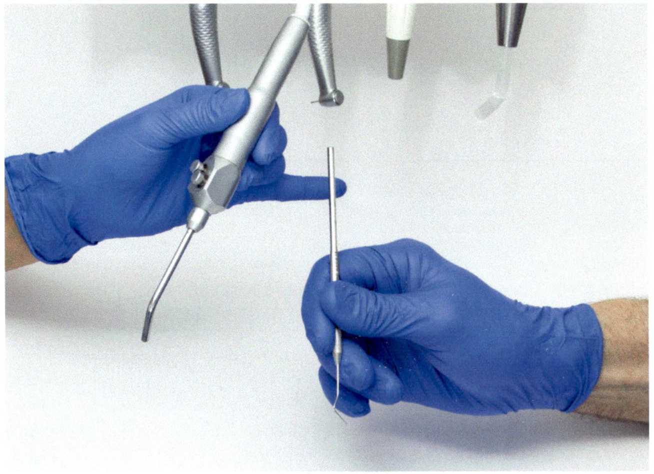

Fig 6–61 The assistant is ready for the next instrument with the little finger open.

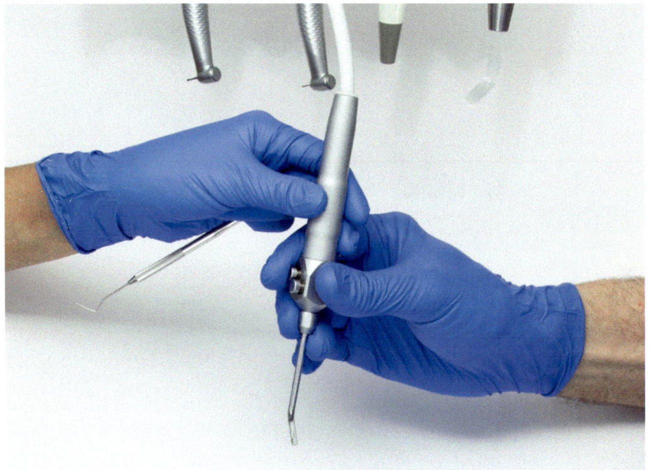

Fig 6–62 The assistant takes the used instrument in the "security position" and transfers the 3-in-1 syringe to the dentist.

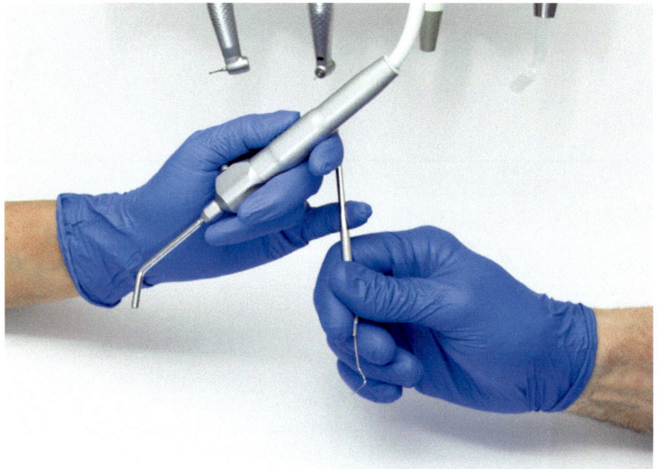

Fig 6–63 When the dentist has used the 3-in-1 syringe, the assistant takes the unit instrument with the index and thumb, then transfers the hand instruments to the dentist from the little finger position.

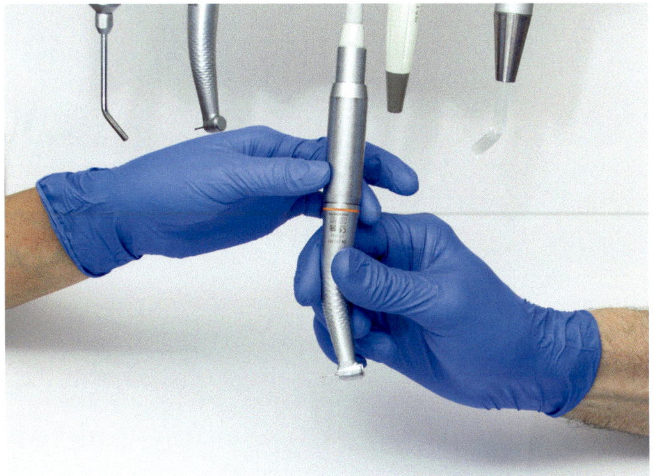

Fig 6–64 The assistant transfers the unit instrument back to the dentist. The assistant is ready with the next unit instrument with an open little finger.

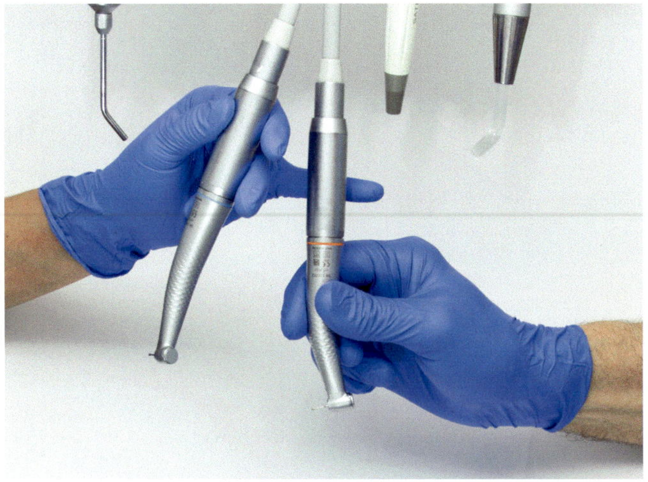

Fig 6–65 The assistant has the next instrument ready, while taking the used one.

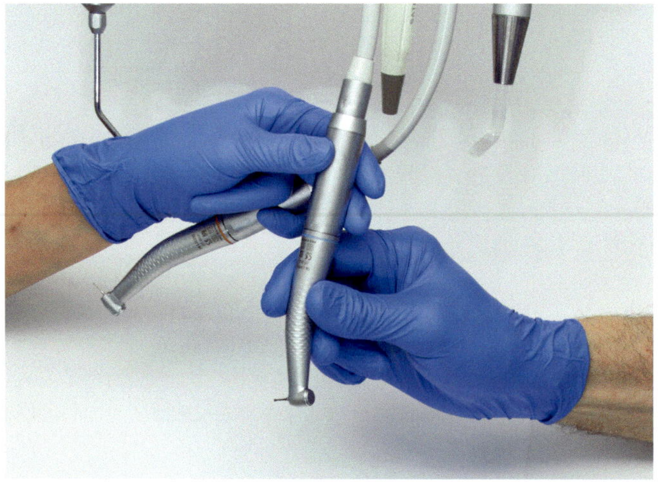

Fig 6–66 The assistant transfers the next unit instrument to the dentist using the "security position."

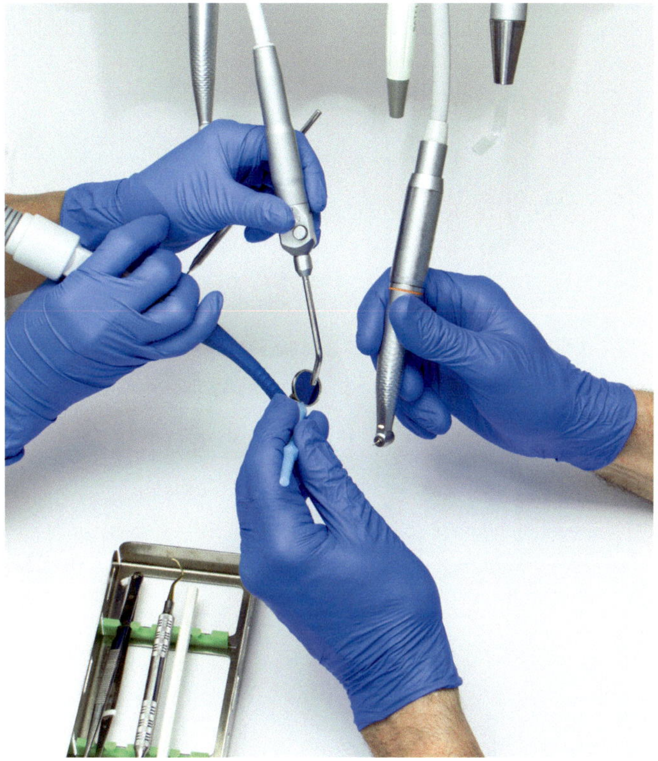

Fig 6–67 The assistant uses a large aspiration tube for retraction; the small aspiration tube is in the retromolar area on the opposite side. The dentist is working with a mounted contra-angle and a mirror, which the assistant dries while holding a probe in the left hand little finger.

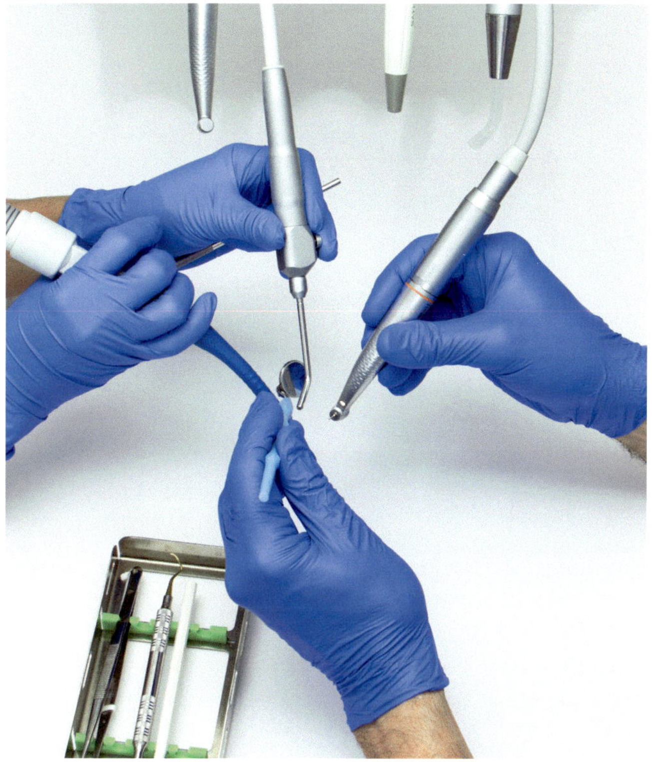

Fig 6–68 The assistant uses a large aspiration tube for retraction, while the dentist uses the unit instrument. If the unit does not have an automatic chip blow feature, the assistant dries the cavity with shaking movements and afterwards returns the syringe to the unit position.

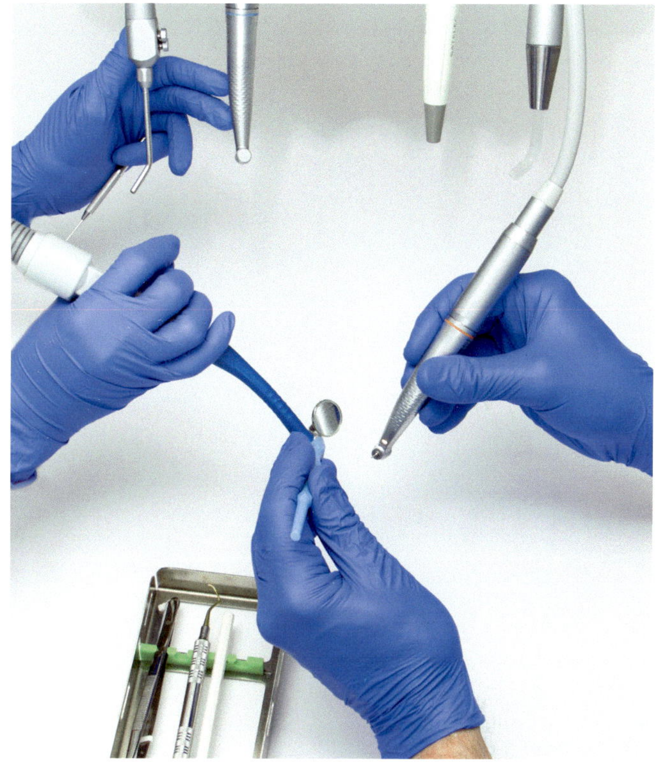

Fig 6–69 The assistant continues to use a large aspiration tube for retraction; the 3-in-1 syringe is placed back on the unit.

In this case, the dental unit does not have an automatic chip blow to dry the cavity after the unit instrument is stopped. Therefore, the assistant has to dry the cavity with "shaking vibrations and maximum air," just after the unit instrument is finished with.

Now the 3-in-1 syringe is placed back on the dental unit support, and the assistant takes the dentist's unit instruments with the left hand, and transfers the probe instead (for the entire procedure, see Figs 6–67 to 6–75).

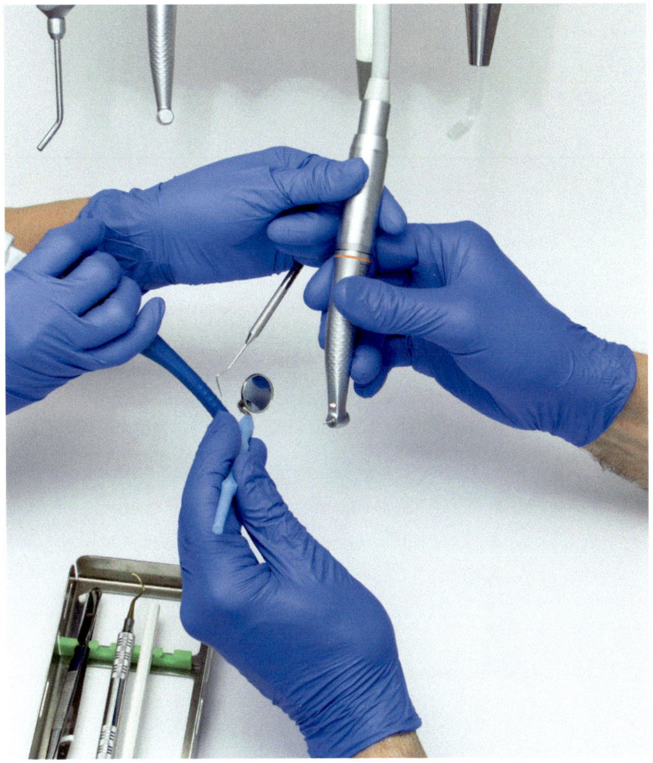

Fig 6–70 The large aspiration tube is used for retraction by the assistant, while taking the micromotor with mounted contra-angle with the left index and thumb.

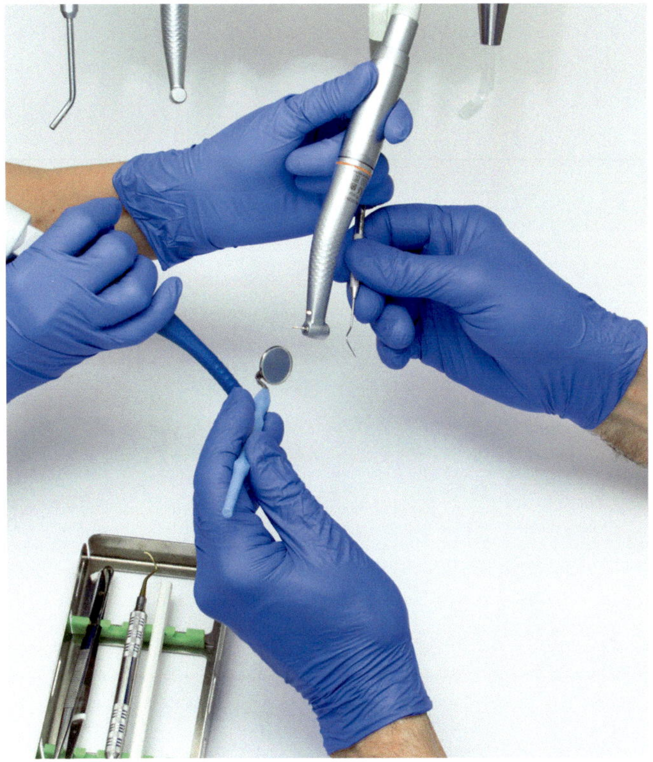

Fig 6–71 The assistant uses a large aspiration tube, while the unit instrument is moved using the "security position" at the same time as the probe is moved to the dentist from the little finger position.

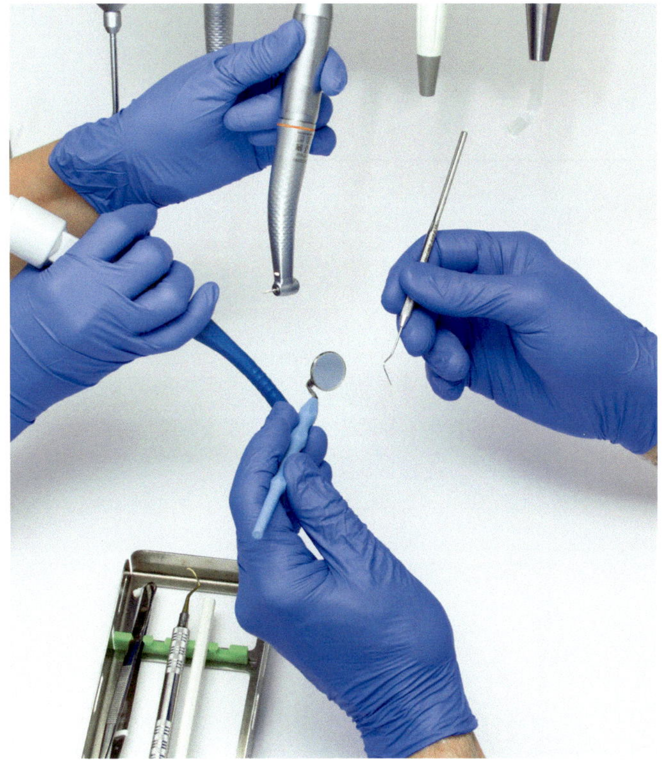

Fig 6–72 The assistant uses the large aspiration tube for retraction while the dentist uses a probe. She is ready to take the probe again and replace it with the contra-angle.

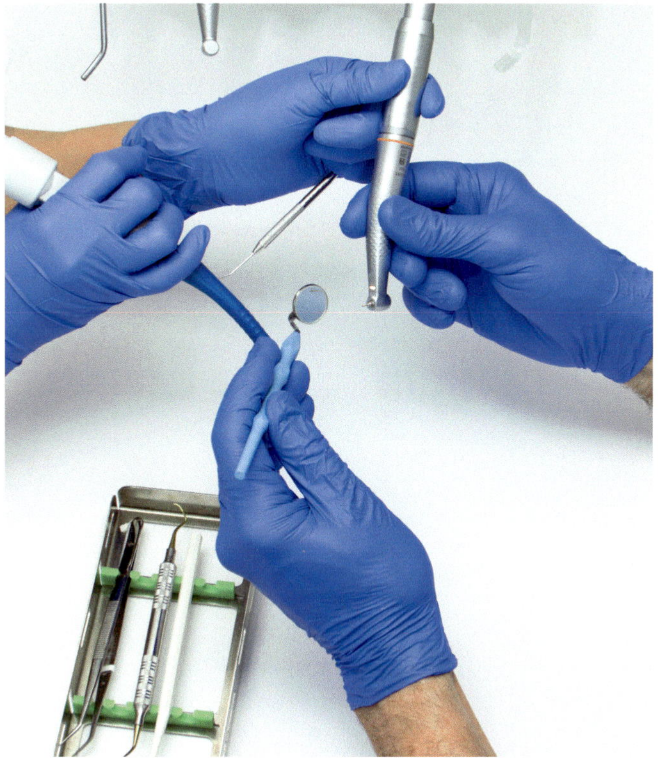

Fig 6–73 The assistant replaces the contra-angle on the micromotor.

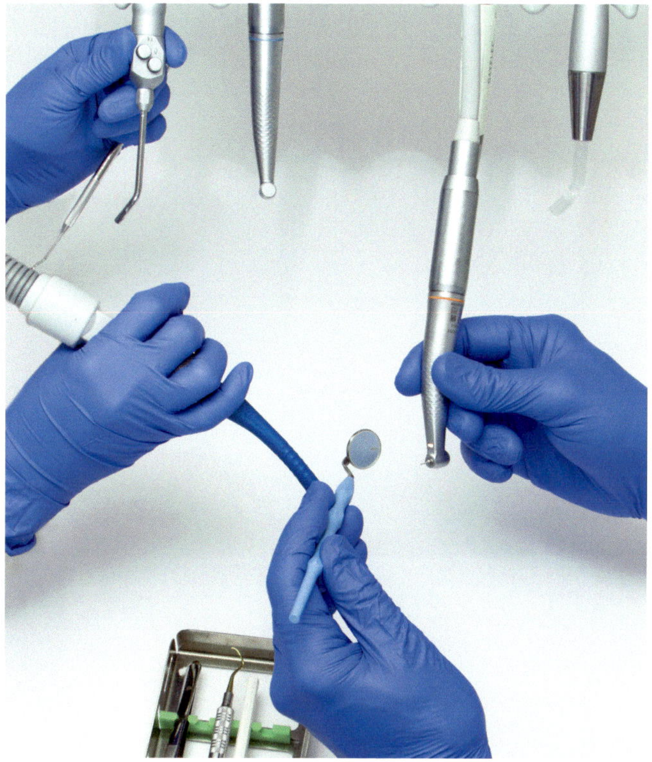

Fig 6–74 The assistant keeps the probe on the little finger and takes the 3-in-1 syringe.

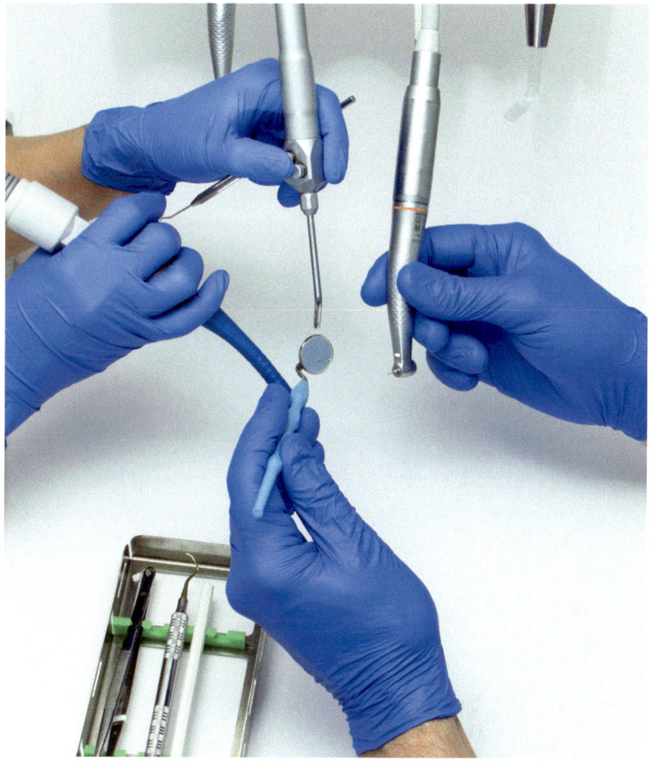

Fig 6–75 Blowing the mirror dry.

Changing burs, diamonds, and polishers

When preparing for a treatment, the assistant mounts the diamonds and burs on the contra-angles according to the protocol for the actual treatment.

During the treatment, the assistant may find time to change burs, diamonds, or polishers for later use. However, if an immediate change has to be done, Figs 6–76 to 6–78 describe a proposal.

The dentist checks the burs are correctly mounted, and work is continued.

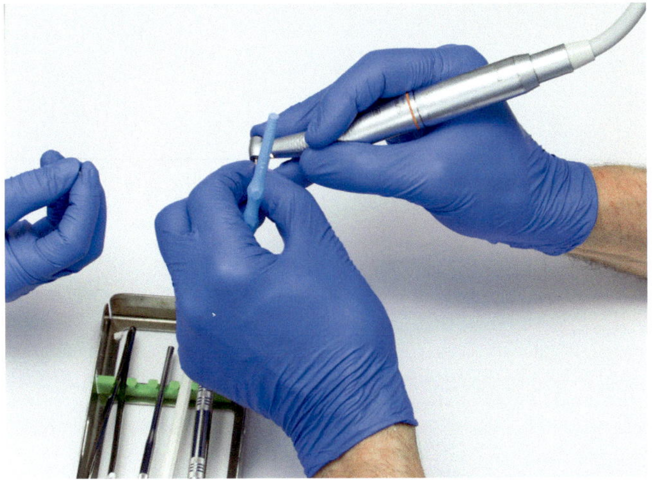

Fig 6–76 The assistant is ready with a new bur, while the dentist transfers the used bur with the left hand.

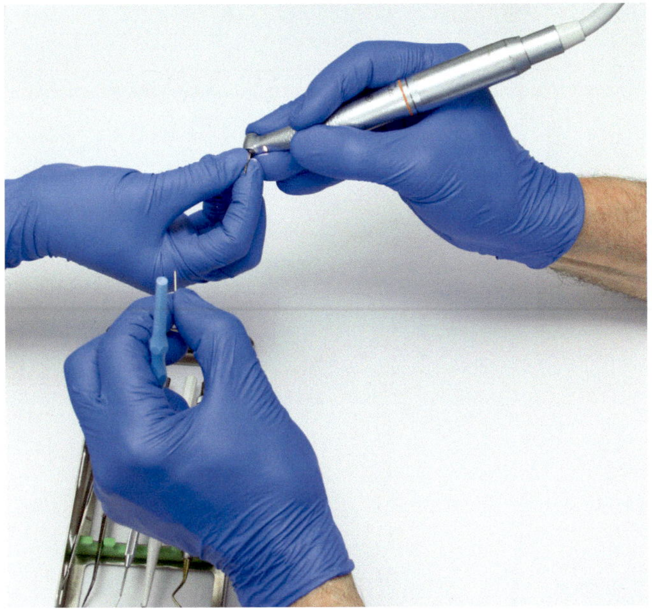

Fig 6–77 The assistant places a new bur in the contra-angle, while the dentist passes her the used bur.

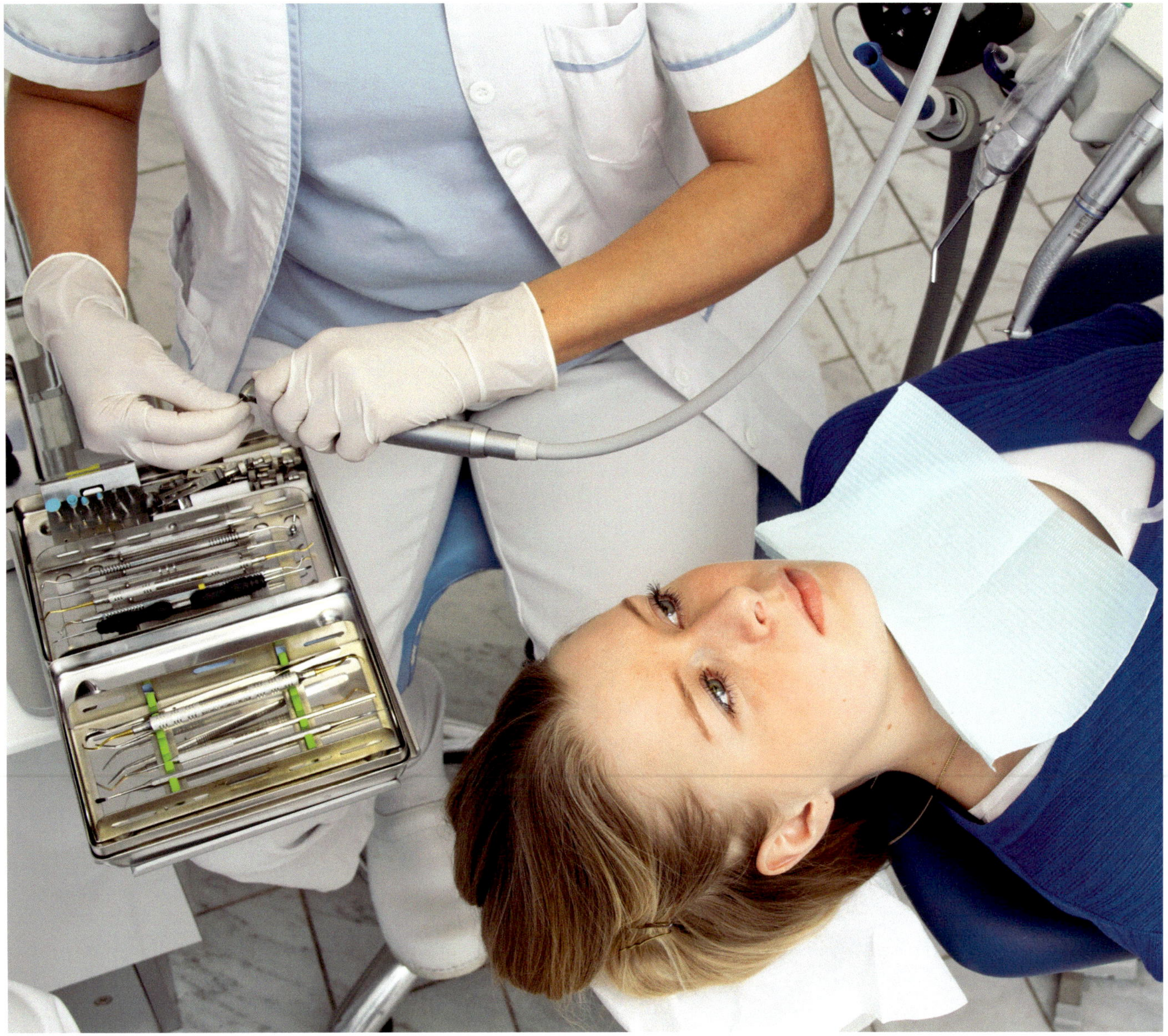

Fig 6–78 The assistant changes the burs and diamonds herself.

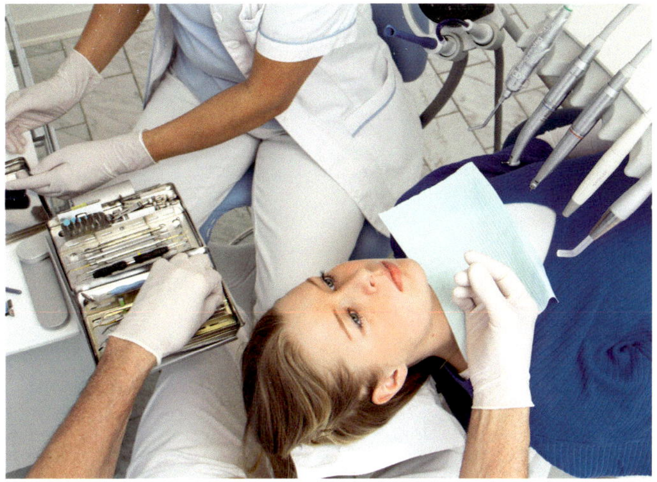

Fig 6–79 The dentist takes the hand instrument with the left hand at the right end of the hand instrument grip, using the left thumb and the index finger.

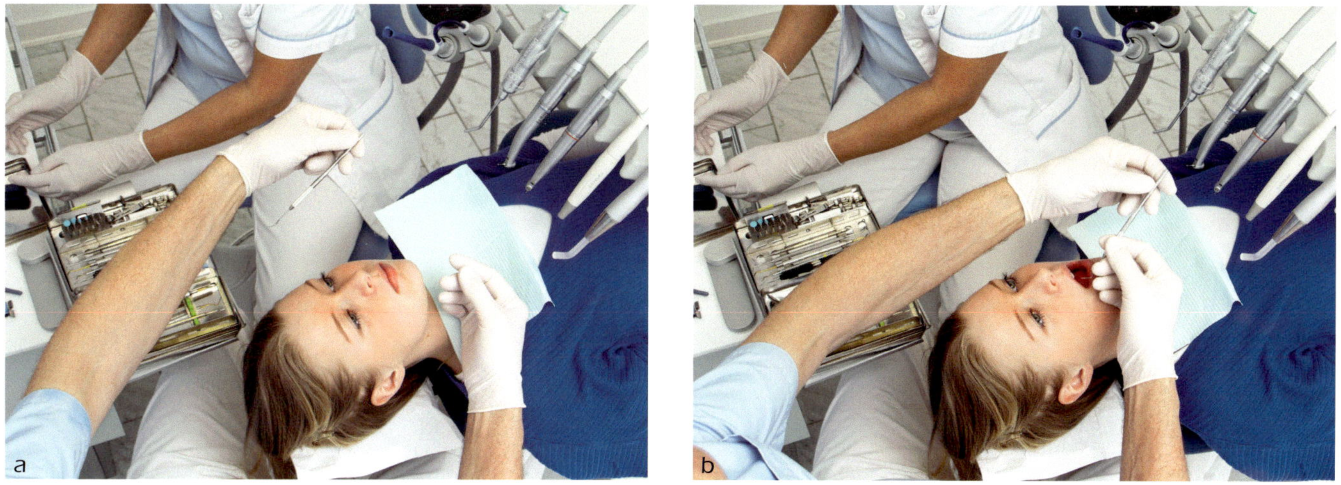

Fig 6–80 (a and b) The instrument is transferred.

WHAT HAPPENS IF THE ASSISTANT IS OCCUPIED?

SOLO left–right hand instrument transfer

The hand instruments can easily be taken by the dentist themselves. It is a matter of training, just like everything else in this book. A well-trained instrument change takes about 1 second.

The hand instrument is picked up with the dentist's left hand as shown in Fig 6–79, and is transferred in a low curve so the patient cannot see the instrument. The instrument is transferred (Fig 6–80), with the hand twisted a little so the palm is moved upwards (Fig 6–81). Note that it is the left hand's middle finger that is receiving the used instrument (Figs 6–82 and 6–83).

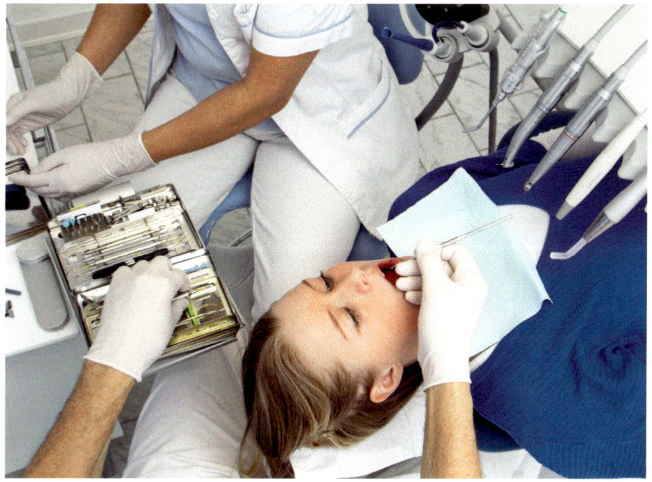

Fig 6–81 For transfer of the next instrument, the hand is twisted a little so that the palm is moved upwards. The instruments are kept parallel, and the middle finger is ready for receiving the used instrument.

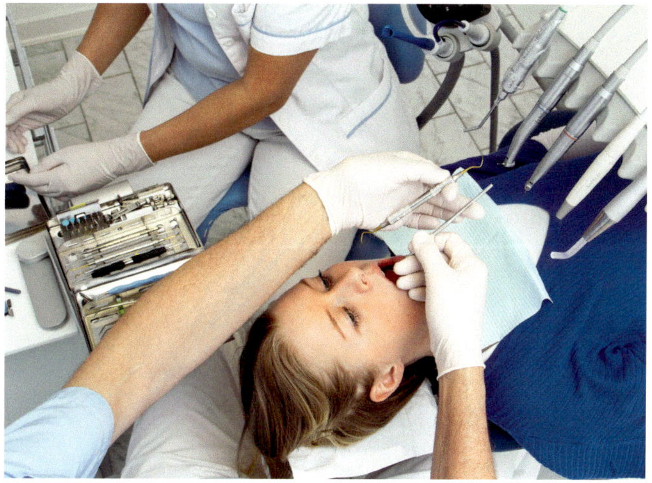

Fig 6–82 The used instrument is taken with the left hand's middle finger.

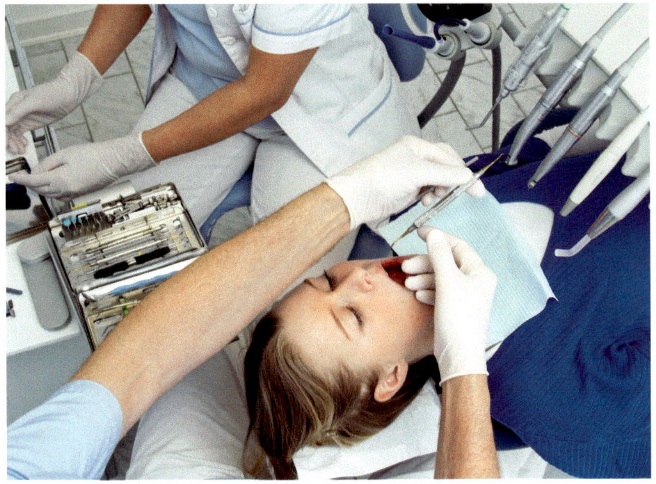

Fig 6–83 The new instrument is placed in the right hand, ready for use.

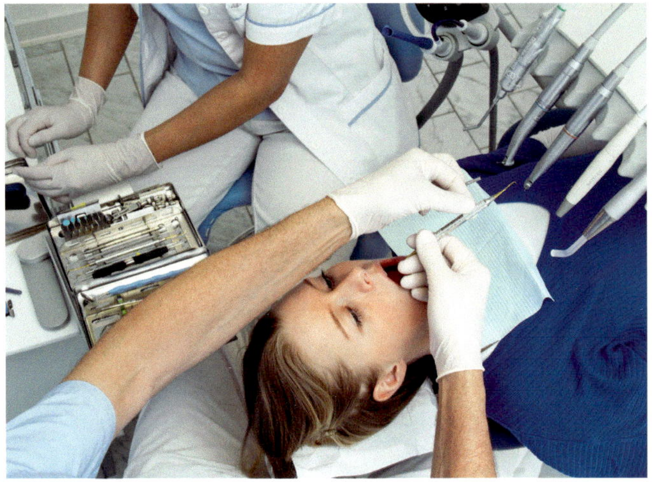

Fig 6–84 The instrument is transferred to the left.

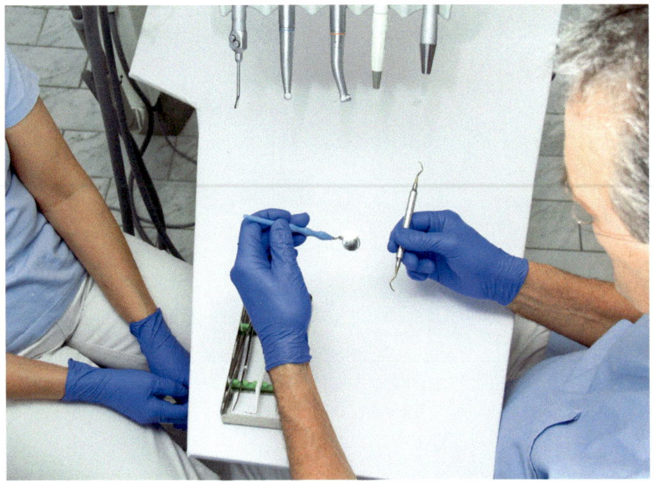

Fig 6–85 The mirror and hand instrument in action.

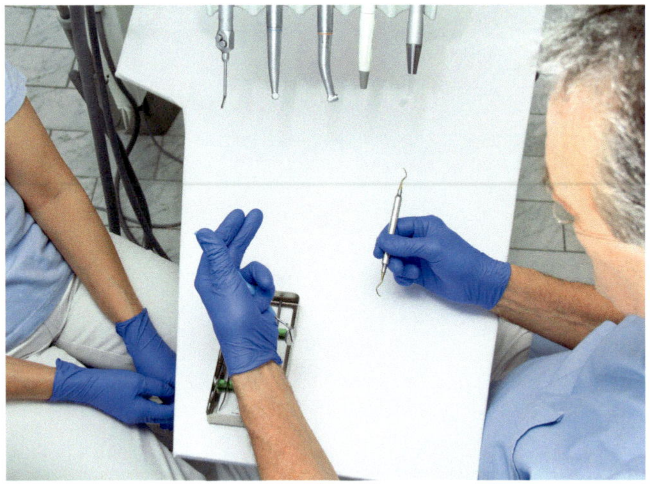

Fig 6–86 The mirror is kept in a resting position, supported by the left hand ring and little fingers.

The used instrument is transferred left to the tray without being turned around (Fig 6–84). See Figs 6–85 to 6–92 to see the procedure done with a mirror.

It is in most cases necessary to "study" the illustrations a few minutes before practicing the technique, and you have to repeat it about 100 times to get the routine before patient treatment. A well-practiced left–right hand instrument change takes less than 1 second.

For further high end teamwork and assistance applied by:

- Composite (page 195)
- Amalgam (page 202)
- Crown and bridge procedures (page 206)
- Endodontics (page 208)
- Scaling and polishing (page 215).

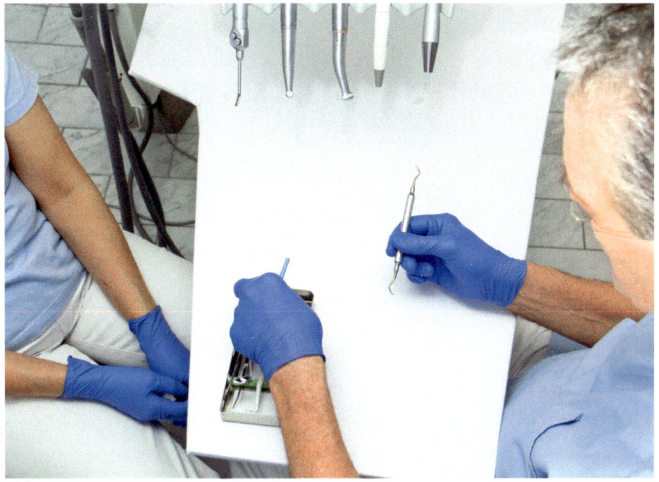

Fig 6–87 Picking up the next instrument from the tray.

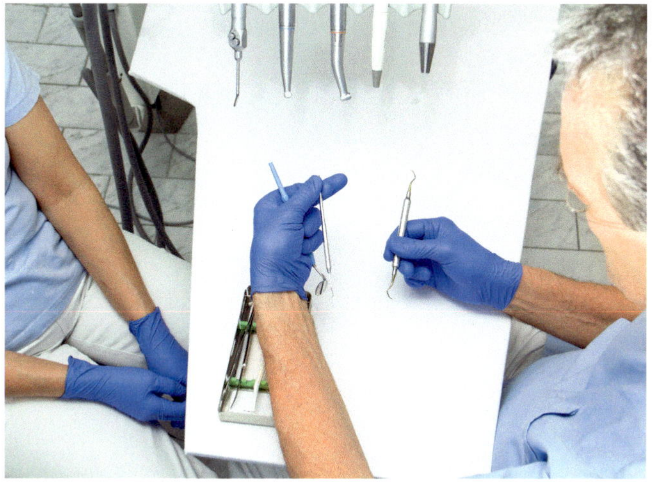

Fig 6–88 The middle finger is ready for changing the next instrument.

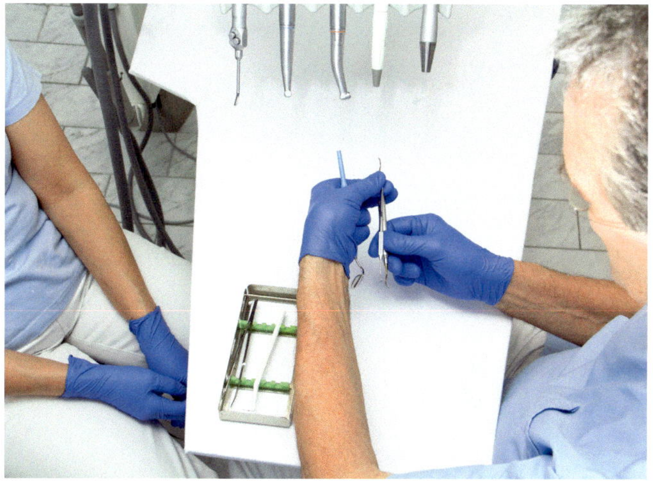

Fig 6–89 The instrument change is performed.

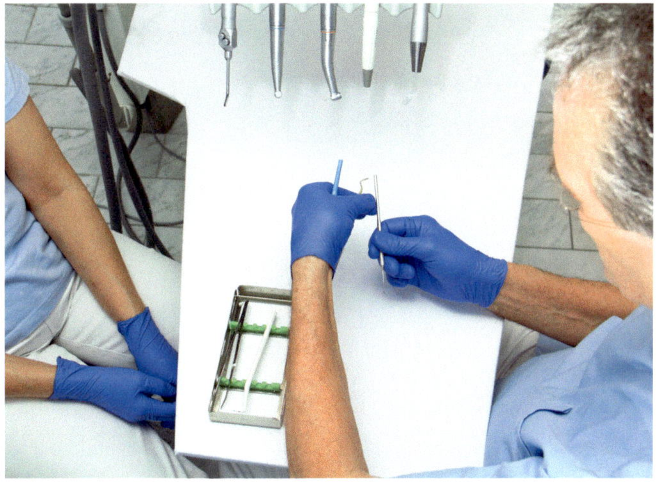

Fig 6–90 The instrument change is finished.

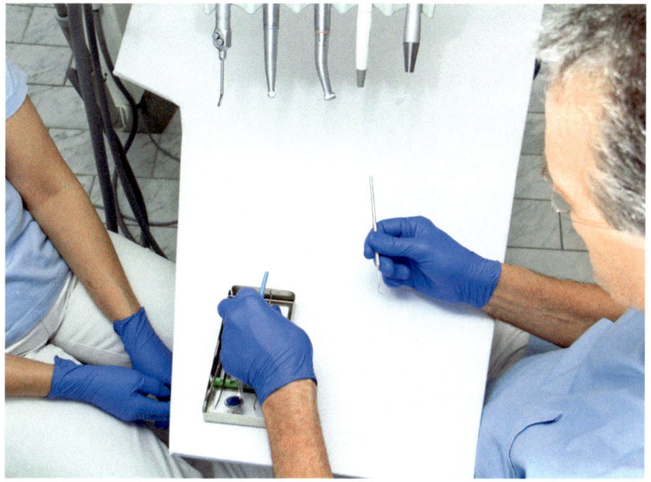

Fig 6–91 Transporting the used instrument back to the tray.

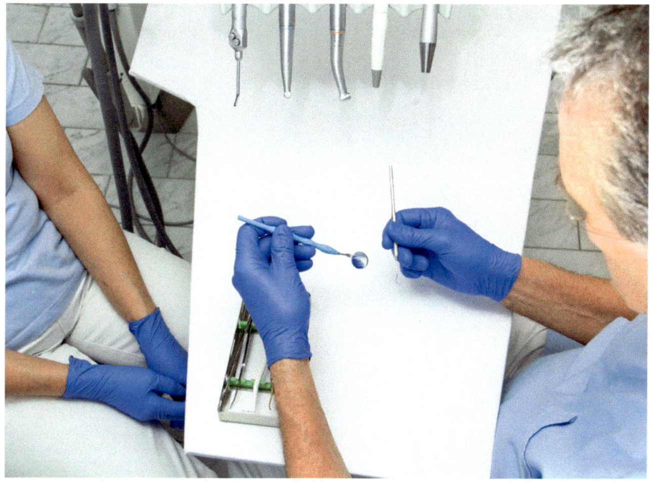

Fig 6–92 The mirror's transition from the resting to working position.

THE ASSISTANT'S TRAINING PROGRAM

The assistant's skills for aspiration, retraction, rinsing and the different four-handed techniques are all trained by repetition of the movement sequence. The number of repetitions differs but in most cases, a count of 100 to 200 times per skill applies. The training is performed during simulated treatment situations, either with a phantom head or by a volunteer "patient," where no real treatment is made.

The time for basic training of the skills is several hours (yes that is correct!). In hands-on training courses, 1 day of training for high-end assistance and teamwork is sufficient for to take all skills into use the next day.

When the skills are well-trained, one does not need to think any more about it. Being guided by protocols while working means that the assistant can predict each step for a work procedure, and is informed some seconds beforehand if the dentist wants to deviate from the protocols.

The assistant can survey the protocols in use and support the dentist by proposals for the next step, before the dentist has thought about it. The assistant's supervision of the protocols for both parties can be an important element in the quality supervision of the dental practice. This is an important upgrading of the assistant's role and activities.

THE DENTIST'S EXPERIENCE

The hands are dancing when all elements play together:

- Perfect vision in fine working postures.
- Trained hands of dentist to achieve fine working postures, precision work and simplification of movements.
- Protocol-guided work – so the major part of the time the work is performed "automatically."
- Protocols are a quality security system.
- Unit instruments, suction holder and the hand instrument tray support four-handed dentistry.
- Four-handed skills are perfectly trained.
- The dentist can maintain undisturbed concentration without the needing to look away or reach.

The principles above make the dentist's work much more relaxing. Concentration can be maintained. The eyes can be kept on the task as long as needed and as long as it is convenient. The hands stay by the patient's mouth and in accordance with the protocol for the hand and unit instruments, and the materials are placed in the hand of the dentist ready for immediate use. The dentist's job is much more relaxing, much less tiring, and takes less, or much less time to do.

Chapter 7

THE PATIENT EXPERIENCE

A CARING APPROACH

Patients are often anxious and very sensitive when in the treatment room. A comforting and caring environment are very important, as the patient is also a sensitive observer of your practice.

SOFT OR HARD HANDS

Touching another person is an intense communication that creates strong emotions. Touching in the facial region is normally restricted to family or those closest to us, and is not accepted outside this situation.

When the dentist touches the patient for an examination or treatment, as well as being a clinical necessity this is at the same time a communication, and a very intensive one at that to a patient who can often be anxious and very sensitive. The face, lips, mouth and tongue are the most sensitive parts of our body, so we have to bear this in mind.

We touch the patient in order to support our hands, and in order to retract soft tissues to enable visual inspection of an actual tooth, or surface of a tooth.

The touch

The first touch conveys an emotional message. Let's imagine the patient is now ready for examination or treatment. If the first touch for extracting the lips or cheeks is made with a sudden retracting movement, the patient may experience this as unpleasant or dominant. In interviews, patients have described this encounter as the dentist having "a hard hand."

Therefore it is important to be very attentive to the emotional values connected to the touching involved in dental treatment. The patient needs a bit of a time in order to feel used to the contact (eg, for a treatment) in order to accept it.

Soft touching

After a light initial touch, a little 0.7-second delay is made. The patient will feel the contact and now has time to both feel the contact and to accept it. After this minipause, the movement is continued, fulfilling the objective as support for fingers, retraction, etc.

Examples:

- *Adjustment of head of the patient.* A slight soft touch with the hand on the cheek, before guiding the patient's head into position.
- *Retraction of cheek.* A soft touch with suction tube before starting retraction.
- *Hand support for dentist.* A soft touch before the final support position is established.

When working, the dentist's hands are securely and stably supported, and the patient feels distinct and precise micromovements that convey the feeling of every movement being conscious and planned. The patient feels the assistant's supporting attention, gently keeping the lips, cheek or tongue away.

FACE-TO-FACE DISTANCE

Around us we have a personal territory, through which only closest relatives may pass. The radius of this varies between different cultures, and may be around 50 to 60 cm.

As a stranger, should you pass the boundary of a person's personal territory, it is often perceived as an aggressive or dominant action and can create strong emotions. This is why the dentist must take care. As dentists, we are moving "head and hands" wide into the patient's personal territory and must therefore be aware of the patient's emotions in order to prepare them, look friendly and be kind. Protocol-guided, highly trained teamwork enables the dentist to maintain relaxed concentration. Solutions to potential "problems" are presented, often before the problems are perceived.

When the dentist and assistant are working in a well-trained team, with supportive teamwork and a four-handed dentistry, the patient is an observer the whole time. When anxious, the patient is often very sensitive and all senses are "open." The patient will see the dentist's face very closely and right before their eyes (approx 35 cm distance). The patient will see the dentist's head in a state of relaxed concentration, keeping the eyes on the task in the mouth of the patient without having to look or move away.

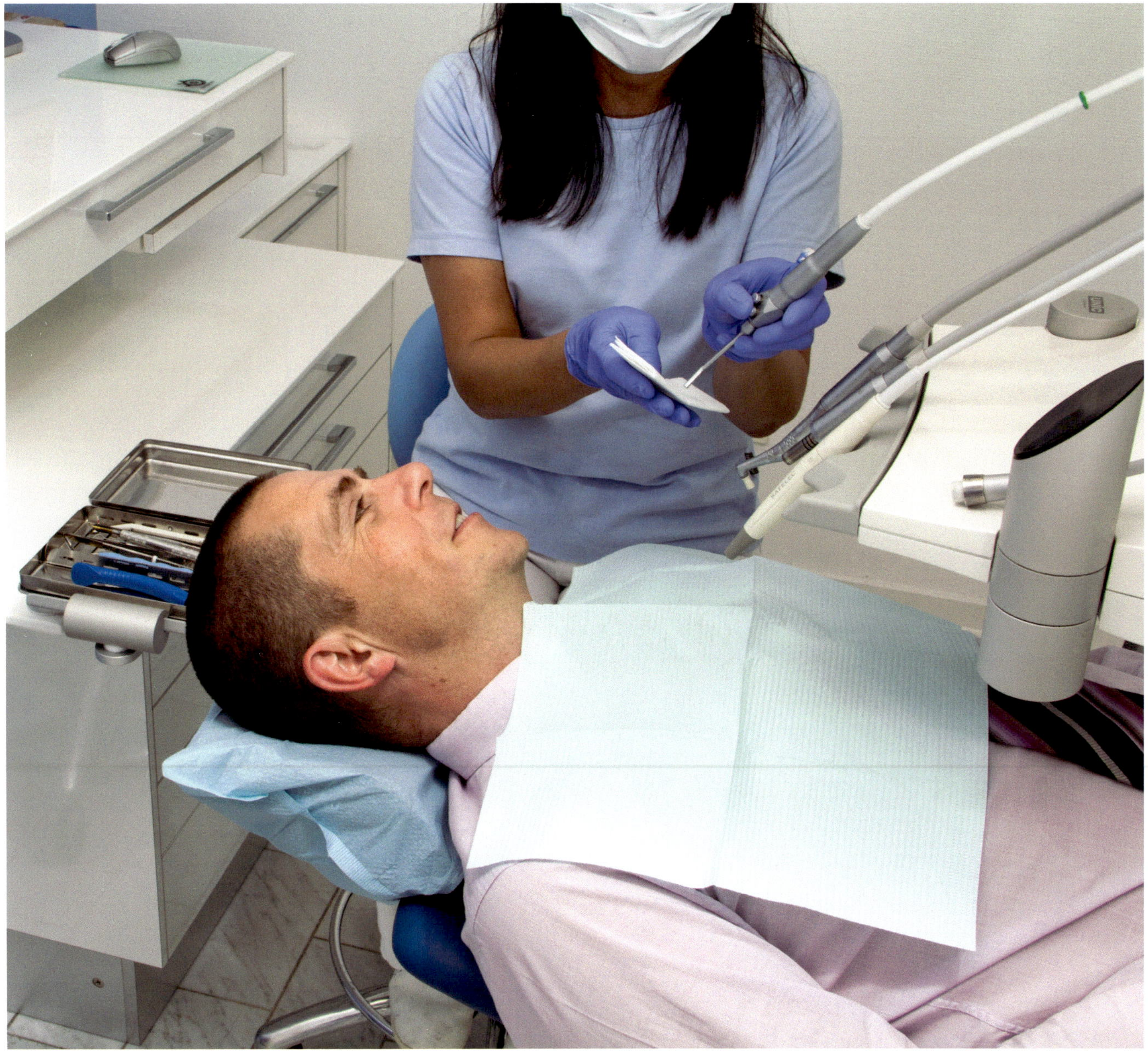

Fig 7–1 A serviette is wetted.

The dentist's face

The dentist face should look as presentable as possible and well groomed, with the knowledge that the patients will see the neck and face of dentist from below. Discrete makeup for female dentists is recommended. In patient interviews, it is often commented that male dentists should particularly take a little more extra care.

Patients have suggested the use of a nose hair cutter and cutting the hair in the ears, adjustment of the eyebrows, daily shaving (especially on neck) and sometimes the "deep cleaning" of skin. The smell associated with smoking is unpleasant for a large number of non-smokers.

The dentist's face-to-face distance

Over time, becoming used to the close proximity of patients' faces can cause the dentist to become desensitized to the emotional impact of this close contact. Both dentist and assistant should be aware of this. At such a short distance, a friendly and caring facial expression is much appreciated by the patient.

AMBIENCE

The patients are also very sensitive to the relationship between dentist and assistant. Their pleasant interaction is very important for the patient's experience. When working with well-trained protocol-guided teamwork, the number of the small requests from the dentist of "give me this or that" is very much reduced, and is replaced by "automatism." This confirms the impression of competence by the team and creates a relaxed atmosphere. Although the hands are working fast, precise, well planned and coordinated, the relationship between the dentist and assistant is relaxed. A friendly, warm interaction is experienced as being very positive by the patients.

A satisfied exit

A serviette with an impermeable back protects the patient's clothes. The dentist has another small serviette placed on top of this. It is used for cleaning water from the patient's skin, or for cleaning the mirror (Fig 7–1).

When the treatment is finished, the patient's mouth is carefully rinsed with spray and a large suction tip. The objective is to offer comfort and care for the patient. The rinsing ensures that no blood is left in the mouth, which can later color the cuspidor rinsing water. The assistant has a small serviette slightly wetted with water for a careful cleaning of the lips and mouth surroundings. This is the last soft touch and if done carefully, the patients will appreciate it and feel good as a result. Or for example, you might use an attractive blue water cup and an extra serviette, which the patients will appreciate and comment on (Fig 7–2).

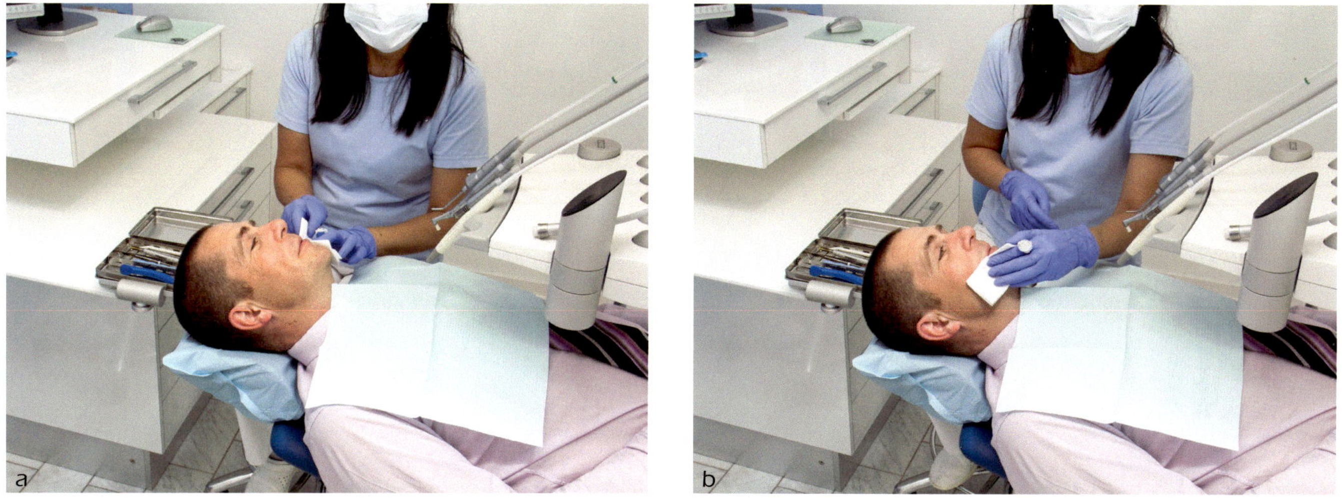

Fig 7–2 (a and b) Careful cleaning of the patient afterwards.

One could also use a mini-towel heated in a microwave oven, as per business class flights. Some practices have also placed a little cleansing cream with attractive scent on the serviette, knowing that scents influence feelings.

When the patient has rinsed, they will leave the practice sensing the scent. In particular, men have said that this exit service is a nice touch.

Chapter 8

THE WORKSTATION

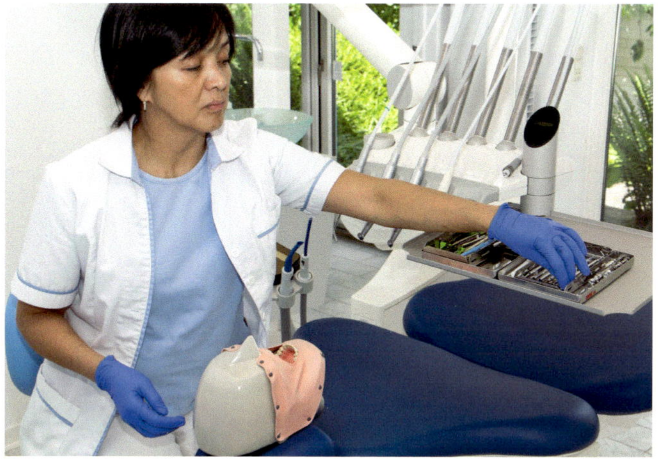

Fig 8–1 Assistant tries to take a hand instrument from a hand instrument table, on the right side of the patient.

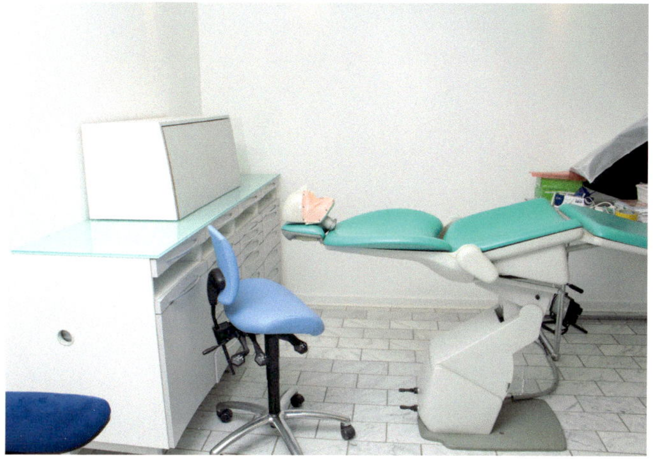

Fig 8–2 Only 45 cm of free space is available behind the patient chair.

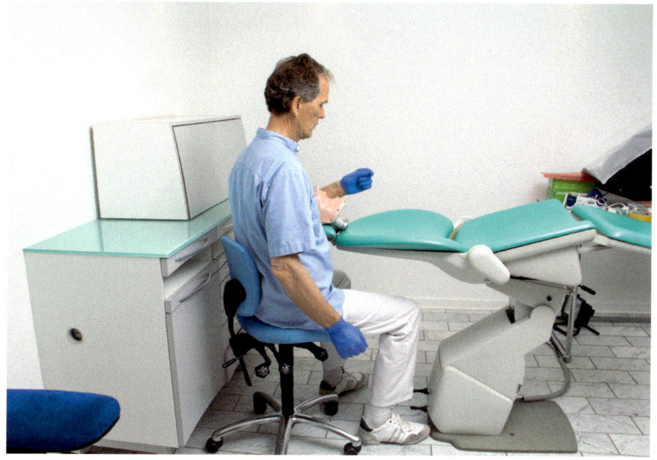

Fig 8–3 There is no space for the dentist to work in a 12 o'clock position when needed, due to the direction of vision on the left side.

TREATMENT ROOM CABINETRY

The design of the treatment room cabinetry has great influence on the work of the dentist and assistant. It may either support or seriously disturb their work.

Up to this point, the following parts of the assistant's complete workplace have been described: the patient chair, the assistant's and dentist's stools, unit instruments, suction holder and hand instrument table. The assistant also needs a workplate and storage area for hand instruments and materials, as well as an organization concept for these.

The assistant's cabinetry

Behind the patient chair, a line of cabinetry modules with drawers is placed. Most cabinet arrangements lack acceptable functionality and have not been redesigned for decades. In fact, many workplaces were better many years ago than how they are now. Looking at most dysfunctional workplaces, one has the impression that the mental model for the arrangement of work modules is a kitchen however, with special inserts in the drawers.

Working methods are often performed without awareness, and therefore even obviously impractical working methods may be repeated for decades, creating poor work postures, and loss of time and energy (Fig 8–1).

One such example is if the hand instrument tray is not placed between the assistant and the dentist. The assistant has difficulty in reaching the instruments, "amputating" her ability to assist. Another is when the hand instrument table is placed over the patient, leaving no space for the unit instruments or for the assistant to pass them to the dentist, as part of a team. Placing it on the dental unit is not an ideal solution either.

A space of 40 to 45 cm between the patient chair headrest and the cabinets behind does not allow enough space to enable the dentist to work in a 12 o'clock position (Figs 8–2 and 8–3). This means that the dentist has to twist the neck and back to look at the left side of the patient's teeth. (There has to be at least 60 cm between the headrest and the modules behind the patient chair.

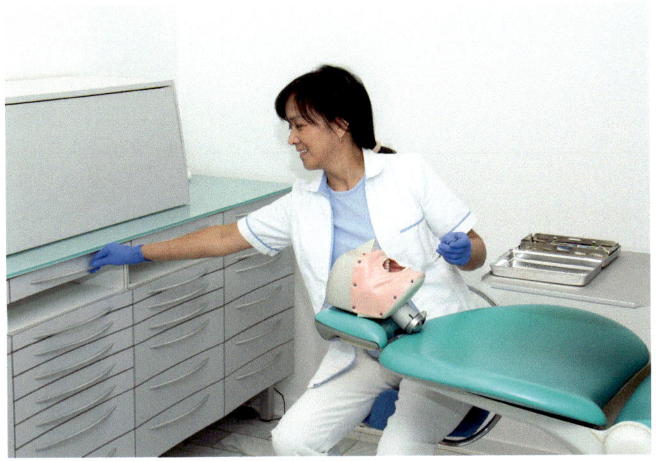

Fig 8–4 No tabletop within reach.

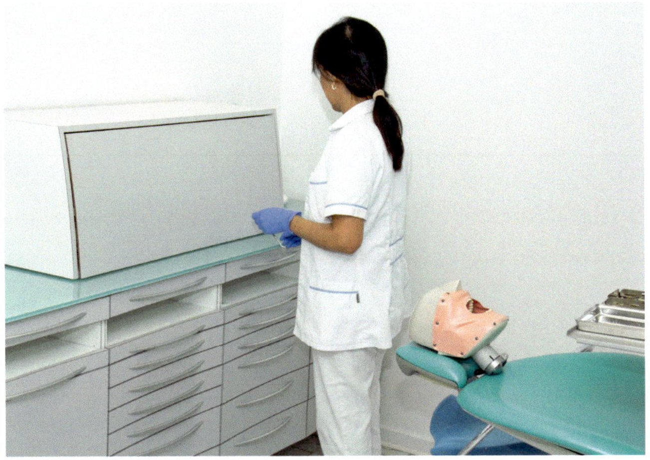

Fig 8–5 The assistant stands up for mixing.

No tabletop or work table for the sitting assistant

For working in a sitting position, there has to be a tabletop about 75 to 80 cm above the floor. A kitchen table of 90 cm cannot be used as a worktable for a sitting person (Fig 8–4).

The assistant must be able to use the working table without needing to move away on her stool. The reach of the arms of the assistant decides where materials, etc, are placed. The front of the tabletop must – for these reasons – be placed 20 cm behind (and to the side from) the headrest of the patient chair.

Not enough storage space within reach

The assistant has to repeatedly move away from the patient, with the result that assistance for the treatment is seriously disturbed (Fig 8–5).

No materials in the treatment room

In some regions or countries, one may see a dental practice where the materials are not stored at the chairside (excepting a few). The materials and hand instruments are arranged individually for each patient in the sterilization room on large plastic trays, according to the planned treatment.

But things may often go differently as planned. If something unplanned for happens, the assistant must go the sterilization room to collect the necessary materials and instruments on a tray or in a tub. This is not a flexible system. The assistant will often have to leave the patient, so the dentist loses assistance, along with having interruptions and disturbances of workflow. With a humoristic touch, one could call it "jogging assistant organization."

A WORKSTATION – INSTEAD OF "DRAWER MODULES"

The basic principle to apply for a good workstation is that it must be adapted to and support the best working methods, and not the reverse.

A good workstation must support organization, assistance and undisturbed concentration. However, many cabinetry combinations obstruct organization, assistance and concentration.

Priority of work by patient

A workplace should support the work of the dentist and assistant in their four-handed collaboration, with the objective of focusing all activities towards the patient. Therefore, the workplace is an integrated part of the total workflow and its organization, including materials and instruments.

The value of the workplace is decided by its ability to support and simplify, and to eliminate any activities that distract the dentist's and assistant's focus away from the patient. It should also avoid the need for the assistant to leave the dentist, even for unplanned deviations in the workplace. This is a deduction from basic principle number 6.

The functional measures of the workstation

Here is a plan of the workstation with correct measurements, according to the work objectives:

The measurements for the workstation are decided by the space necessary to allow the dentist to work in different positions between 9 and 12 o'clock without limitations, as well as allowing the assistant to reach any instruments or materials needed, without moving away from the patient (Fig 8–6).

The work tabletop

The assistant – and occasionally the dentist – needs a work tabletop. In Fig 8–7 you can see the exact positioning and measurements needed for the tabletop. This position allows the dentist the space for a 12 o'clock position, and is at the same time very close to the assistant. With just a slight turn on her stool, she can reach and prepare materials at the tabletop.

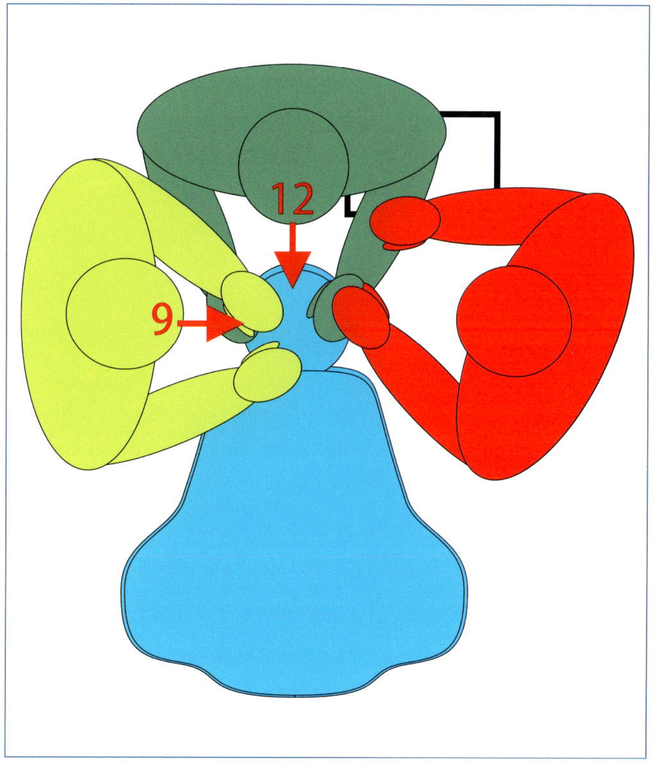

Fig 8–6 It is important there is enough space around the patient's chair so that the dentist can work in all clock positions (9, 10, 11 12).

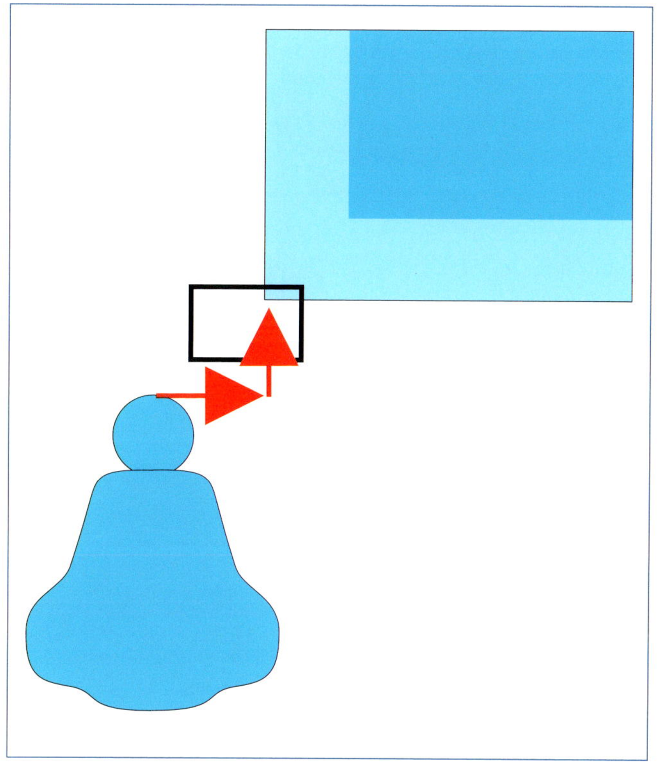

Fig 8–7 Exact position and measures needed for the working tabletop.

TEN RULES FOR THE ASSISTANT'S WORKSTATION

The workstation in the treatment room has a large influence on the work of the dentist and assistant, even more than the dental unit. (For a SOLO working space, see page 162.)

The first two demands are related to the dental unit:

1. The assistant has access to the unit instruments placed between the dentist and assistant, over the patient. The multifunction syringe is closest to the assistant. (An ergonomic unit consists of a multifunction syringe, two micromotors and a scaler, all held by a balanced unit instrument support.)
2. The suction tube holder is on the left of the assistant, close to the multifunction syringe.

The following eight demands are related to the workstation:

1. The hand instrument table should be between the dentist and assistant, close to the upper left of the patient's head.
2. A large tabletop for the preparation of materials, close to the hand instrument table.

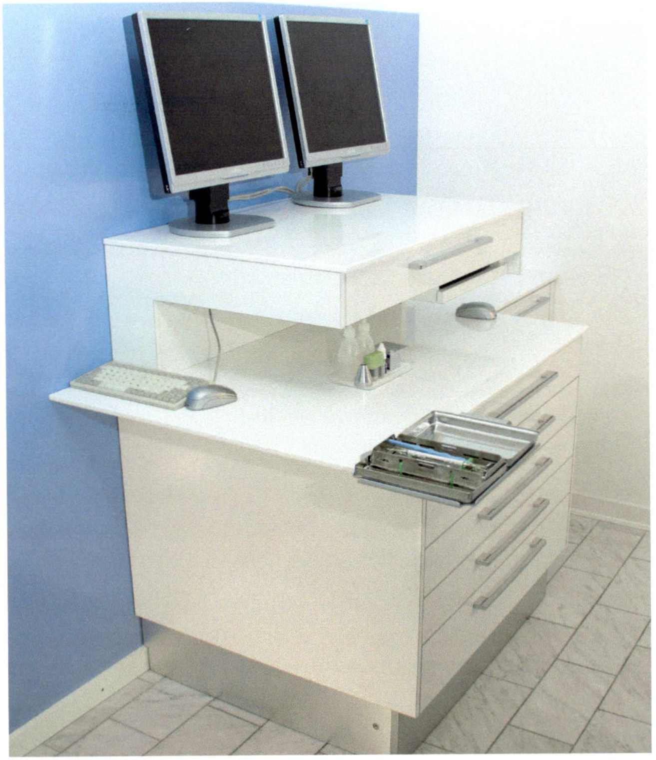

Fig 8–8 The MEGASPACE workstation, developed in 2012.

3. The hand instrument cassette system is supported and incorporates a storage area for hand instruments.
4. Preparations for all treatments (except for surgery) can be made without leaving the workstation.
5. The "most important drawer" (see page 153).
6. A place for the material trays in use and for storage.
7. A computer workspace for the assistant.
8. DUO–SOLO work supported.

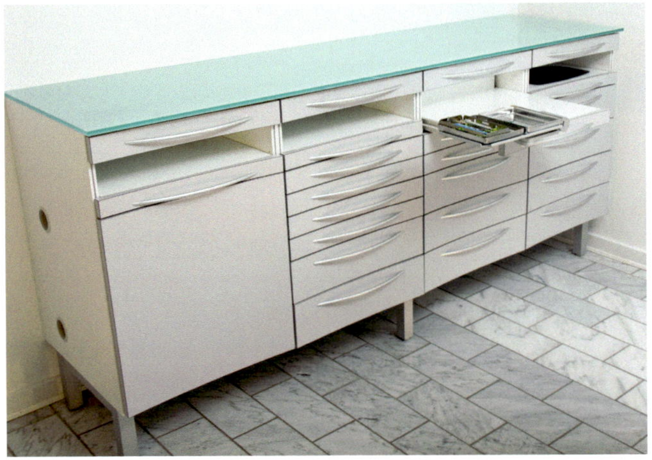

Fig 8–9 The WORKSTATION 2, from 2000.

Next we will take a look at three workstations fulfilling these requirements. All were developed by the author in order to create workplaces that are an integrated part of the organization of materials and instruments, and enable an efficient workflow by preparing and using them in the treatment of patients.

The MEGASPACE was developed in 2012 for *Dancing Hands* and is very concentrated and functional, with a 2.3 m^2 storage place very close to the patient. It's a good workplace both for assistant and dentist (Fig 8–8).

It should comply with all requirements and functional measures. A good super-organized workstation (such as MEGASPACE) may save an hour a day. Transferred to economic turnover, this may increase income too, so you could effectively buy one workspace every 4 to 8 weeks!

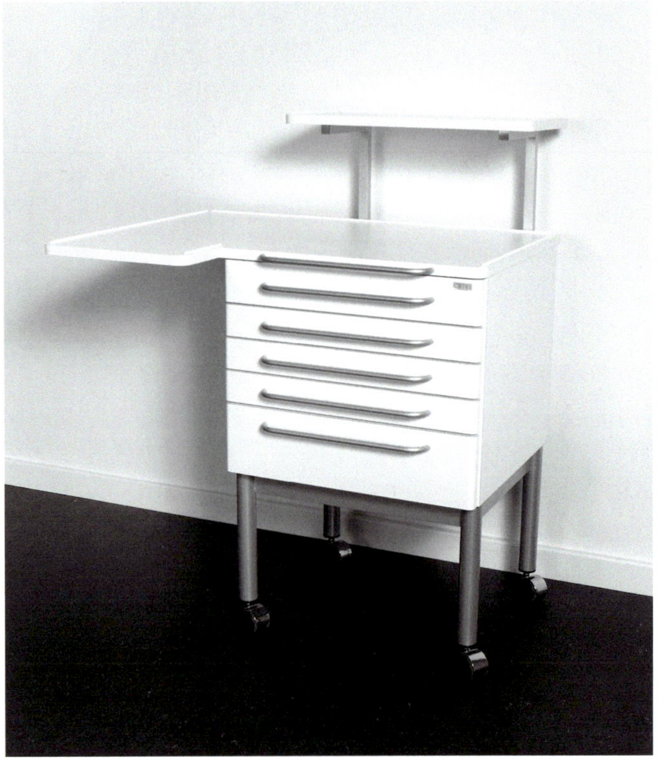

Fig 8–10 The WORKSTATION 3, from 1975.

The WORKSTATION 2 is a year 2000 version of an ergonomic workstation (Fig 8–9). It complies with all working requirements and functional measures.

The WORKSTATION 3 from 1975 is still an acceptable solution, if available space is small and the workplace has to be mobile (Fig 8–10). The storage area in drawers is small and has to be completed with other modules. It complies with functional measures and workplace demands as previously described.

THE MEGASPACE ALL-IN-ONE WORKSTATION

For more detailed information (16 pages) go to www.netergonomie.com, English/Megaspace

For *Dancing Hands* – working as DUO and DUO–SOLO

For *Dancing Hands*, the author has developed a new workstation for assistant and dentist, representing a synthesis of the knowledge and competence communicated in this book. It is an update to and a support to contemporary dentistry.

Why was MEGASPACE developed?

As described in previous chapters, there are several dental units and patient chairs that support ergonomic working methods and four-handed dentistry. But there are almost no workplaces that comply with the functionality as described in this section. Theoretical ergonomics are not enough; ergonomics must be transferred to practice.

The name "MEGASPACE" was coined because there is no other workstation with so much space in such a compact unit (Fig 8–11). It has a 2.3 m^2 storage area (equal to 23 standard dental cabinet drawers!) and almost a 1 m^2 worktable within reach of the dentist and assistant.

As the name "Megaspace" is already registered (by Mercedes!), the full and correct name of the workstation is "MEGASPACE by Skovsgaard."

MEGASPACE combines important features:

- Precise measurements of the space for dentists and assistants working in a team.
- The hand instrument table is between dentist and assistant, close to the upper left part of the patient's head.
- A large tabletop for the preparation of materials close to the hand instrument table.
- The "most important drawer" in the practice.
- High material density.
- Everything within reach for the assistant.
- Optimal support for high-end assistance.
- Supports working DUO as well as DUO/SOLO.
- The dentist can work alone.
- Organization of materials and instruments is supported.
- The hand instrument tray system supported.
- An abundant storing place.
- Preparations for all treatments (except for surgery) can be made very fast and without leaving the workplace.
- Storage and working area for large material trays.
- Computer workspace with screen and keyboard, for both dentist and assistant.
- Enables a fast switch from one treatment to another.
- Small measures.
- Very large working area and abundant space.
- Very little space needed.
- The MEGASPACE is 76 cm deep and 100 cm wide, which is considerably smaller than other workstations.

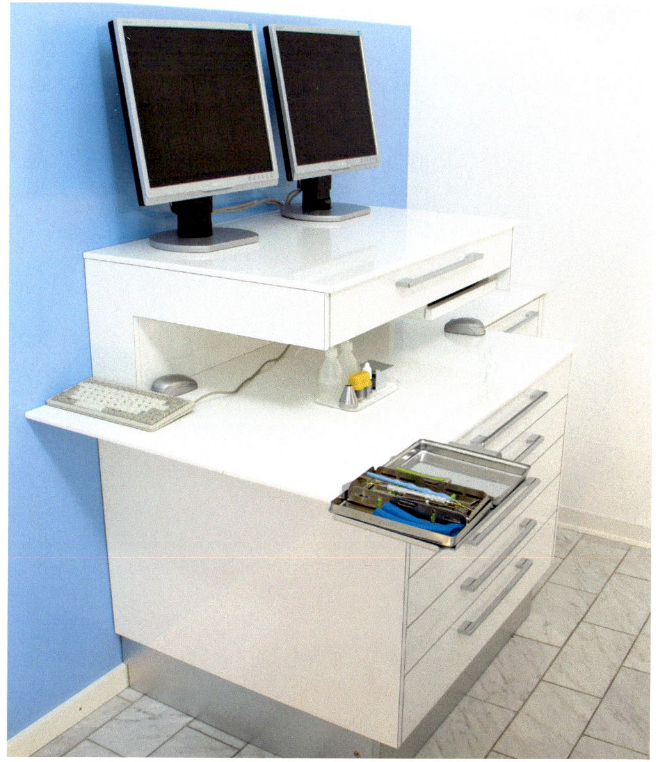

Fig 8–11 MEGASPACE with dentists and assistants workplace.

The MEGASPACE is 100 cm wide, and the assistant needs 50 cm more space on her side. This space can be used for a standard module for hand instrument trays or for a washbasin near the assistant (Figs 8–12 and 8–13).

Above this, a wall module can be placed, for storing paper serviettes, liquid soap, alcogel for hand disinfection, gloves and patient plastic cups.

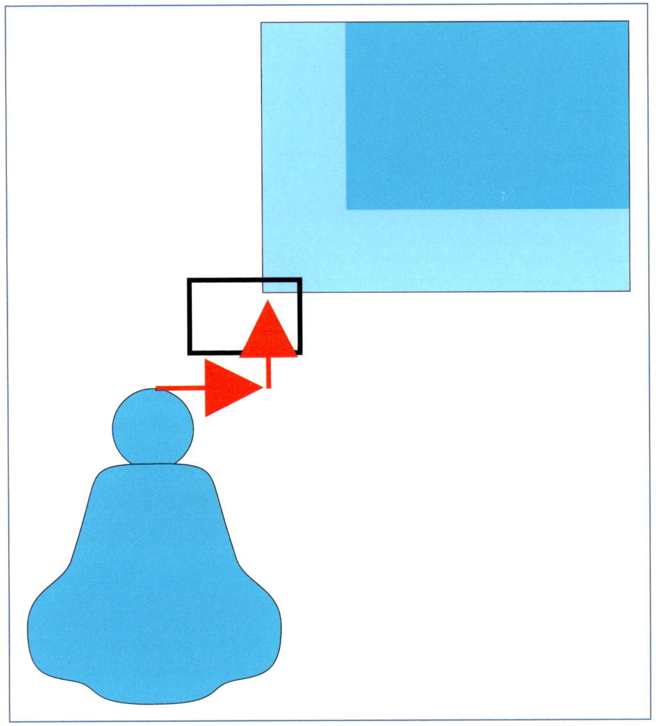

Fig 8–12 Position of the horizontal patient chair headrest, in relation to MEGASPACE.

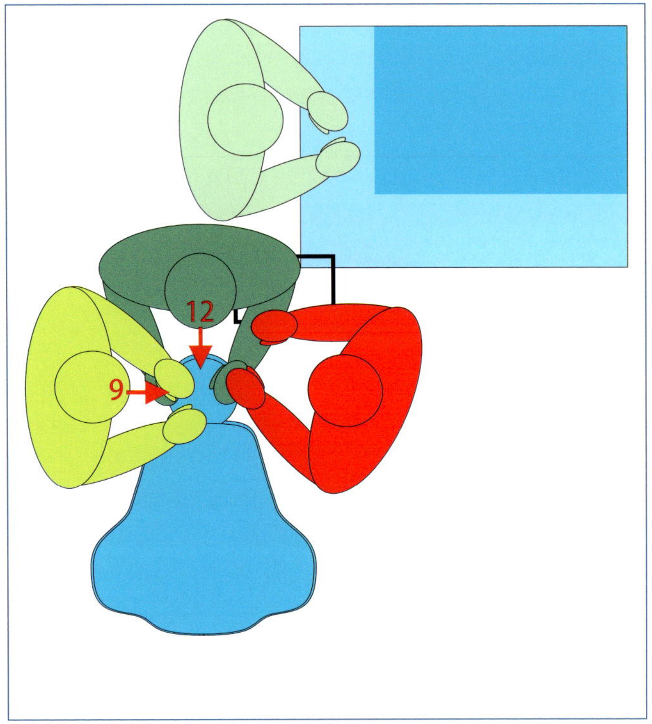

Fig 8–13 Dentist can work in 9 to 12 o clock positions, and also has a work position at the left side of MEGASPACE.

It is very important that the measurements for the MEGASPACE are precise, in relation to the patient chair, and adjusted to the correct working height.

The work tabletop is 75 cm above the floor, and has an effective workspace of half a square meter, with the upper part offering a little less. Altogether, about 1 m^2 working area is available to the assistant and dentist (Fig 8–14).

The hand instrument table

The hand instrument table is placed on a mobile arm and a sliding support. If the dentist is working in a 12 o'clock position, then it may be moved towards the assistant.

If the patient is shorter than average, the hand instrument table is moved forwards. The hand instruments are within reach for both assistant and dentist.

The assistant

To assistant's side, there is a worktable 80 cm long (+20 cm sometimes covered by the hand instrument table). While the assistant is aiding the dentist, she can turn slightly to her right side and here she can reach the worktop with her right hand. Materials can be prepared here (Fig 8–15).

A tray with bottles, cement, etc, can be placed under the upper drawer and slidden forward when needed (Fig 8–16).

A small keyboard should be preferred, because then the pull-out plate can be made shorter and leave better visibility to materials on the worktop (Fig 8–17).

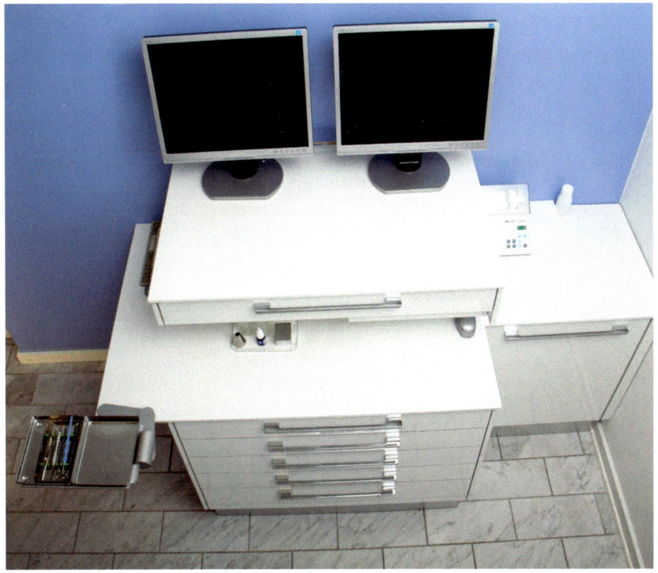

Fig 8–14 Table worktops.

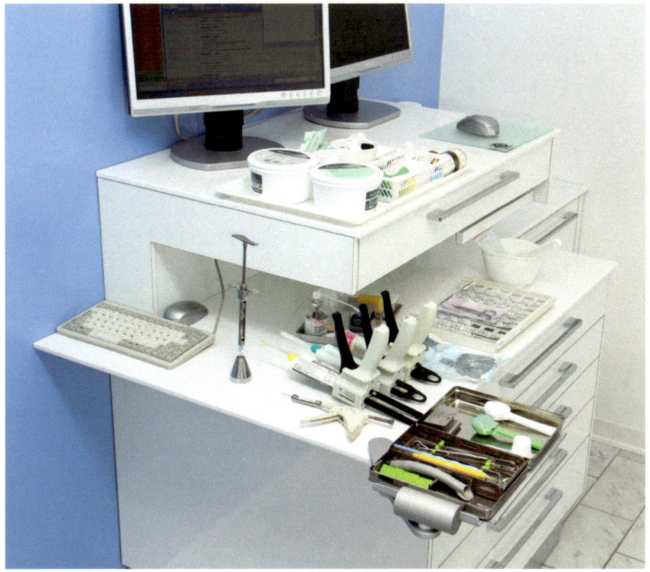

Fig 8–15 Materials for a crown on the working tabletop.

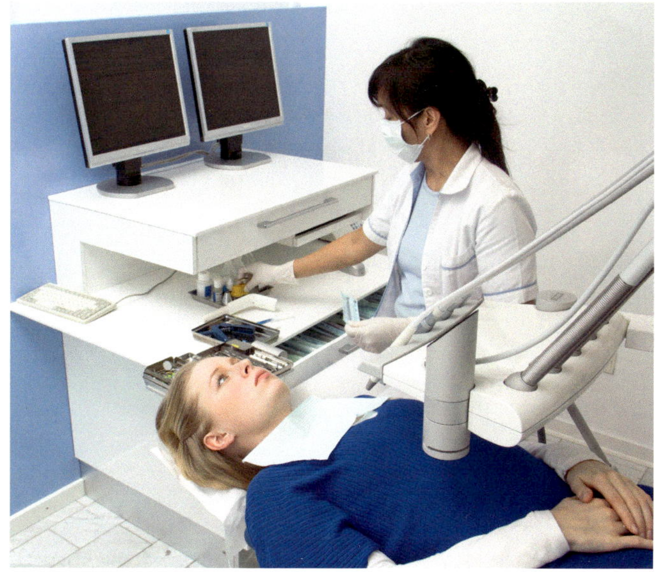

Fig 8–16 Tray with bottles under the top drawer.

DUO–SOLO

The dentist has a workplace of 60 cm (+15 cm sometimes, covered by the hand instrument table). The computer screens are placed on the plate on top of the upper drawer. The dentist's screen may be turned directly towards the dentist, and to share the screen with the assistant, or both may have one each.

The dentist also has to access the working area on top of the upper drawer, eg, for accessing a cordless polymerization lamp (Fig 8–18).

The most important drawer in the practice

This has space equivalent to four standard drawers. Altogether the available storage is 0.36m^2, equal to

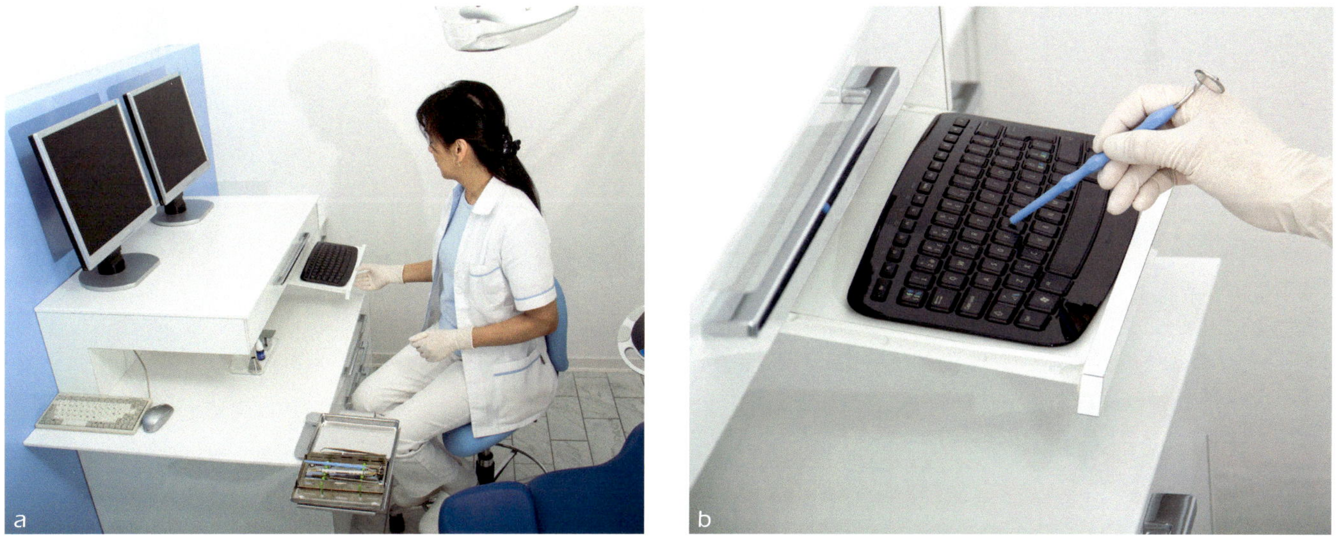

Fig 8–17 (a) The assistant's computer keyboard in a resting position, and (b) in a working position.

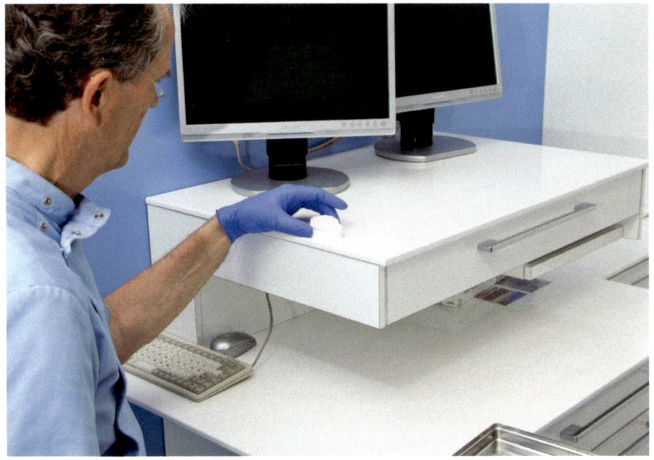

Fig 8–18 The dentist by the tabletop.

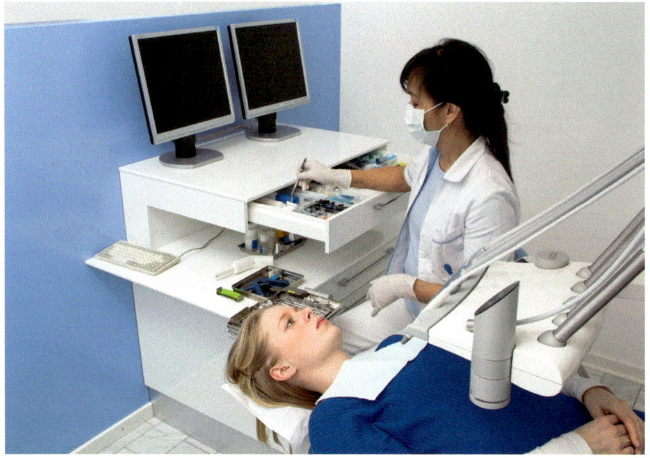

Fig 8–19 The assistant uses tweezers to remove something from the most important drawer.

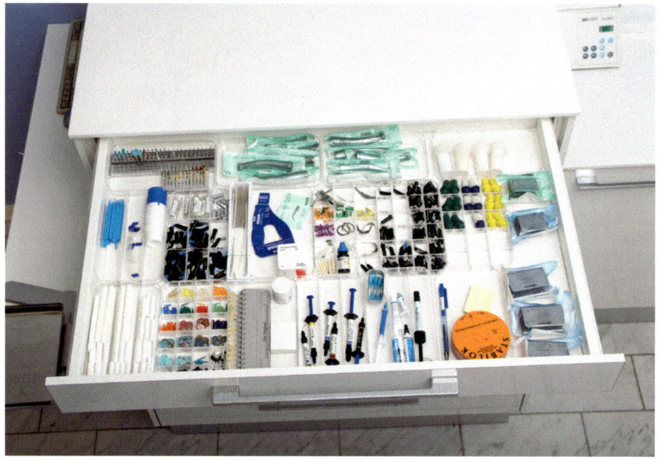

Fig 8–20 The most important drawer of all.

three standard dental drawers' usable storage area (standard opening 35 cm), on a space only 80 cm wide. With the subdividers, the storage area is equivalent to more than four standard drawers – all within reach of the assistant.

This drawer has absolutely the best functionality, because it can easily be opened before or during an examination or treatment to pick up the necessary materials. During the working day, a lot of small materials are used again and again. They are picked up with tweezers (not used in mouth of the patient). This drawer is ideal for all small materials, and used very often (Fig 8–19). Materials and instruments are taken with a pair of sterile tweezers (not used on the patient), in a grip with the instrument sloping down.

The most-often used materials used take highest priority and are therefore positioned to be the most easy to reach. The materials in all drawers are organized with a MATRIX system, according to the frequency of use by the assistant and dentist (see Megaspace description on www.netergonomie.com).

Using the most important drawer

This is used for small materials that are often in use, as well as all for materials for fillings (composite, or amalgam in countries where this is used).

If the reader is familiar with tub systems, the "most important drawer" replaces a "general tub," and a "composite tub," and/or an "amalgam tub," and so on. (Other tubs are replaced with large material trays, much larger than tubs, and with easy to use low marginal edges.) The example in Fig 8–20 shows more than 100 subdivisions of materials. Burs and diamonds may also be picked up by the assistant, and if she is occupied, by the dentist. Burs should be placed in the protected inner part of the drawer, which is less often opened, or in sterilized bur blocks.

Drawers below the worktable

The exterior 15 cm of the drawers are used for the most-often used instruments and materials (Fig 8–21).

Sterile storage of hand instruments

In order to prevent hand instrument contamination with bacteria from the spray's airborne micro droplets, it is recommended that one does not store hand instruments openly on a nondisinfected instrument holder, but in sterilized paper bags, in the drawers.

If hand instruments for the examinations of different treatments are grouped in sterile paper bags, in instrument clips, or in trays, then only supplementary instruments need to be placed in the drawers. They are kept sterilized in sterile paper bags and placed in the drawers, which are subdivided with half size cassette covers.

DUO–SOLO working

When working SOLO, the dentist can reach the closest 40 cm of the drawers, and when the drawers are fully open, can also reach in the inner part (Figs 8–22 and 8–23). When the dentist sometimes works without an assistant, materials and instruments used by the dentist can be placed here.

First drawer

This should contain the supplementing hand instruments, which are not placed in preset cassettes or trays (Fig 8–24).

Replacement hand instruments

These include extra hand instruments of the same type as those in the hand instrument sets.

Using the drawer for large material trays

A material tray is different to a tub with high edges. The low edges of a material tray give an easier sideways access to the materials. A tub cannot be used if placed on the top of the "most important drawer," where the high edges hinder free vision to the content. The large material tray's working position is on top of the most important drawer.

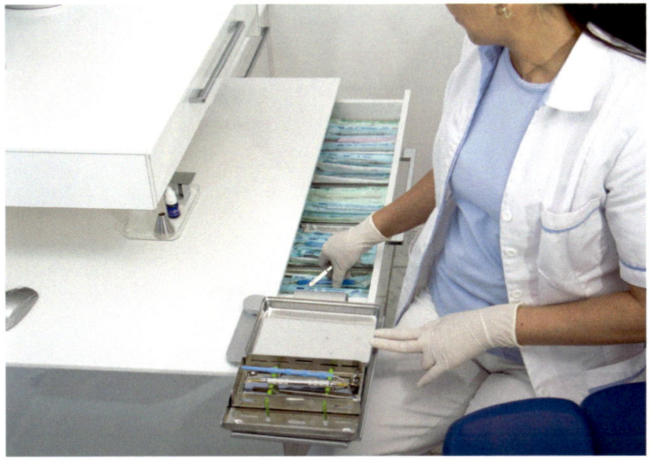

Fig 8–21 The drawer opens 15 cm for picking up instruments during work. Hand instruments are packed in sterile paper.

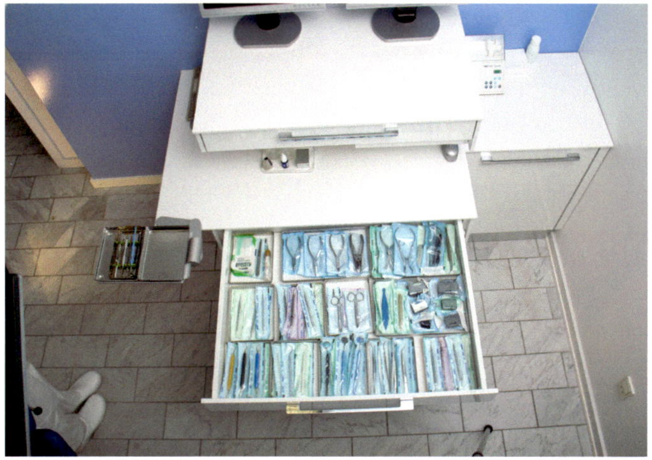

Fig 8–22 The drawer is fully open 60 cm. The inner part of the drawer is used for storage of the seldom-used instruments.

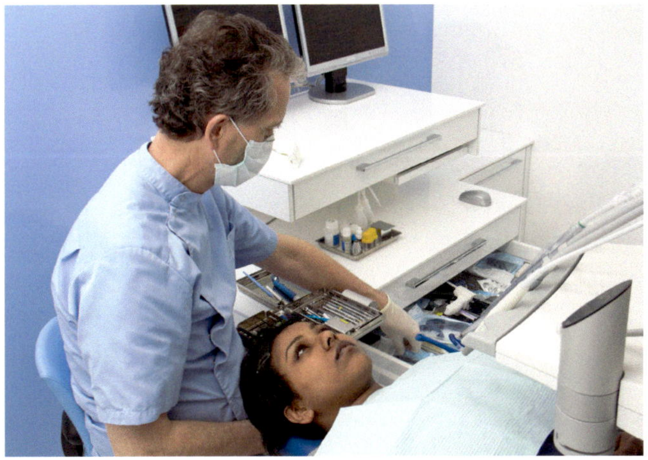

Fig 8–23 The dentist using the lower drawers.

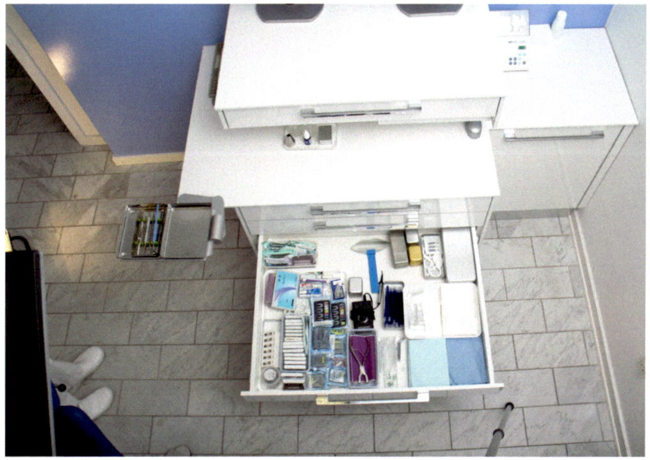

Fig 8–24 A drawer with large material tray. In this case, it is used for endodontics.

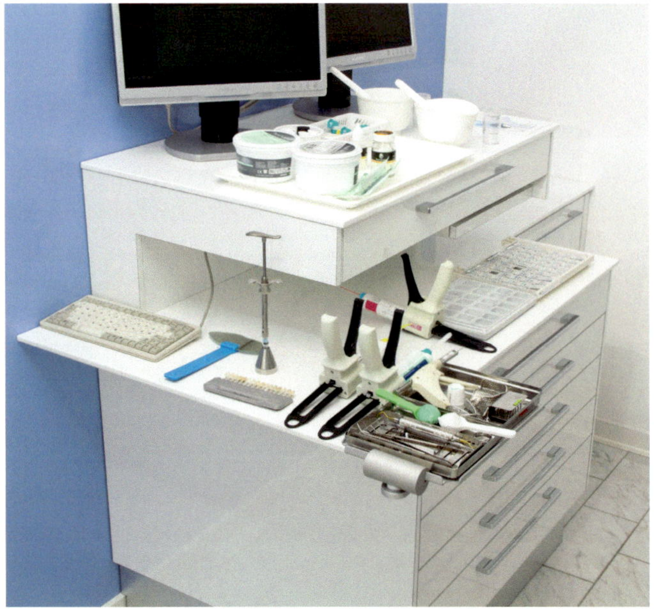

Fig 8–25 Everything is prepared for either crown or bridge procedures – notice how important it is to have the large area provided by the tabletops.

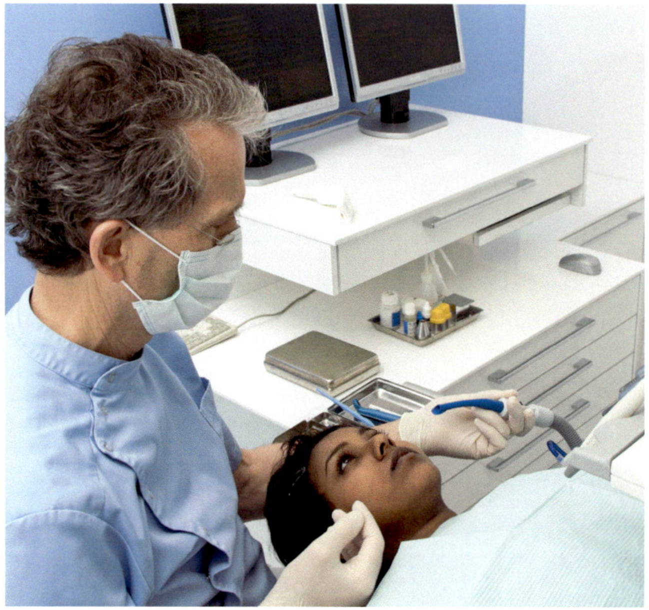

Fig 8–26 The suction holder in the solo working position.

DUO–SOLO – WORKING SOLO SOME OF THE TIME

SOLO work methods

Different variations of DUO–SOLO dentistry is common. In some countries, many dentists only have one assistant (and many have none). The assistant has to take care of so many other tasks that she cannot be continuously present chairside. The dental unit and workstation must be organized so that, when she is present, she can provide optimal assistance for four-handed dentistry (Fig 8–25). (This is described earlier on page 152 [four-handed dentistry].) While working in a mixed DUO and SOLO system, it is essential that the qualities of the duo workplace are not compromised.

Some seem to think that working sometimes with an assistant and sometimes without, means that one does not need to care so much for the workstation. Nothing could be further than the truth. A workstation serving for both DUO and SOLO working methods has to be even more precisely designed than a workstation built only for working DUO. Let's now imagine the assistant is assisting the dentist chairside as described under the description for the working duo, and in the middle of a treatment procedure, the assistant has to leave the dentist to go to reception, where a patient has arrived to pay an invoice.

In the moment she leaves, she places the suction holder closer to the patient's head, where the dentist can take it with his left hand (Fig 8–26). Now the dentist can take hand instruments from the instrument tray using a left-to-right hand transfer.

The solo left-to-right hand instrument transfer

A well-trained SOLO left-to-right hand instrument transfer is made in less than 1 second. Now the dentist can take hand instruments from the hand instrument cassette in the same position as when the assistant was present.

Unit instruments are taken as usual. The small suction is – as in four-handed dentistry – placed behind the last molar in the opposite side as where is worked. The large aspiration tube again serves for aspiration and retraction. Work postures, clock positions, direction of vision, as well as instrument grips for finger and hand support, are all the same as previously described.

When working SOLO, the dentist only has the left hand for retraction when working with direct vision, and therefore has no hand available for retraction when working with a mirror (Figs 8–27 to 8–44).

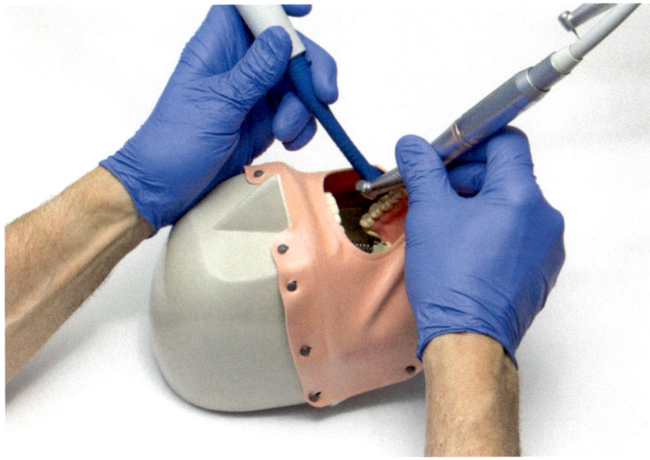

Fig 8–27 Working on occlusal side of left mandibular teeth (and with the same grips on the buccal side, if the dentist sits in a 12 o'clock position).

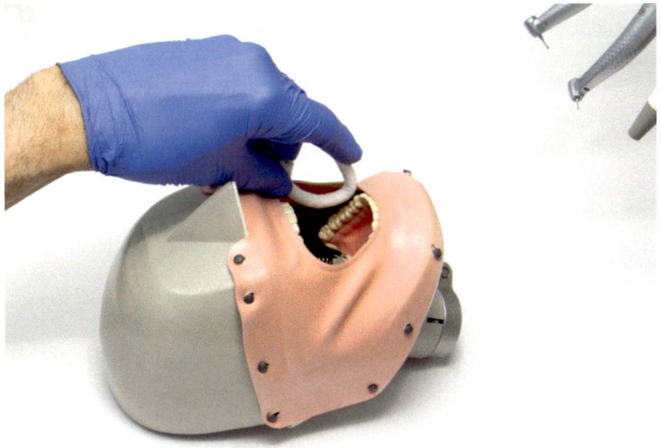

Fig 8–28 A buccal retraction on the mandibular left side, with a Parotis cotton roll (the longest and thinnest of the four versions). The roll is bent over at the tip, as seen here.

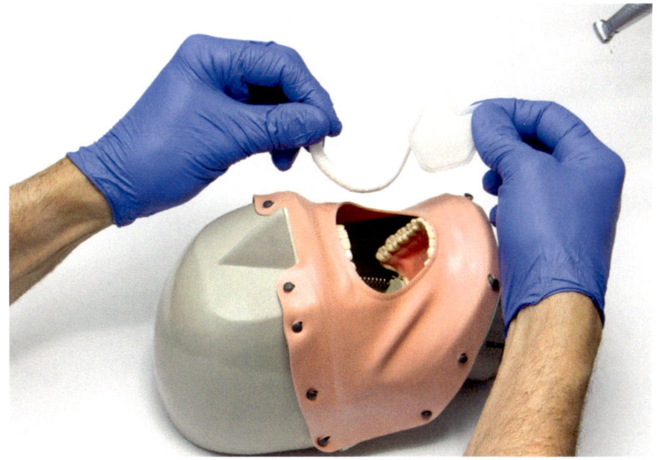

Fig 8–29 The Parotis cotton roll may be supplemented by a dry tip for retracting a voluminous cheek mucosa.

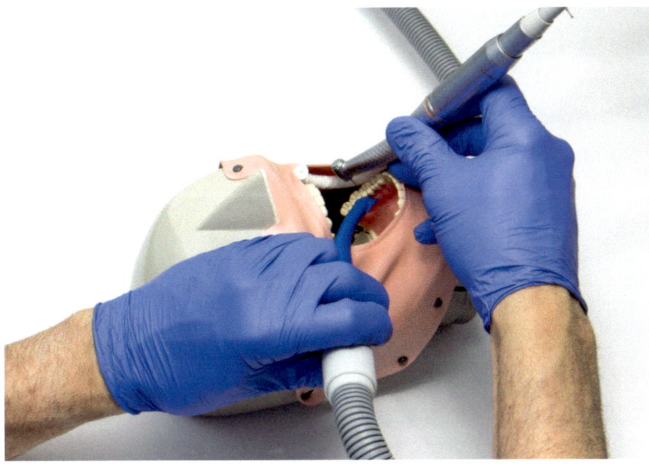

Fig 8–30 Occlusal and lingual aspects of the mandibular left side. The dentist holds the large suction tip in his left hand and uses it for retracting the patient's tongue.

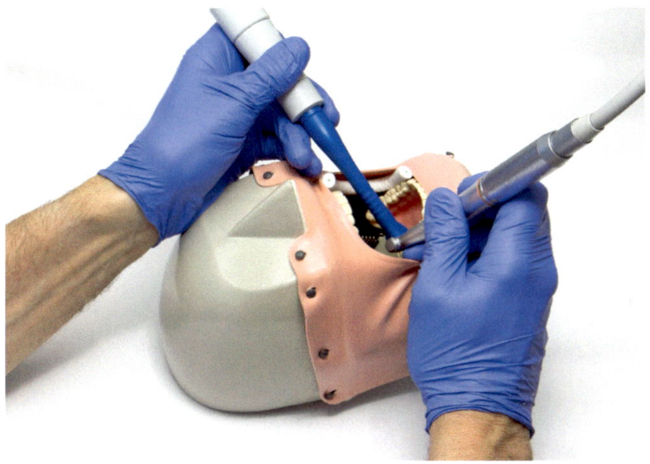

Fig 8–31 Occlusal and lingual aspects of the mandibular right side. The dentist retracts the tongue with the aspiration tube.

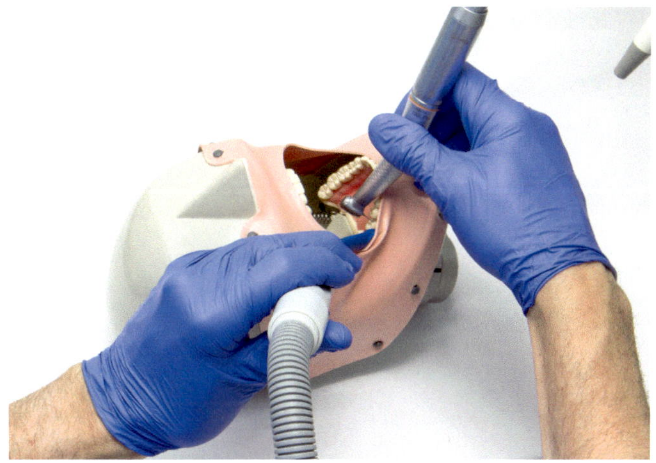

Fig 8–32 Occlusal and buccal aspects of the mandibular right side. The dentist retracts the patient's chin with the aspiration tube.

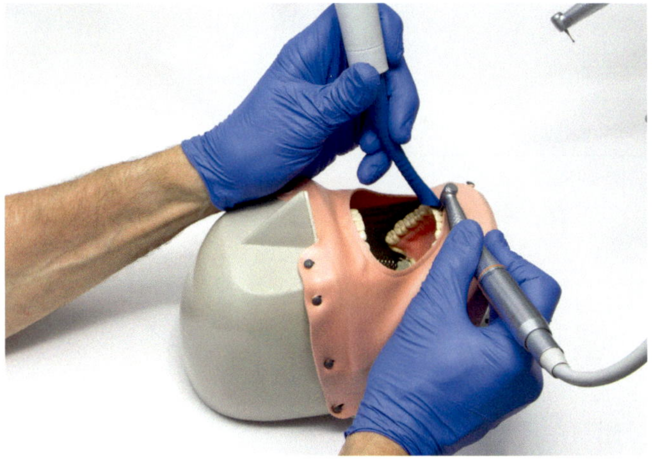

Fig 8–33 The suction tube may be held lingually or buccally in the mandibular incisor region, if the lips are not too forceful.

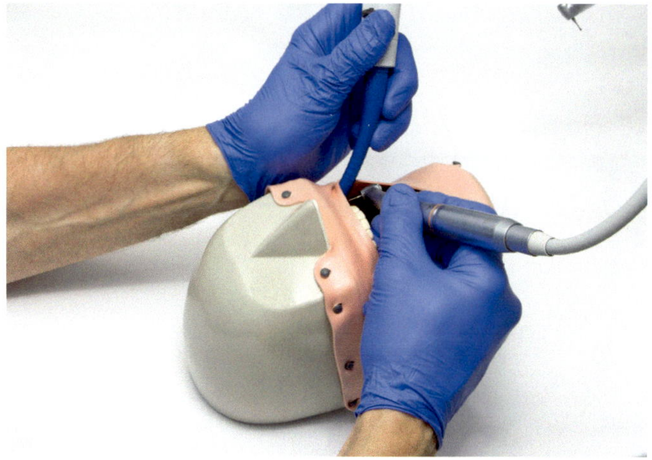

Fig 8–34 Maxilla left side – buccal surface: the dentist holds the large aspiration tube with his left hand, with the patient's head turned to the right. This gives the dentist direct vision.

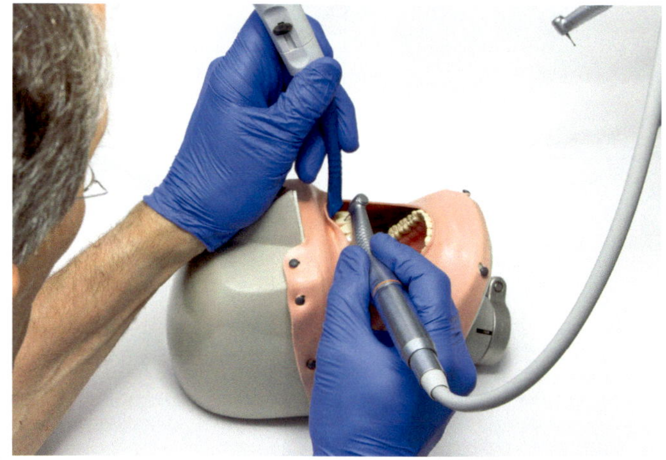

Fig 8–35 The labial maxillary incisors.

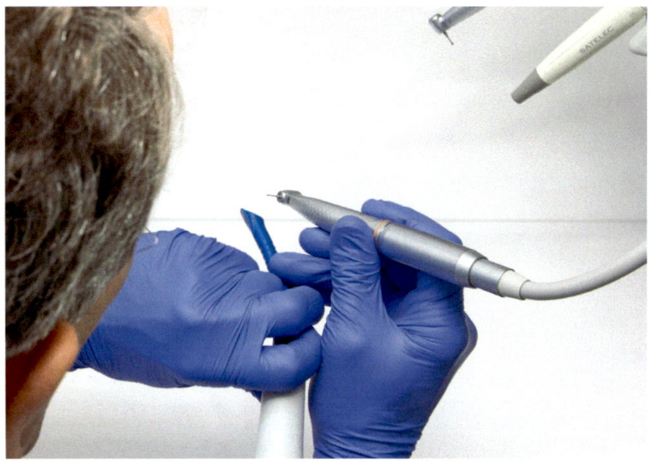

Fig 8–36 The right maxilla, buccal aspect: the right hand is supported by the left, which holds the aspiration tube ready for retraction and aspiration.

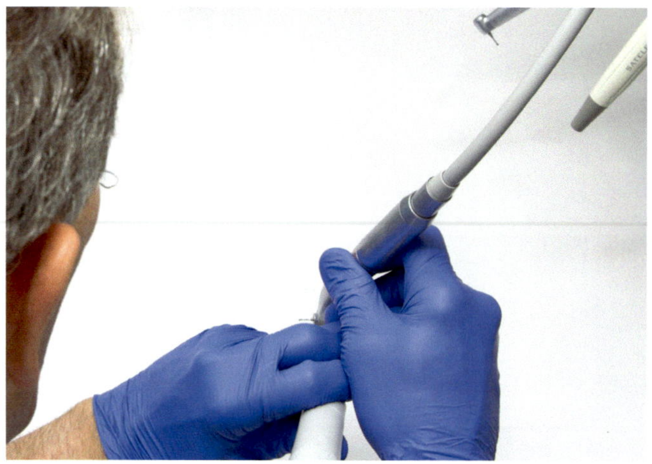

Fig 8–37 The same posture as Fig 8–36, but with the hands ready to be positioned in the mouth of the patient.

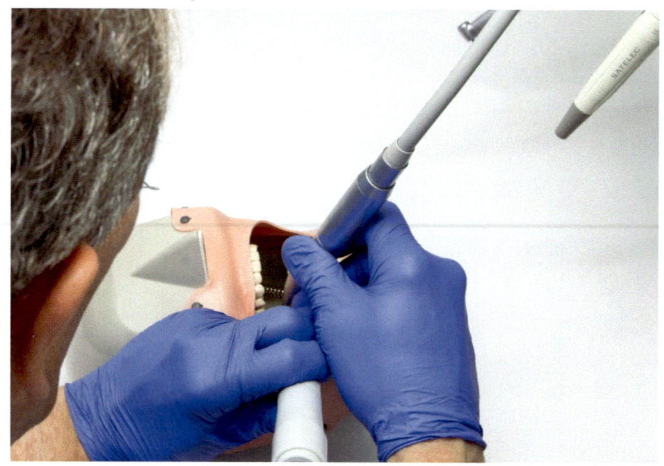

Fig 8–38 The left hand is now supported by the patient's cheekbone and retracts carefully. The right hand is supported by the left hand. If the patient can move the head some way backwards, it improves the direct vision.

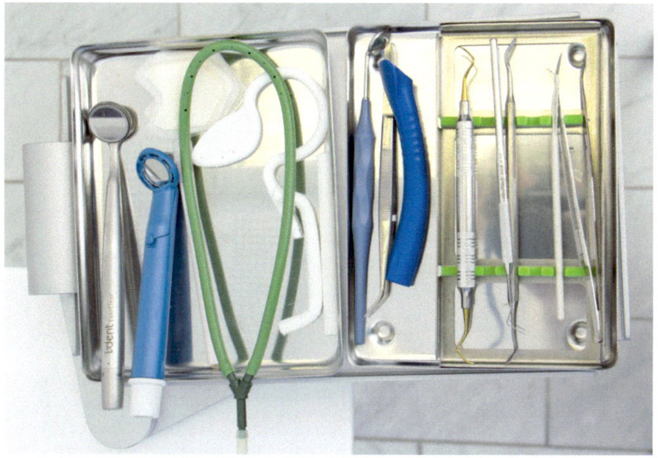

Fig 8–39 Supporting tools for SOLO dentistry: the Everclear mirror with built-in motodrive; Rotromir suction with rotating mirror; dry tip; vacuseptor flexible tube system; tongue retraction suction; Parotis cotton rolls (see www.netergonomie.com).

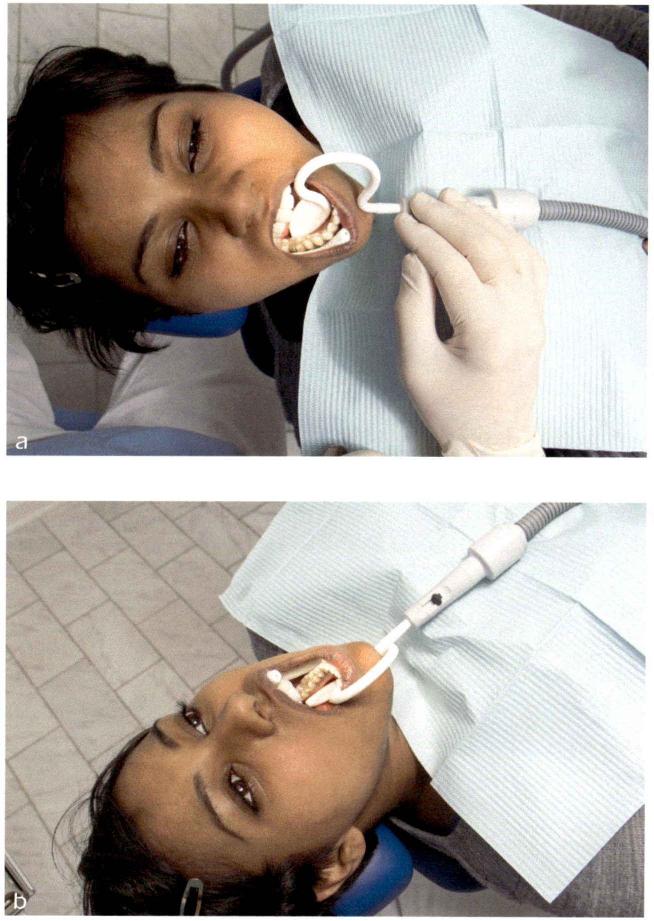

Fig 8–40 (a) When the working area needs to be kept dry, a small suction tube (which may hurt a little) combined with a Parotis cotton roll (b) (the thin and long version) keeps the tongue away.

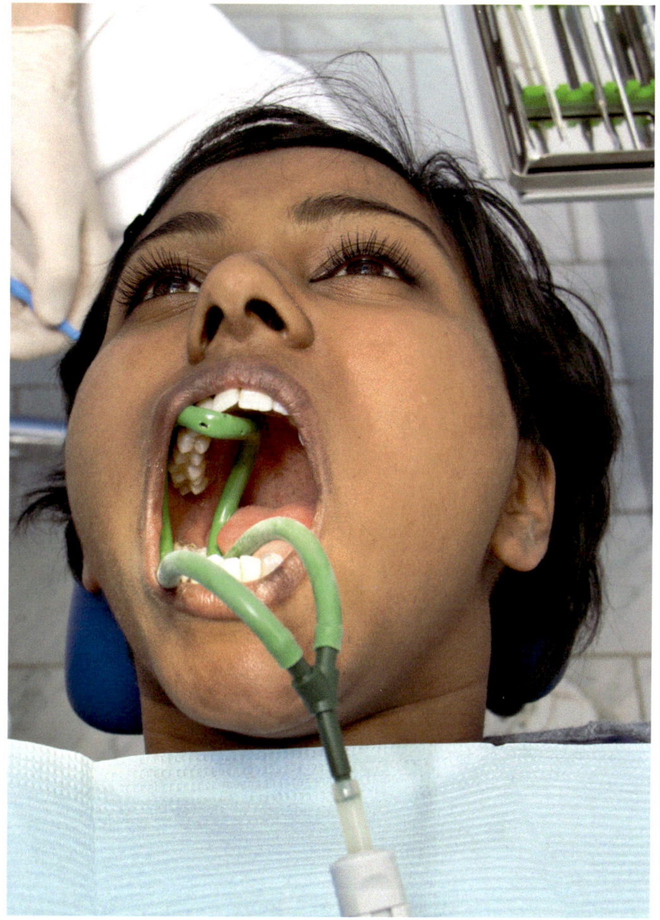

Fig 8–41 Left and right side of maxilla, on the mesial, occlusal and distal surfaces: retraction and aspiration with Vacuseptor (www.netergonomie.com), a perforated rubber tube connected with an adapter for a large amount of suction. Inside the rubber tube, there is a flexible and formable metal thread, so that the tube can be adapted to the interior and exterior sides of the teeth being treated, to provide retraction and aspiration.

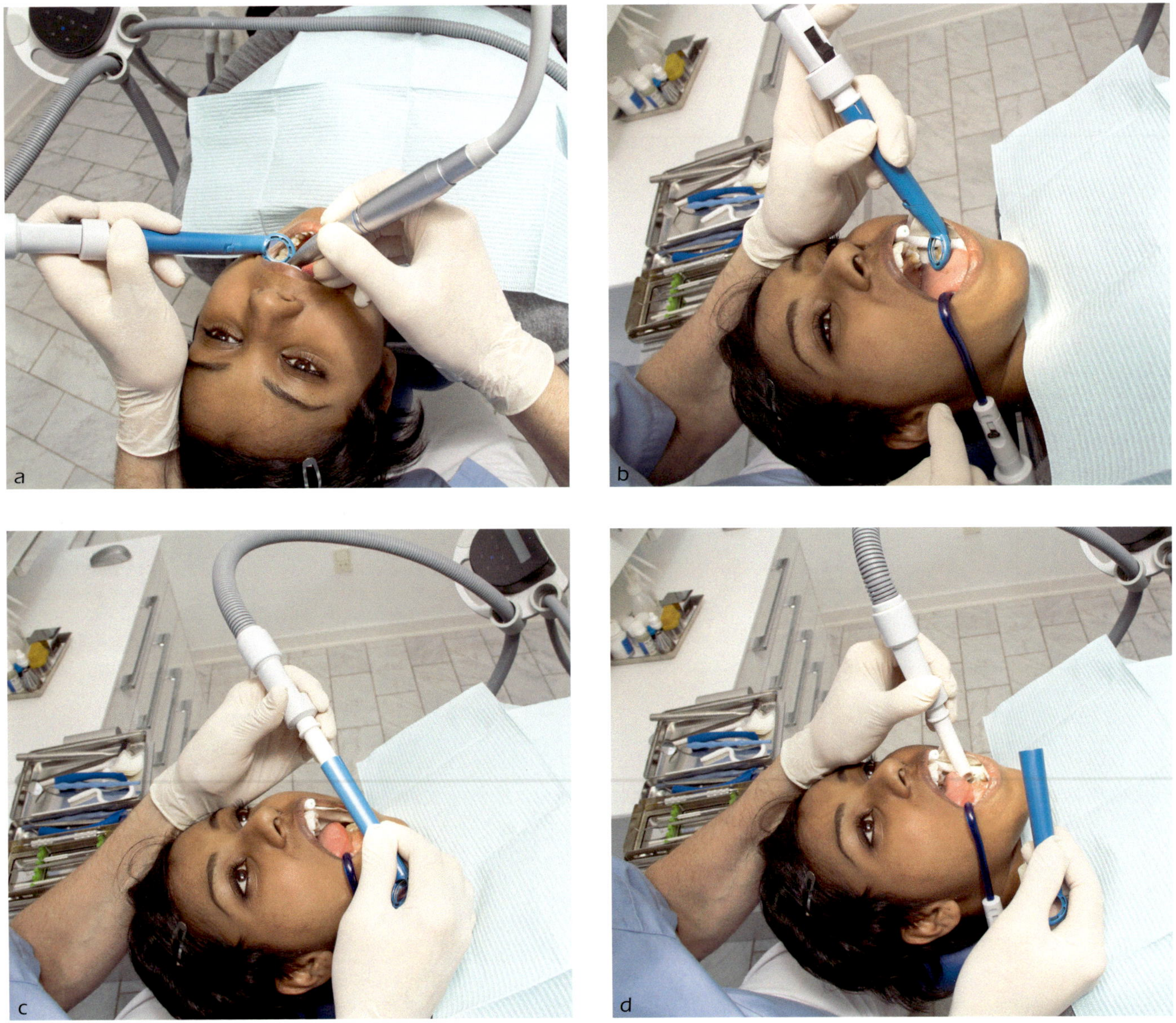

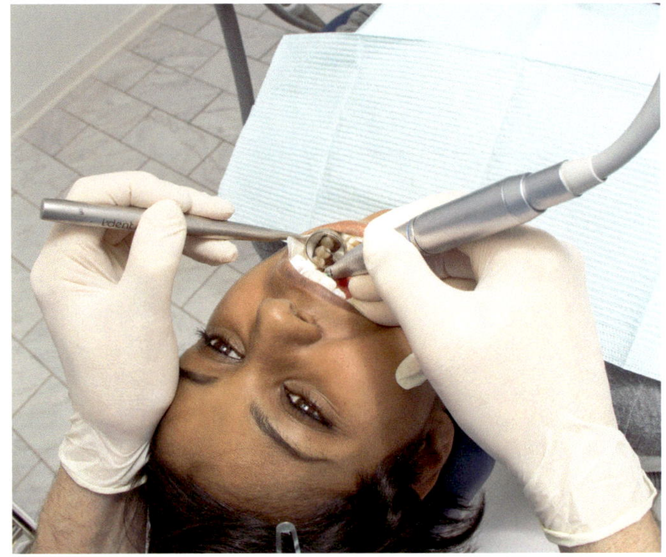

Fig 8–43 Here is another solution: the Everclear mirror contains a brushless sterilizable electromotor, making it rotate very fast. The shaft contains a rechargeable battery. Altogether it is a very elegant (and expensive) solution.

Fig 8–42 (a to d) Another solution is the Rotromir system (www.netergonomie.com), a kind of aspiration tube, where the passing air rotates a built-in mirror so fast that it is kept dry. A sound like an old air-rotor can be heard, so for prolonged use, ear protectors should be used. When more aspiration is necessary, the inner part of the tube is used.

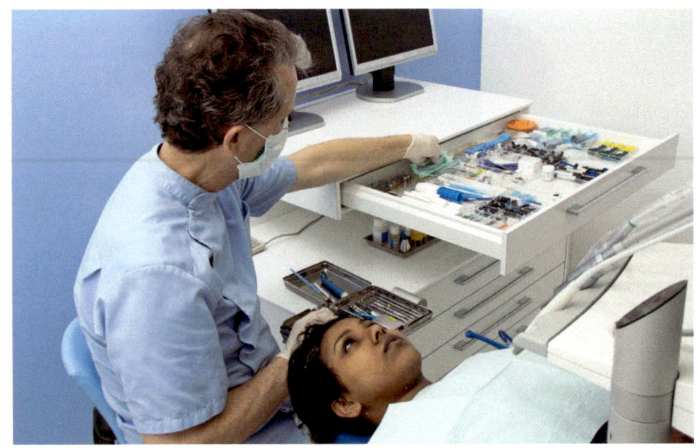

Fig 8–44 The dentist using tweezers for picking up small materials in the "most important drawer."

The DUO–SOLO workstation – MEGASPACE

The most important drawer for the dentist is the uppermost one. They can easily reach materials from about 40 cm, by using tweezers in the same way the assistant does.

In this drawer materials are placed, which the dentist may need to take themselves when alone. With the lower drawers, the dentist can reach within 20 cm (Fig 8–45).

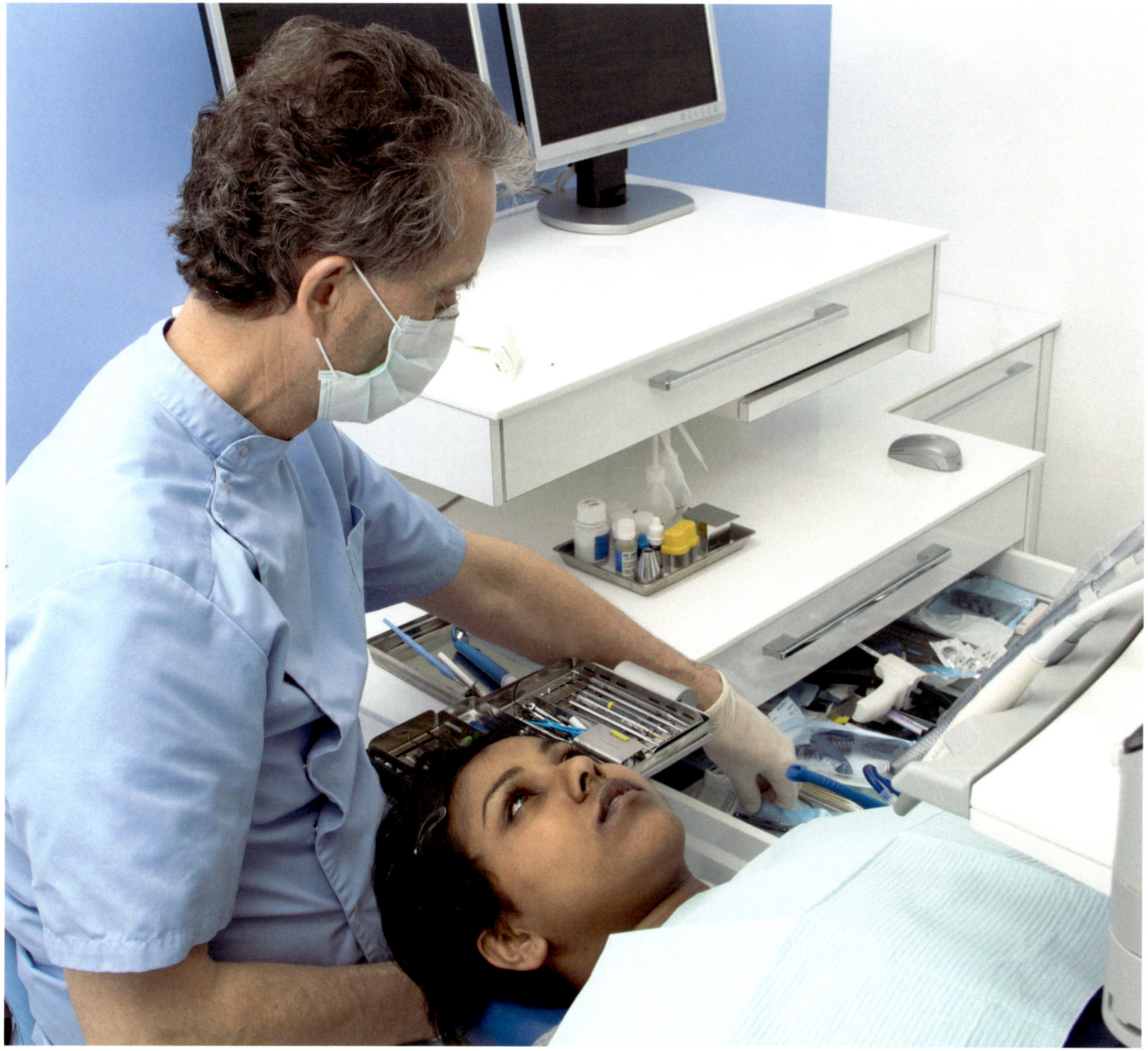

Fig 8–45 The dentist taking the injection syringe from the second lower drawer.

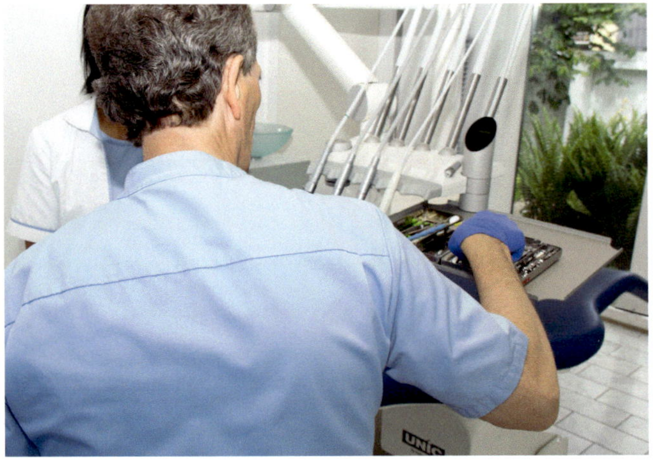

Fig 8–46 The hand instrument tray at the right side of the dental unit (the unit is placed slightly to the left). The hand instrument grip has the thumb coming from below, while the suction holder is closer to the dentist's left hand.

ALL SOLO

Dentist working alone – hygienist also SOLO

The working methods for working SOLO are described previously, under the DUO–SOLO working methods.

If the workplace is designed for possible later work with assistant, then the workplace is laid out the same as for DUO–SOLO work (see page 156).

One difference for entirely SOLO working today is the use of a hand instrument tray, placed beside the unit instruments over the patient. The dental unit may be placed slightly to the left. The

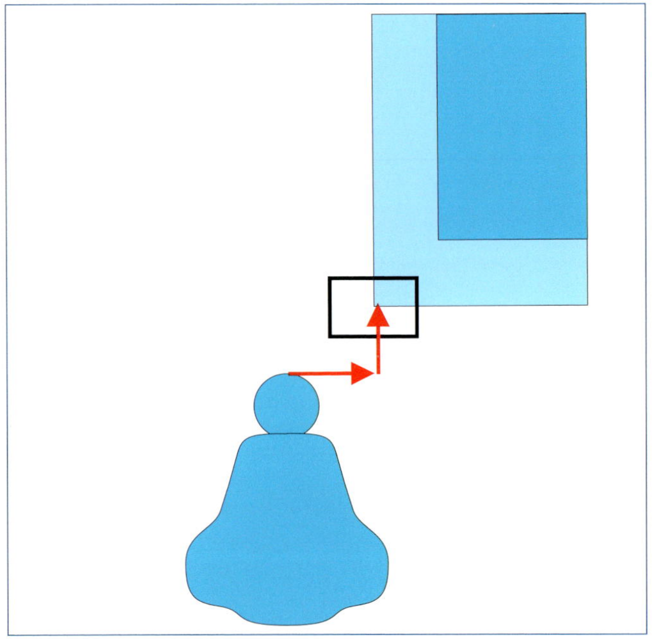

Fig 8–47 The MEGASPACE is mirrored and in an entirely "solo" working position. The hand instrument table is on the right side.

hand instruments are taken with a grip, so the dentist's elbow does not need to be elevated (Fig 8–46).

The hand instrument grip passes the edge of the tray and enables the dentist to take the instrument with the thumb below the instrument.

MEGASPACE in an all-SOLO position

In some countries, many dentists work alone not only during chairside procedures, but also in the practice.

The dentist will also take on all the duties usually carried out by a receptionist: using the telephone and making appointments, bookkeeping and all the tasks involved in sterilization and examinations, treatments, preventive procedures, etc. They are actually taking on all of the procedures and responsibilities for the practice. One reason for this may be that there may not be many patients per dentist in the region, or it might be based on old habits and traditions.

- SOLO – The chairside procedures for a dentist working without an assistant are described earlier on this page.
- DUO/SOLO – Working methods for the workplace for when sometimes working with an assistant and sometimes without, is described on page 156.

In a dental practice with one or more assistants, the assistant may compensate for a physical practice design where the instruments and materials are not organized in the closest proximity to the patient. She moves around in order to "collect" instruments and materials from where they are stored.

However, if the dentist is working completely alone, an unpractical organization will be a heavy burden on the dentist, who has so many tasks to perform. So how should the workplace, treatment room and practice be designed, if the dentist is alone and does not want to have an assistant in future? Firstly and most importantly, all instruments and materials must now be within reach of the dentist.

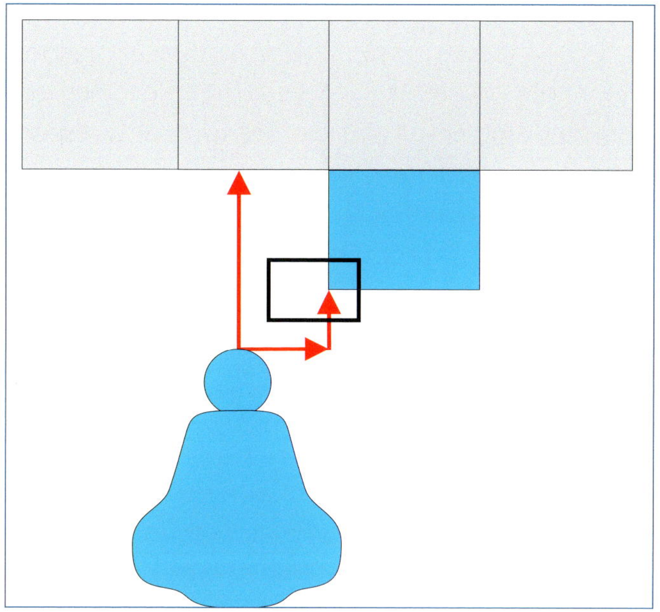

Fig 8–48 The measurements of the WORKSTATION 2.

Therefore, the MEGASPACE is turned 90 degrees clockwise and is "mirrored." The extension of the tabletop with the hand instrument table is placed opposite the standard MEGASPACE (Fig 8–47). If the room for sterilization and storage is placed within short and direct access to the treatment room, the dentist will have short and efficient "runways." The reception should also be as close as possible to the treatment room.

How to buy MEGASPACE

If you would be interested in finding out more about MEGASPACE and how to purchase one, please send an email to dancinghands@mail.dk

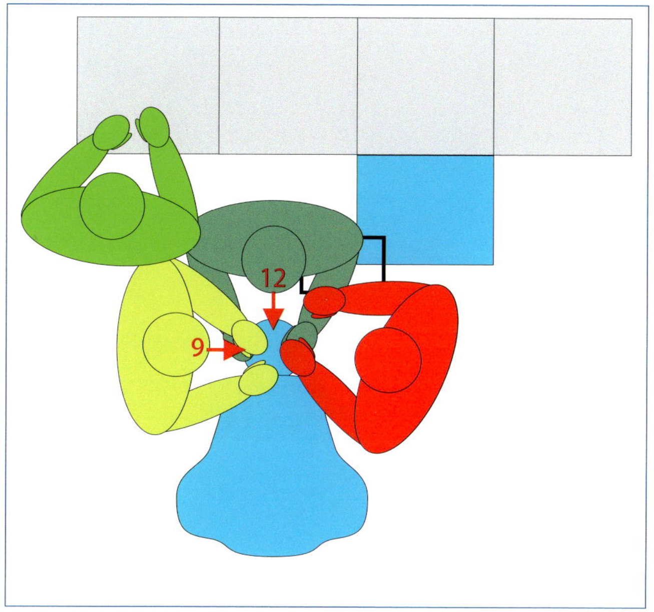

Fig 8–49 Workspace for the dentist and assistant.

WORKSTATION 2

Working as a duo and solo

Whereas the MEGASPACE is the author's most recent workplace design, the WORKSTATION 2 is 10 years older (and is also designed by the author). It fulfills the same functional work demands as the MEGASPACE.

Measurements

The dentist can sit in working clock positions from 9 to 12 without limitations. The assistant has a hand instrument table workplate, the "most important drawer in the practice," and reachable material trays.

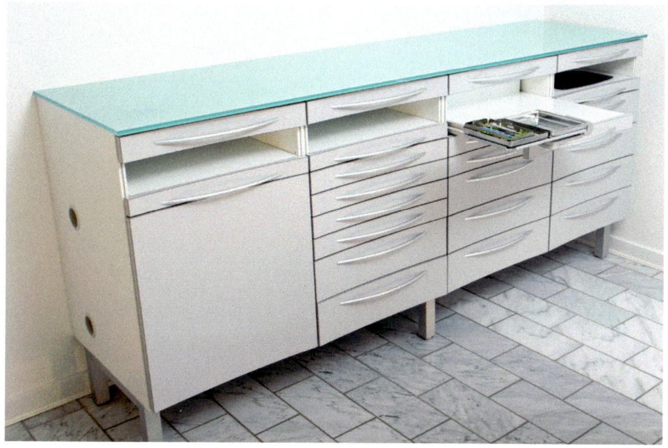

Fig 8–50 WORKSTATION 2.

The measurements for WORKSTATION 2, in relation to the headrest of the patient's chair in a horizontal position and at working height, have to be precise. It fulfills the same criteria as the MEGASPACE, however the "most important drawer" is much smaller in the MEGASPACE. The WORKSTATION 2 is larger than the MEGASPACE, but the content is about the same (Figs 8–49 and 8–50).

The workplate is a pull-out tabletop, is much smaller and the drawers below are not available when it is in a "working position," and the computer keyboard is further away (Fig 8–51).

The hand instrument table – DUO and SOLO

The dentist can occasionally use the pull-out workplate on his side, but this must be pushed in when the dentist is working in the 11 to 12 o'clock position. This drawer is supplemented by drawers to both right and left sides (Figs 8–52 to 8–54).

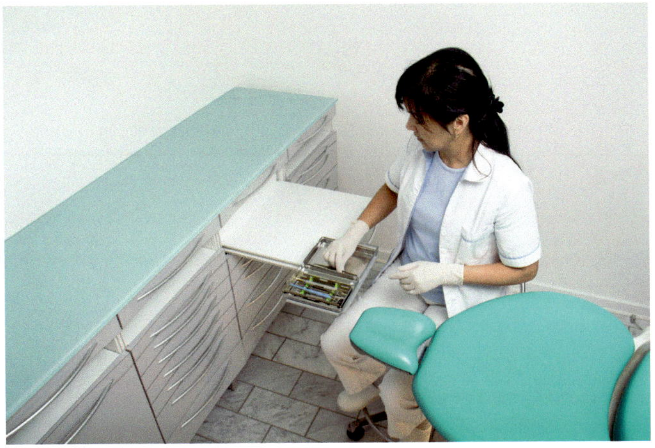

Fig 8–51 The assistant has a pull-out workplate, which also supports the hand instrument table for the hand instrument tray.

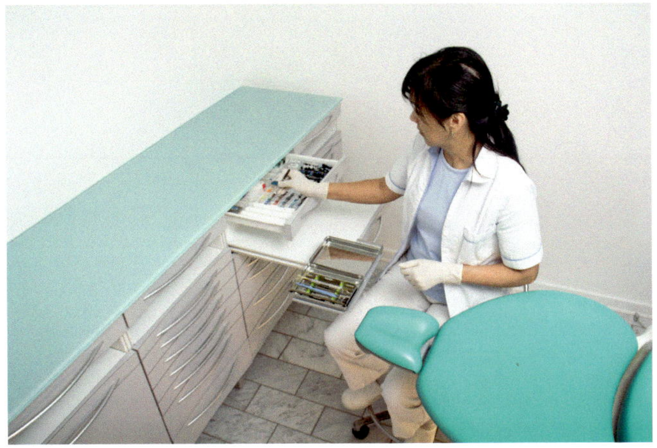

Fig 8–52 "The most important drawer." An important feature is that there is a 10 cm free space above the pull-out workplate, so "the most important drawer" can be opened with materials still on the workplate.

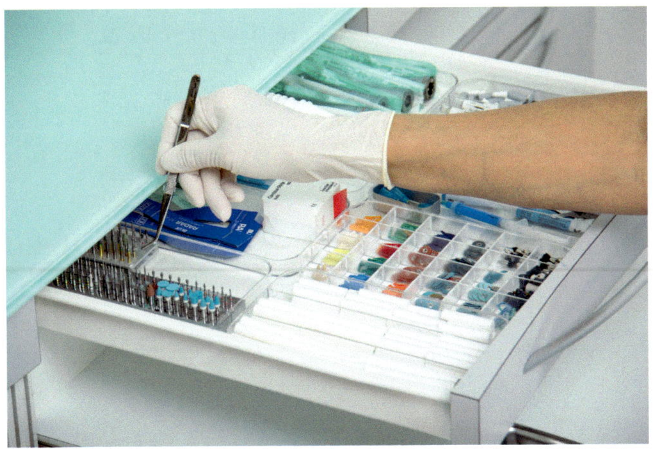

Fig 8–53 This drawer is supplemented by drawers to both right and left sides.

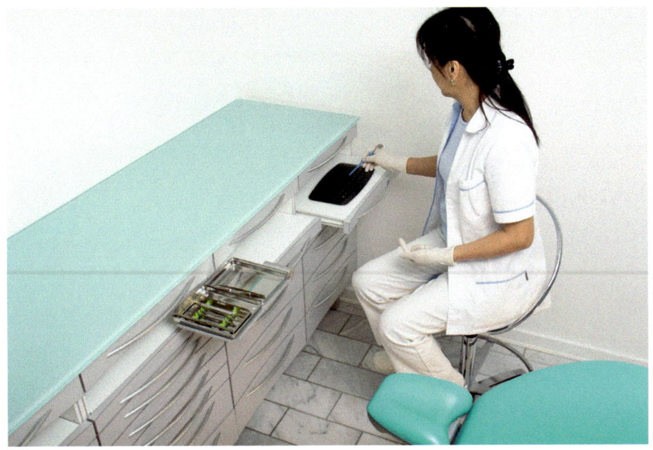

Fig 8–54 The assistant's keyboard is placed on the right pull-out workplate and the computer screen above it. On the very left module, at the dentist's side there is a pull-out workplate with a keyboard for the dentist and a computer screen above. The secondary workplate (upper one) on top of the most important drawer. The material trays are placed here when not in use.

WORKSTATION 3

The WORKSTATION 3 is a mobile cabinet with an extended tabletop and an integrated place for hand instrument trays.

This workplace will also have the same ergonometrics, and is proportioned in relation to the patient's chair as the two workplaces described above (when it is placed correctly in relation to the headrest of the horizontal backrest of the patient chair) (Fig 8–55).

The extended workplate has a support for the hand instrument tray and a working area directly beside it. Material trays of moderate size can be placed on the workplate. The dentist can use this extended workplace on their side. WORKPLACE 3 was designed by the author 40 years ago, and is still a fine support for four-handed dentistry, although the storage space is very limited.

The assistant can partially put her legs under the left side of the tabletop, and there is a place for the instruments and materials for most treatments. However for the preparation of treatments with many items, the large material tray must be placed on an adjacent tabletop.

The instrument tray support is integrated and extended 15 cm towards the front. The dentist can use the left side of the tabletop and there is a place for the dentist's legs under the tabletop. The storage area can be extended if you mount a shelf, 30 cm deep, 15 cm above the back part of the tabletop.

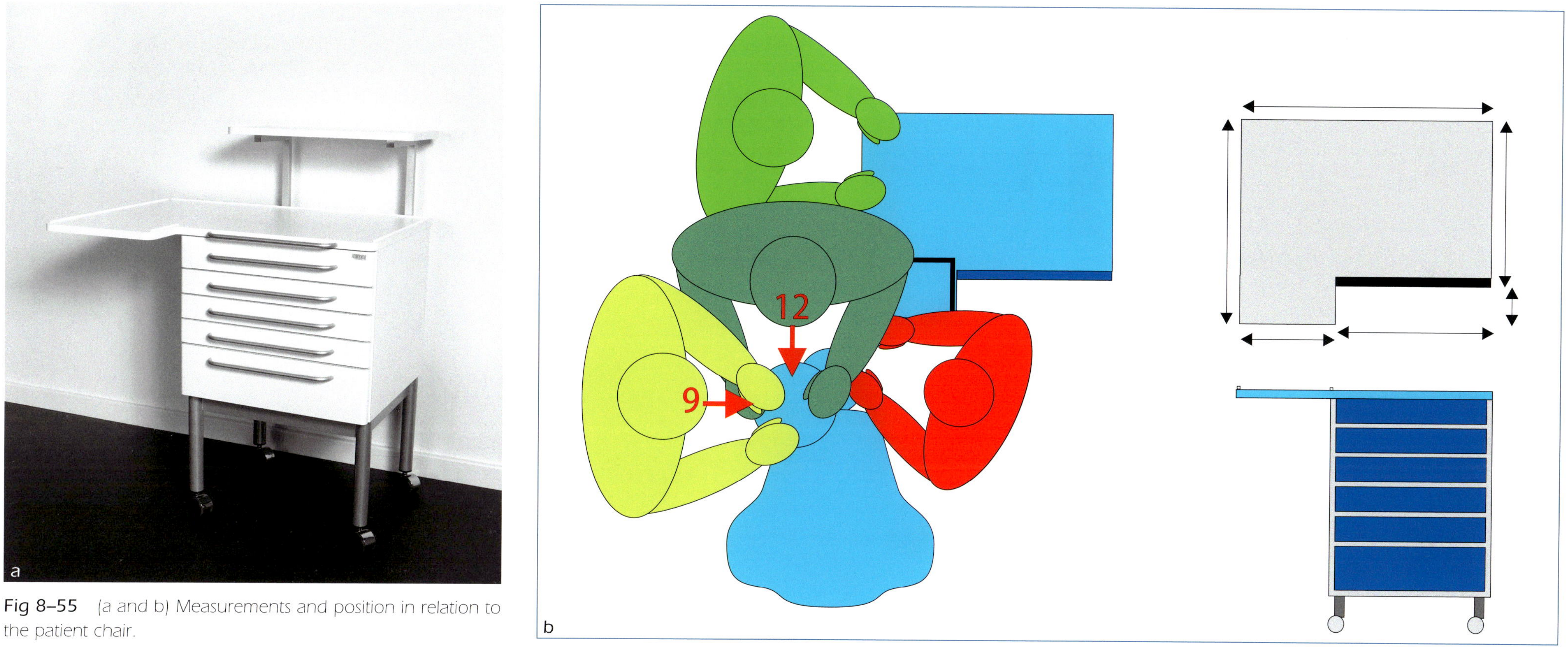

Fig 8–55 (a and b) Measurements and position in relation to the patient chair.

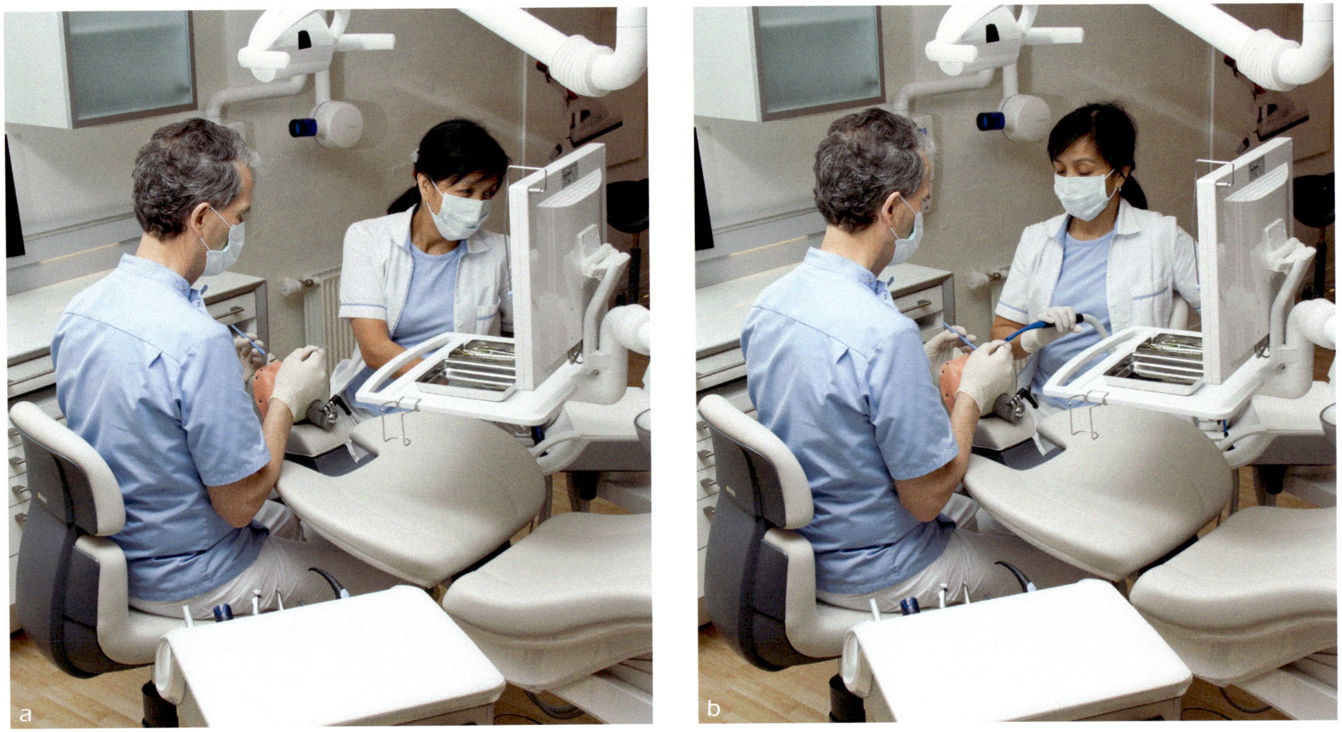

Fig 8–56 The large suction tube is picked up with the left hand (a) and transferred to the right (b).

MODIFICATIONS FOR ASSISTANCE WHEN WORKING WITH A DENTAL UNIT ON THE PATIENT'S RIGHT SIDE

Unit instruments on the right side do not support high-end assistance, and compensatory methods have to be used.

Position of hand instruments

When the unit instruments are placed on the right side of the patient, this position is often combined with a hand instrument table placed over the patient.

When the patient is reclined in a horizontal position, the patient is elevated so the distance of the dentist's eye level to the patient's mouth is about 30 to 33 cm, or if precision vision is not needed, maybe 40 cm. The dentist will work with an upwards-inclined forearm. The taller the dentist, the more upward and inclined the forearms. If the hand instrument table is placed over the patient, it will have a very high positioning, where it is difficult for the assistant to pick up instruments. The hand instrument table positioning over the patient will only be acceptable for the assistant to use if the dentist is short. If the dental unit or chair is combined with a MEGASPACE, then the hand instrument table is used here.

To conclude, unless the dentist is of below-average height (eye-to-elbow distance), the hand instrument tray should be placed at the upper left side of the patient's head. Using a workstation such as MEGASPACE or the WORKSTATION 2 or 3 enables the integration of both hand instruments and materials in four-handed assistance.

Suction holder

The suction holder is often placed to the left and behind from the assistant, who is facing the patient. The large suction tube cannot be taken directly with the right hand, but must be taken first with the left hand, and then transferred to the right.

The 3-in-1 syringe

If this is also placed in part at the left and back of the assistant, then the assistant has to twist herself to take it. A holder for the 3-in-1 syringe, mounted at the assistant's side of the instrument table over the patient, provides a much better functionality.

The unit instruments

The dentist must be able to choose different clock positions according to the direction of vision. This means that the dentist must be able to sit in a

9 o'clock position in the cases where this position ensures the best posture. The foot controller must therefore be placed at the left side of the patient's chair base, while the unit instruments are on the right side of the patient. But what is the best way to integrate unit instruments in four-handed dentistry, with the objective that the dentist retains concentration, without having to look away or reach?

This can only fully be obtained if two assistants are present chairside. The second assistant is standing (or sitting) on the right side of the dentist and prepares the unit instruments and passes them to the right hand of the dentist. The dentist does not need to look away, twist the body or reach, keeping both hands and eyes on the focus of work. Working with two assistants is a solution that was used many years ago, but is not a realistic option for most dentists anymore. A partial solution is illustrated in Figs 8–57 to 8–60:

The micromotor with contra-angle can be placed in a resting position on the hand instrument table, so it can be reached by the assistant and be integrated in a four-handed alternating transfer between the contra-angle and probe. This is a very common situation. In doing so, it is probably easier that the assistant changes the micromotor's contra-angle when another one is needed. This is simpler than the dentist returning the used micromotor with contra-angle to the holder on the dental unit, and taking a micromotor with another contra-angle.

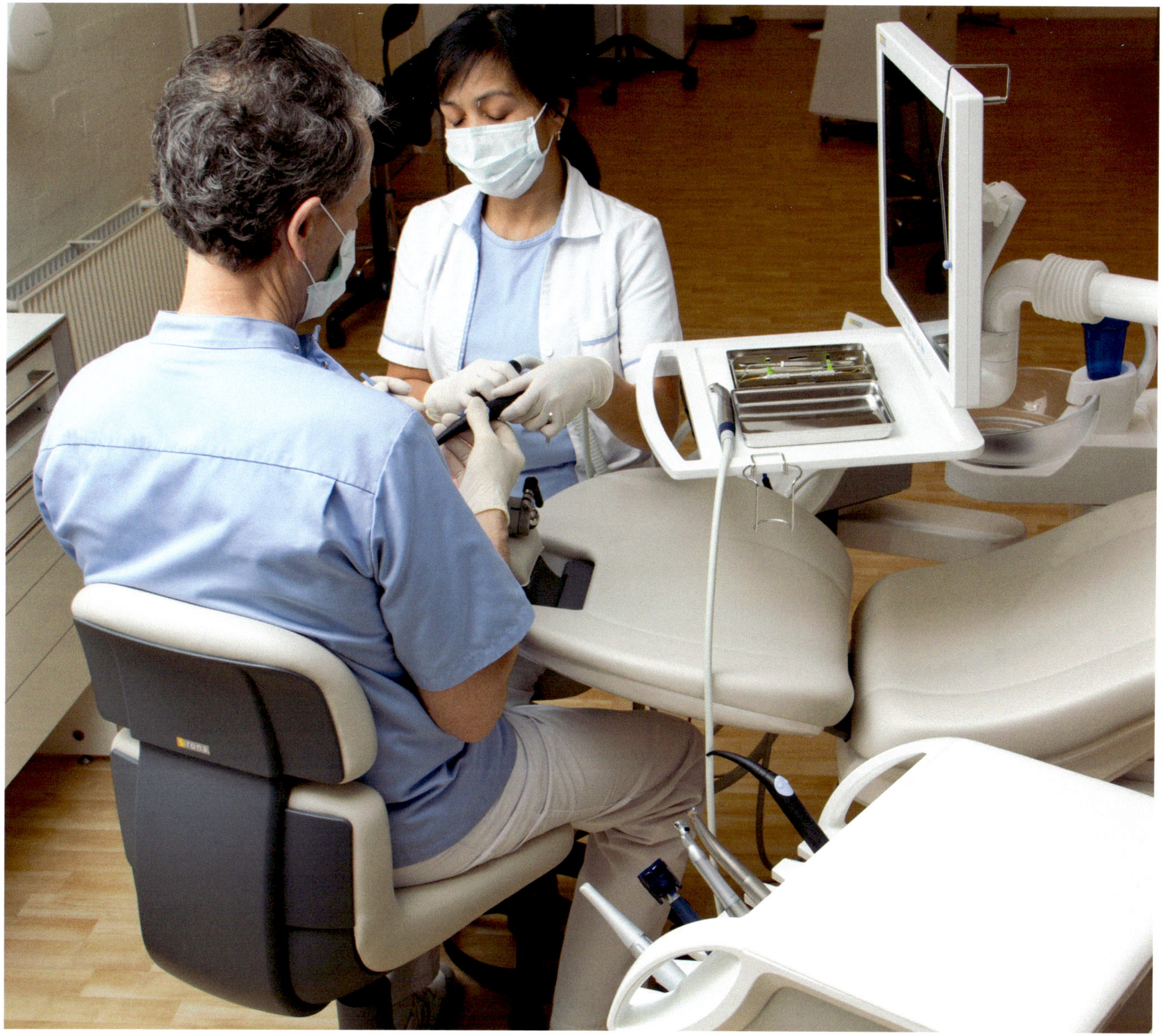

Fig 8–57 The micromotor is placed on the tray where the assistant can take it and pass it to the dentist's hand - and if needed change between probe and micromotor.

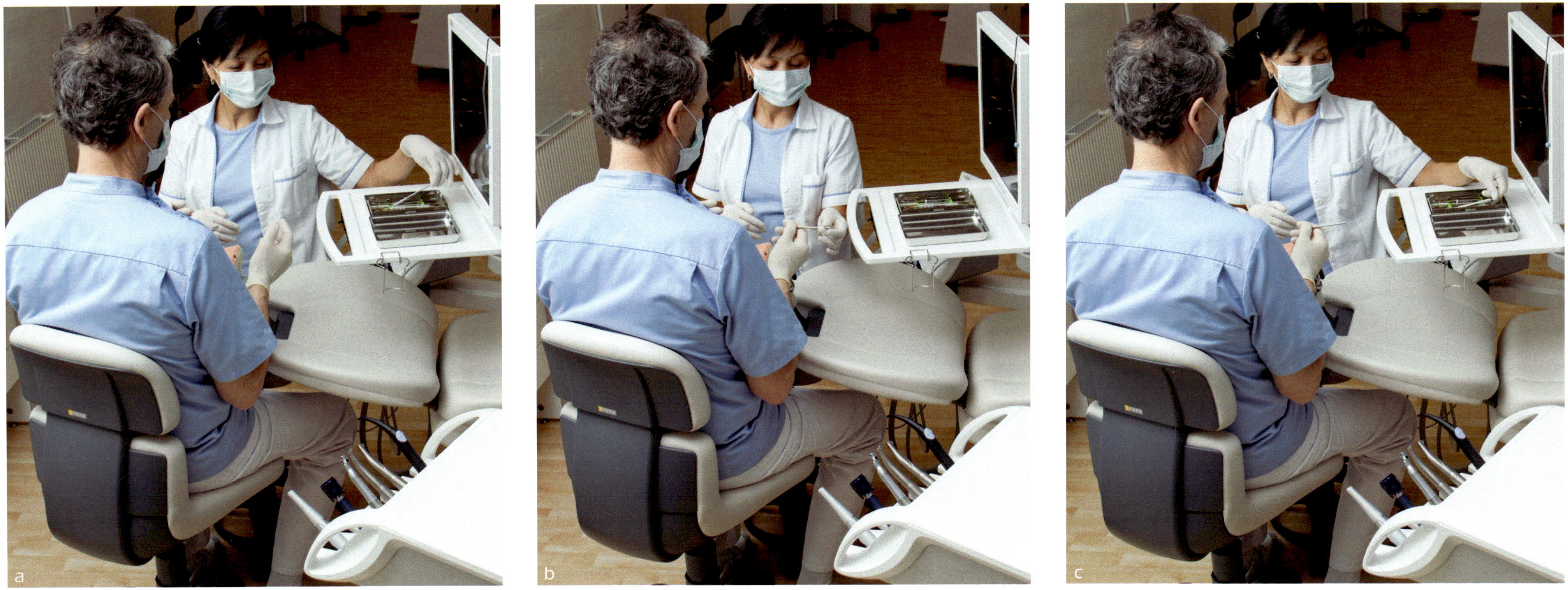

Fig 8–58 (a) The assistant takes a hand instrument... (b) ...and passes it to the dentist. (c) The assistant takes the next instrument.

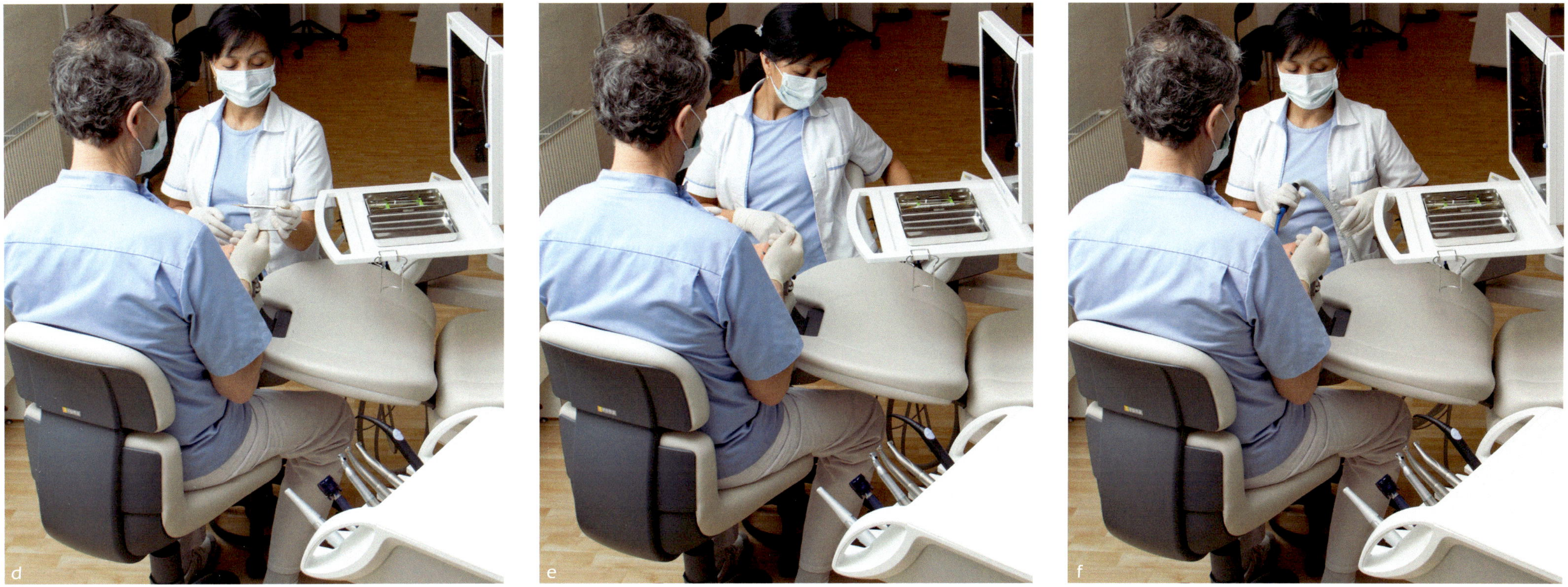

Fig 8–58 (cont) (d) The used instrument is taken and next instrument transferred to the dentist. (e) The assistant now takes the aspiration tube with her left hand, and (f) then passes it to her right hand.

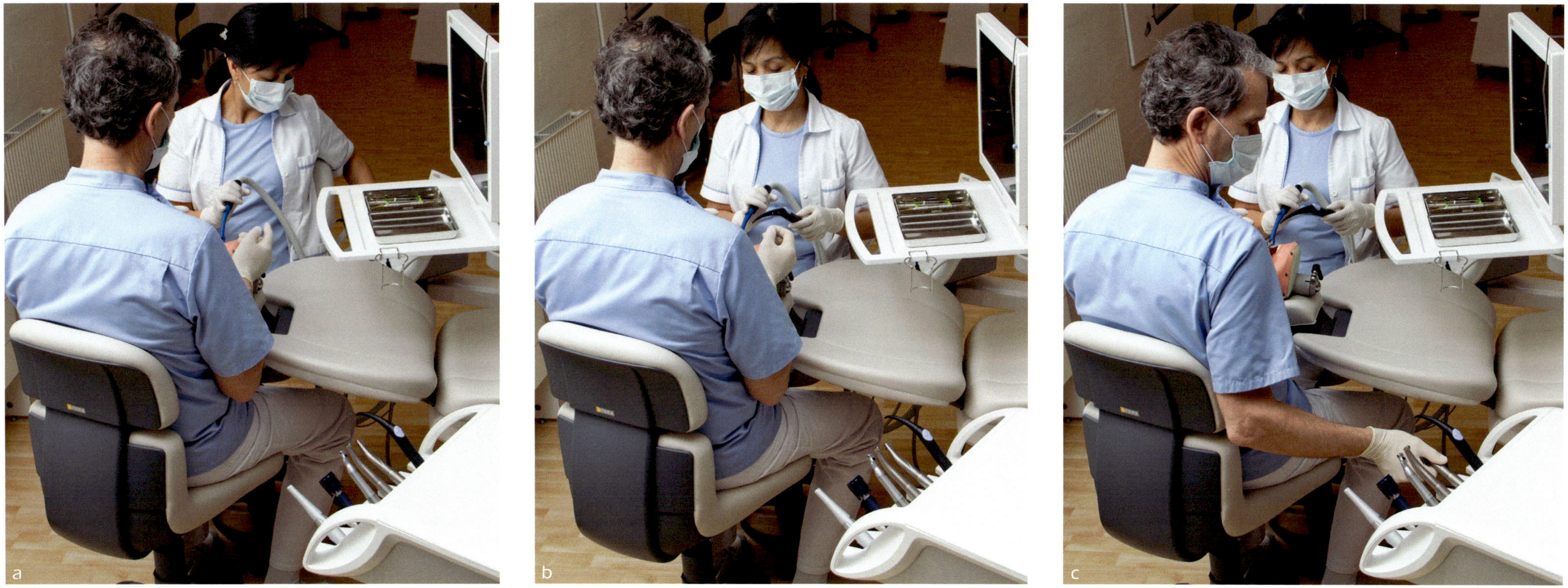

Fig 8–59 *(a) The assistant takes the 3-in-1 syringe. (b) It is then ready to use by the dentist. (c) The dentist takes the micromotor with red contra-angle.*

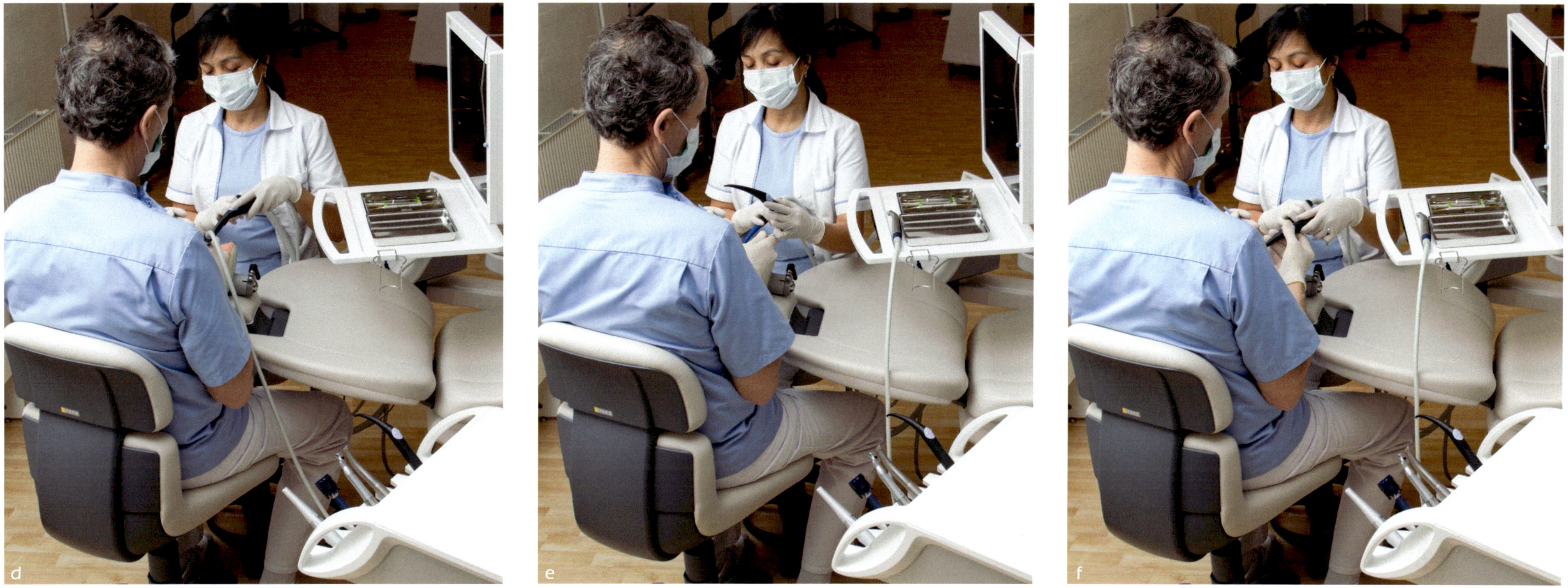

Fig 8–59 (cont) (d) The assistant is drying the mirror, in preparation for use in the maxilla. (e) The dentist has placed the micromotor on the hand instrument table, taken a hand instrument and then finished using it. The assistant takes the used hand instrument, and (f) passes the 3-in-1 syringe to the dentist.

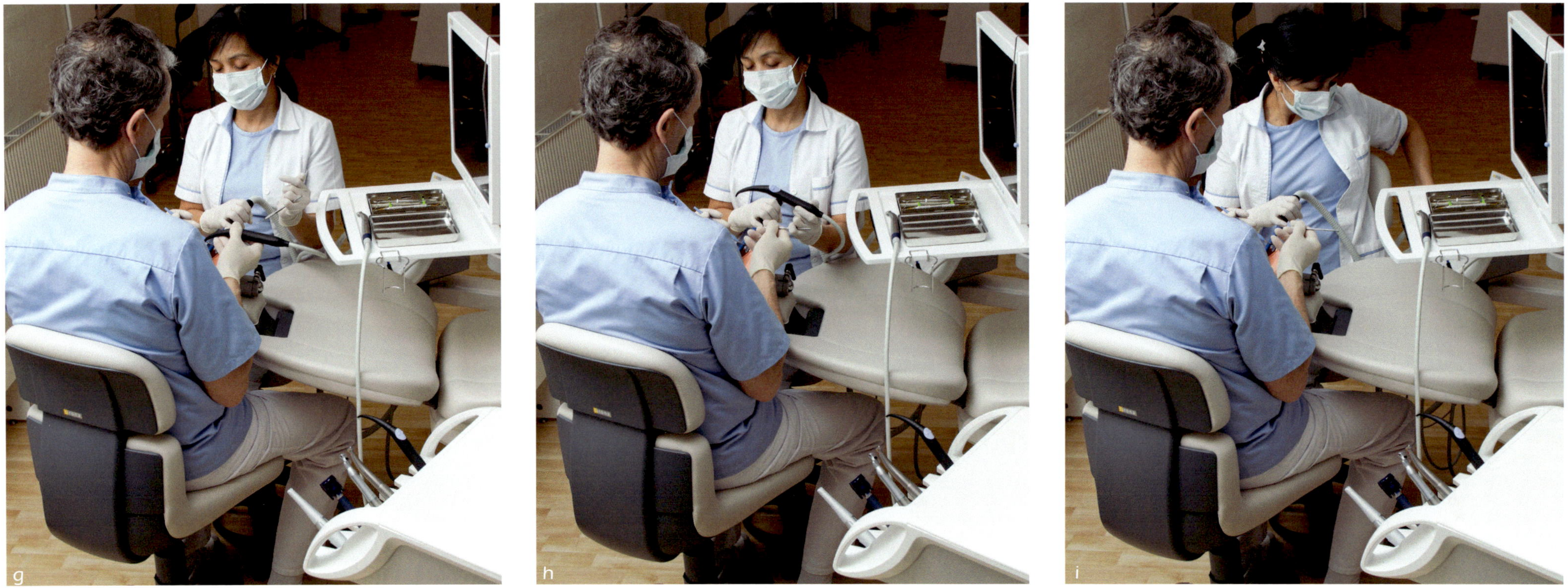

Fig 8–59 (cont) (g) The dentist has finished using the 3-in-1 syringe. The assistant is ready with the hand instrument in her little finger. (h) The assistant takes the 3-in-1 syringe and places the hand instrument in the dentist's hand. (i) The 3-in-1 syringe is placed back on the holder.

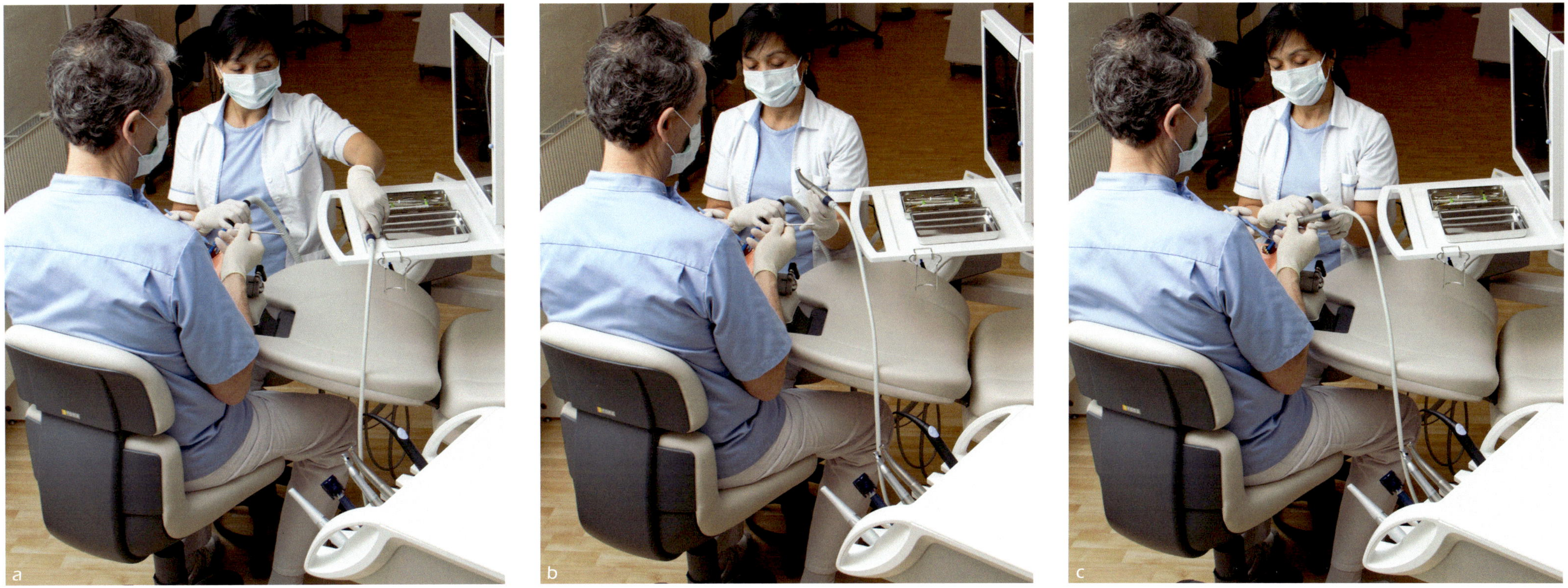

Fig 8–60 (a) The dentist has finished using the hand instrument, and the assistant is picking up the micromotor placed on the hand instrument tray. All the time, the assistant keeps the aspiration tube in her right hand. (b) The assistant takes the used instrument and is ready to transfer the micromotor to the dentist's hand. (c) The dentist is working with a new unit instrument.

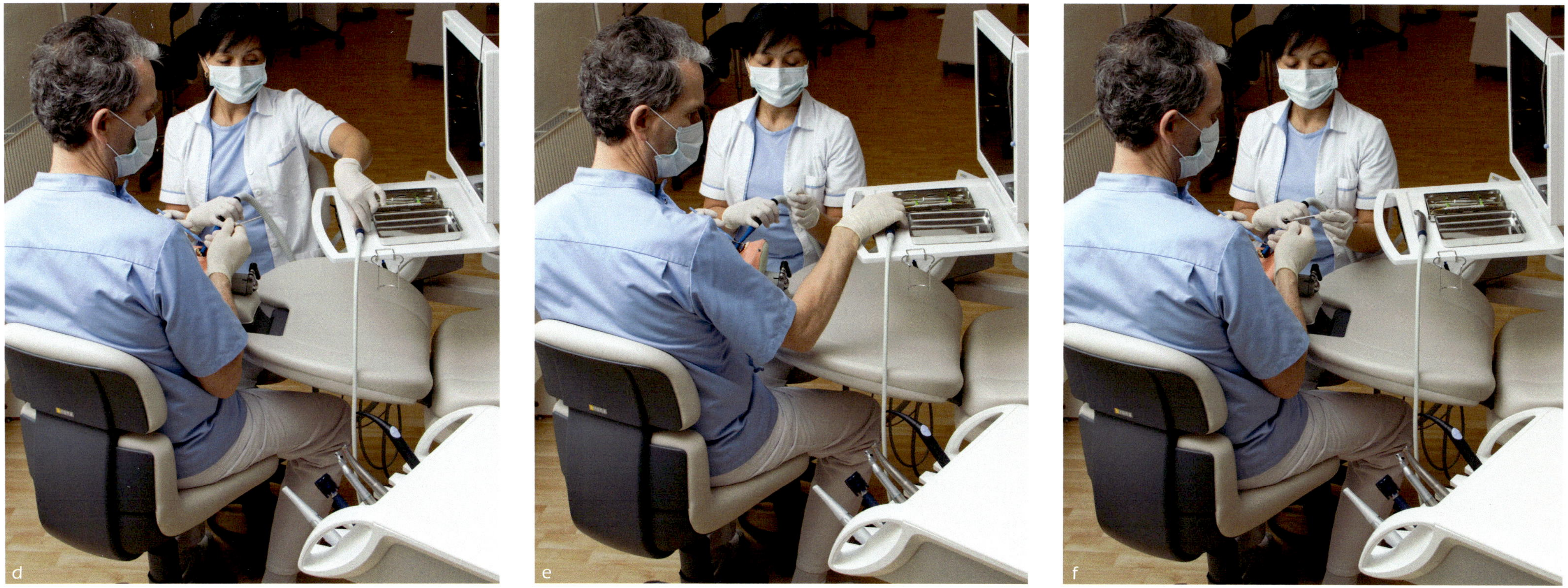

Fig 8–60 (cont) (d) The micromotor is again placed on the hand instrument table. (e) The dentist can now take the micromotor himself if the assistant is occupied. The dentist does not need to twist the spine to take the unit instrument (while sitting in a 9 to 10 o'clock position). (f) Using these modifications, one unit instrument at a time can be reached by both dentist and assistant, and be integrated into the assistance methods.

TEAM DENTISTRY

Modifications for the dental unit in a 12 o'clock position

This arrangement of unit instruments is very rare in Europe, due to its lack of functionality. (The author was not able to find one to photograph for this book either!) The dental unit may, depending on its position in relation to the headrest of the horizontal patient chair, hinder the dentist from being able to work in a 12 o'clock position, when this position is necessary to have direct vision to the left side of the teeth.

The dentist cannot grasp the unit instruments with his right hand, so the unit instruments have to be transferred to the dentist by the assistant. As the unit instrument tube is fixed behind the patient, the tube has to pass around the head of the patient, in most cases on the assistant's side.

If the dentist needs to take a unit instrument themselves, he must take it first with the left hand and pass it to the right hand, while arranging the unit instrument tube over the legs on their side. Aspiration tubes may be taken by the assistant's right hand and kept there for use. The hand instrument table needs to be placed further away, so it may not be possible for the dentist to grasp a hand instrument unaided. Alternating a four-handed shift between a unit instrument and hand instrument is also possible. In general, the dentist will be very dependent on the assistant, and working SOLO is not an easy solution.

Chapter 9

ORGANIZATION OF HAND INSTRUMENTS AND MATERIALS

HAND INSTRUMENT SYSTEM ORGANIZATION

The organization of the hand instruments must be adapted to the best work methods, and not the reverse.

Organizing and functional grouping for hand instruments

A traditional solution for the organization of hand instruments can be described as follows. Hand instruments are stored in drawers placed on open instrument supports. When the instruments are needed they are picked up from the drawer one by one.

If a treatment, eg, a composite filling, is needed in the same session, then the instruments for this are picked from the drawers as per the above. Then later when the treatment is finished, all hand instruments are collected and carried to the sterilization room. Here, after some time they form a pile of instruments, which may be stored in a pre-disinfection bath in a closed ventilated cabinet, to protect the assistant from breathing in the vapors from the disinfection liquid. The assistant (now wearing thick rubber gloves) takes the instruments and rinses them under cold water, inspecting each one and cleaning when necessary with a little bronze brush and detergent. Then again the instruments are placed approximately in a low pile on an autoclave tray, and sterilized in the autoclave. Then the autoclave tray is carried to the treatment room, the actual drawers are opened, and the instruments are positioned in the drawer holders. If two or more dentists are sharing a practice, the instruments may be mixed and will need to be sorted.

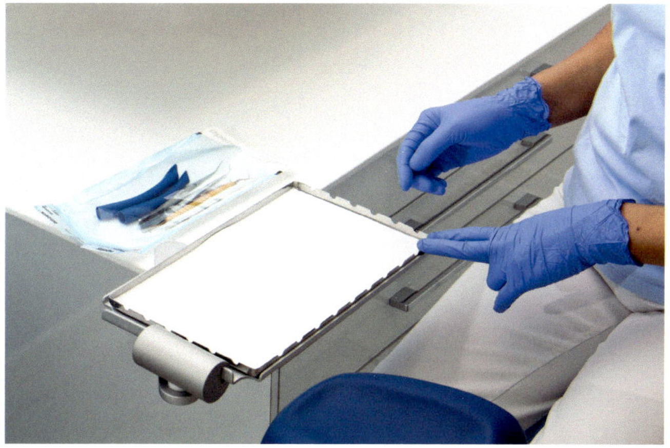

Fig 9–1 Hand instruments ready for the dental examination, in a sterile paper bag.

This procedure is complex and very time consuming. Furthermore, the hand instruments are stored openly in drawers on the instrument supports, which in many cases are not disinfected regularly.

Grouping of hand instruments

Instead of collecting hand instruments one by one, the instruments are organized according to their use. The most simple grouping is to place the hand instruments for a certain procedure in sealed paper bags for sterilization (Fig 9–1).

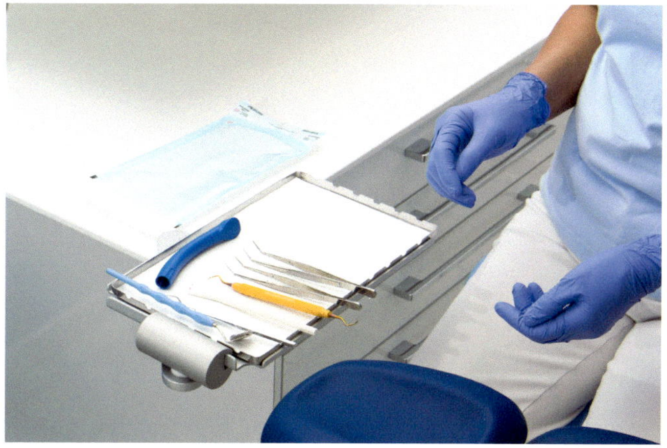

Fig 9–2 Hand instruments on an open tray.

Examples of examination instruments:

- straight probe
- double ended curved probe
- periodontal probe
- two tweezers – one for use in the patient's mouth and one (marked with a colored ring) for picking up cotton rolls and small materials.

The sterile paper bag is opened and the instruments are arranged on a serviette, or better still, on an open tray (Fig 9–2). The chairside assistant cleans the hand instruments that come into contact with materials like liners, cements, composites etc, with a wipe immediately after use, before any hardening. This means that further visual inspection and manual cleaning in the sterilization process is no longer necessary. The instruments for examination are supplemented with the instruments used for treatments.

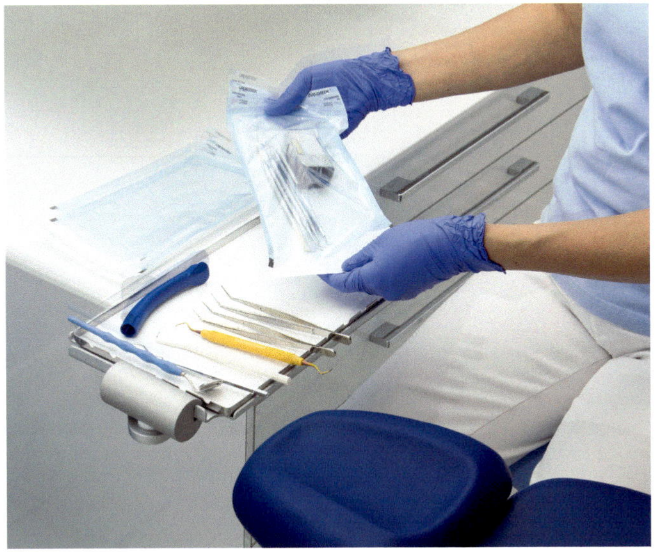

Fig 9–3 Hand instruments for composite in a sterile paper bag.

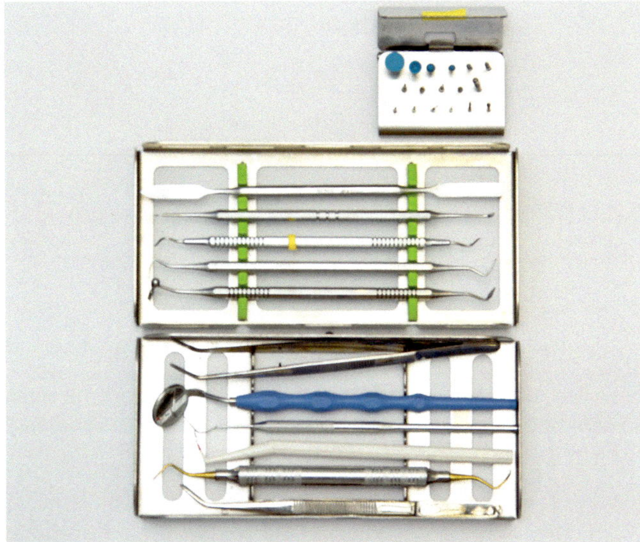

Fig 9–4 Instruments ready for use in an examination on a tray, with composite instruments alongside in a second tray.

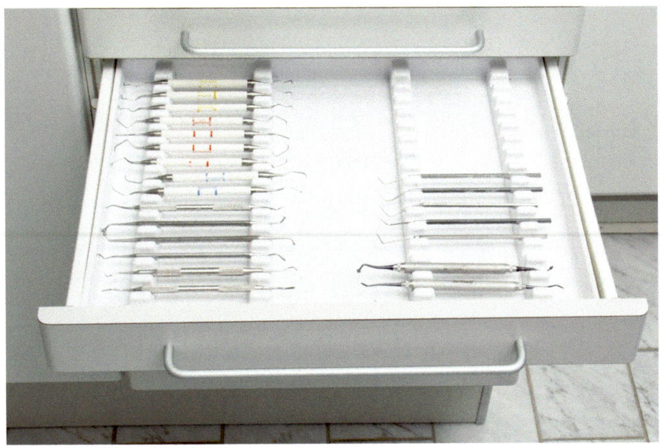

Fig 9–5 Hand instrument storage in a drawer. The plastic insert cannot be sterilized or disinfected in a thermodisinfector. The hand instruments are not stored in a manner that preserves sterility and have to be sterilized regularly, combined with disinfection of the drawer insert.

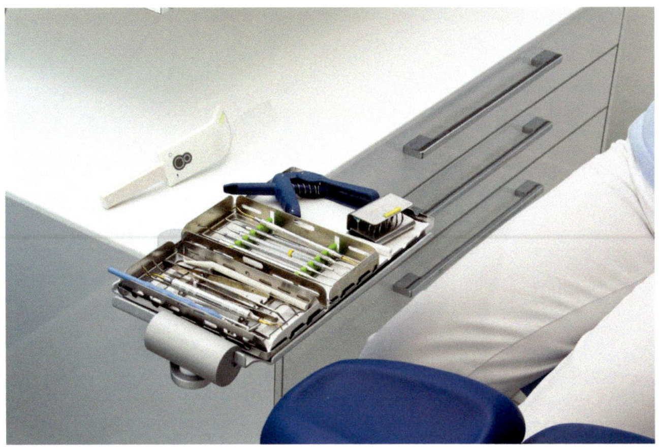

Fig 9–6 Instrument clip for examination and for composite placed on a serviette.

Instruments for treatments

The instruments for a given treatment are also organized in sterile paper bags. If a treatment needs to be performed, then a paper bag containing the required instruments is picked up from a drawer and opened, and the instruments placed on a serviette or tray as shown in Fig 9–3.

After the appointment has finished, the assistant separates the hand instruments used for the examination from those used for the treatment (Figs 9–4 and 9–5). Then each "handful" of instruments is placed in a separate compartment of the instrument washing machine, so they are not mixed.

The hand instrument clip

The use of hand instrument clips is a further improvement for hand instrument organization. It is a clip holder for the instruments, which can be closed when the instruments are not in use. The instruments are always placed in the same sequence in the holder. They may be marked with colored rings, so one can see at a glance if the instruments are placed correctly.

The hand instruments are cleaned chairside with a wipe placed on the instrument holder's metal edge, for materials like liner, cement and composite, before they harden as described on page 179 (Fig 9–6).

When the appointment is finished, the clip is closed and placed directly in fitted holders in the instrument washing machine. After washing, they

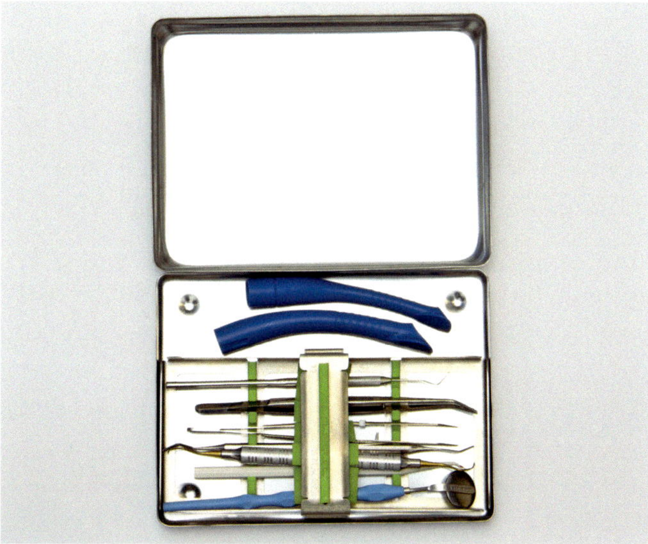

Fig 9–7 A half-size tray with an instrument clip for hand instruments is used for an examination. In the cassette, a large suction tube and a tip for the 3-in-1 syringe is placed too. The clip is closed.

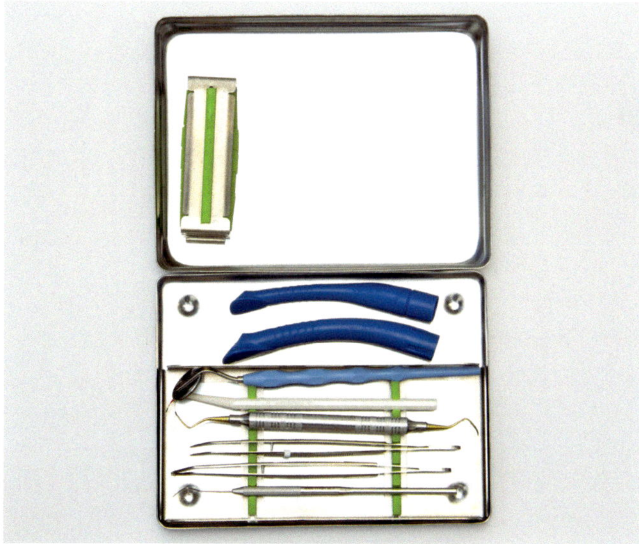

Fig 9–8 The clip is opened.

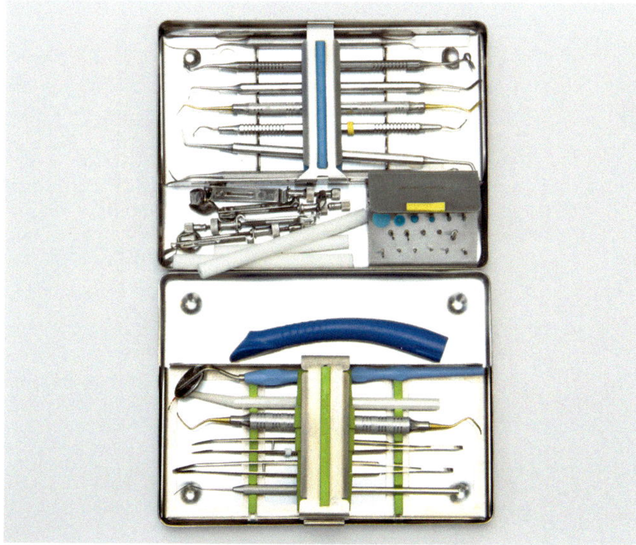

Fig 9–9 An examination cassette and a cassette for composite with an instrument clip for composite instruments, bur stand for composite, matrix systems and cotton rolls.

are placed in a sterilized paper bag, sealed and sterilized. There are a number of different instrument clips on the market; some examples will now follow.

Instrument clips in a cassette with cover

A hand instrument cassette is made of metal, with a bottom and a cover. Aluminium has been used, but cleaning in the instrument washing machine from sterilization corrodes the anodized surface, and after a long time causes visibly heavy discoloration and corrosion. However, stainless steel has become the material of preference. One can, when needed, polish the surface of stainless steel with a polishing paste used for glass ceramics, for example.

Standardized trays are used for grouping hand instruments. They exist in a full size version 28.0 × 18.5 cm, and in a half size version 14 × 18.5 cm. Instrument clips, like those shown above, are placed in the cassette. There is also room for bur stands, etc. When the tray is open, the cover may be used as a supplementary sterile "work surface."

The use of half-trays gives flexibility. The basic tray with instruments for examination is always used, with supplementary trays being an additional option for specific treatments:

- For just examinations, only a basic tray is needed.
- For a composite filling, a composite tray is added to the basic tray.
- If an amalgam filling is made, an amalgam tray is added, etc.

See Figs 9–7 to 9–12 for examples of trays used for surgery. According to your needs, you may have different full- or half-size trays for the treatment room.

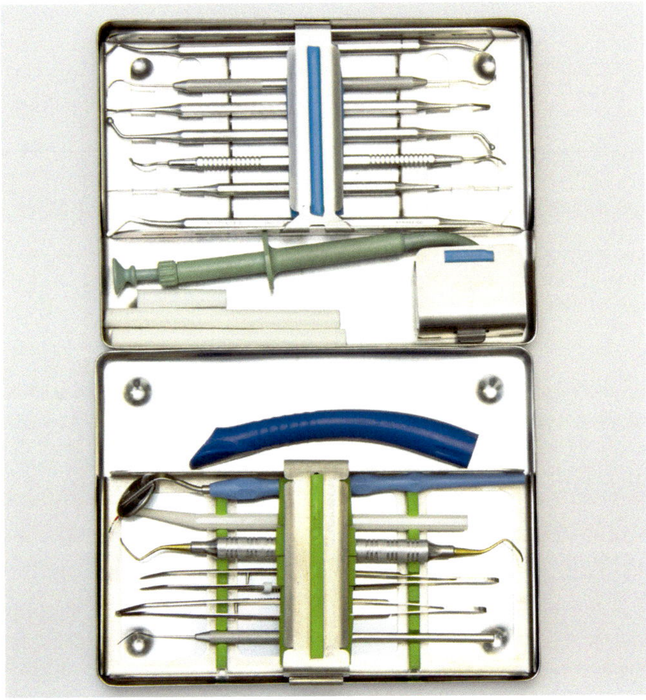

Fig 9–10 An examination cassette and an amalgam cassette (if amalgam is used).

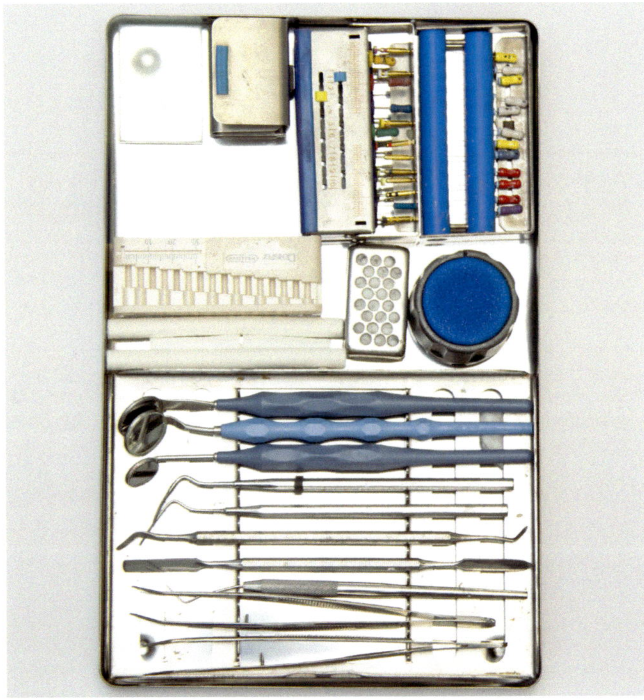

Fig 9–11 An endo cassette with an instrument clip for 10 hand instruments. The collapsible file stands (Nicrominox) are fitted with several files, each of smaller sizes. (The bur stand is also Nicrominox.) The file measuring block is from Maillefer, and the file stand is called an "interim stand" or a fileholder. The endo tray is used together with the large endo-material tray.

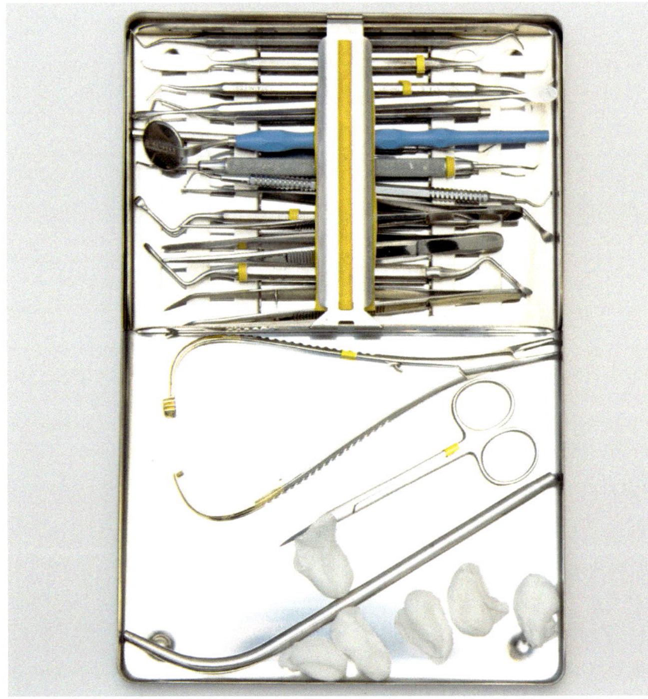

Fig 9–12 A full size surgery cassette.

Half cassette

- composite
- amalgam (if used)
- endodontic treatment
- subgingival scaling
- minor surgery
- suture cut-tray.

Standard cassette

- surgery standard
- periodontal surgery
- "micro" surgery
- elevators and forceps for roots
- rubber dam tray.

Additional hand instruments, which not are present in the instrument clip, are placed in sterilized paper bags, in a drawer (Fig 9–13).

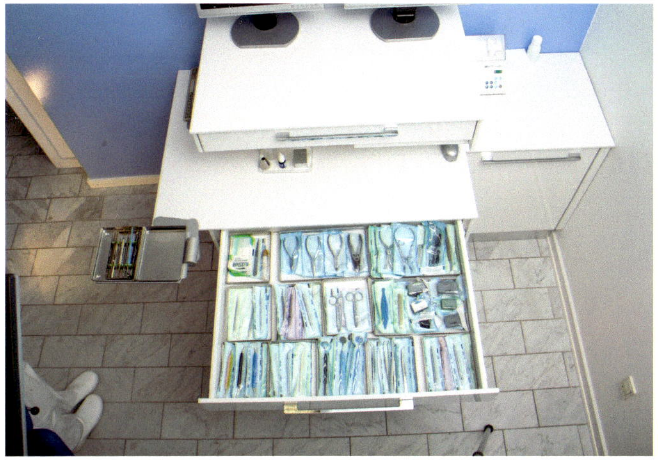

Fig 9–13 Refill of instruments from a drawer.

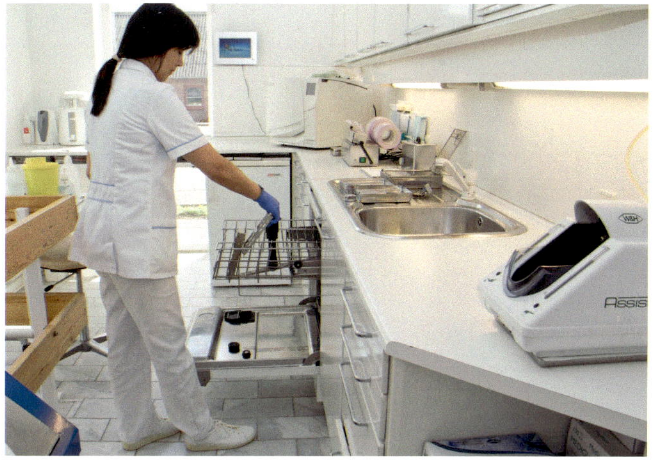

Fig 9–14 Closed instrument clips with hand instruments and cassettes being placed in the instrument washing machine. The segmented pre- and post-vacuum autoclave assures sterilization in the closed cassettes.

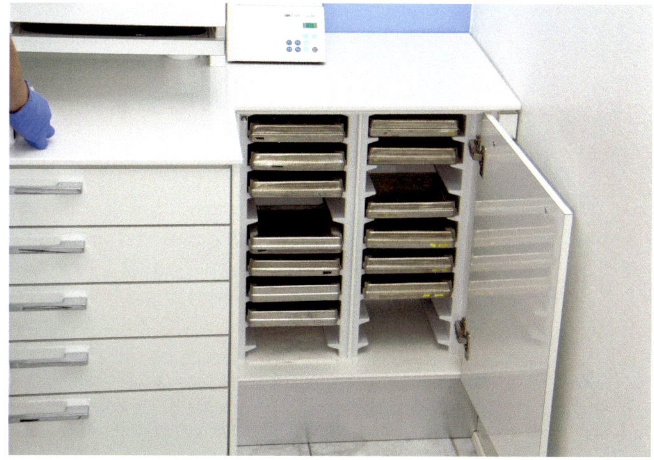

Fig 9–15 The cabinet for cassettes.

Refill of instrument clips from refill drawer

With the MEGASPACE workplace, the second lower drawer refill instruments are placed in sterile paper bags. Extra hand instruments, identical to those in the instrument clips, are stored here (Figs 9–14 to 9–16). If by accident a hand instrument is missing in the instrument clips, then another can be found in this drawer. This also applies if a new mirror is needed, or if an instrument has slipped out from the dentist or assistant's hand and fallen on the floor (Fig 9–17).

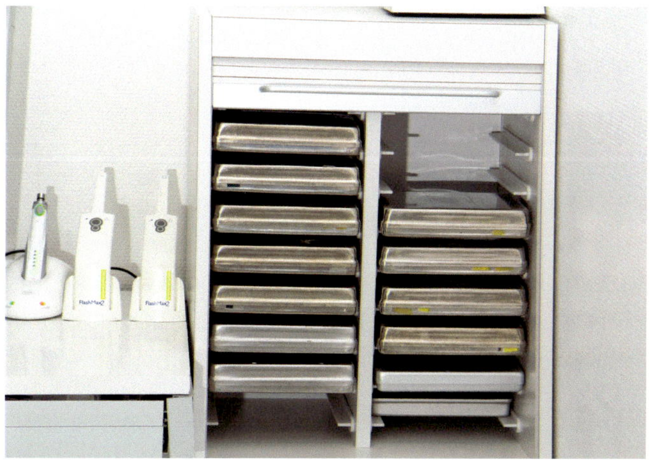

Fig 9–16 The cabinet for cassettes, version 2.

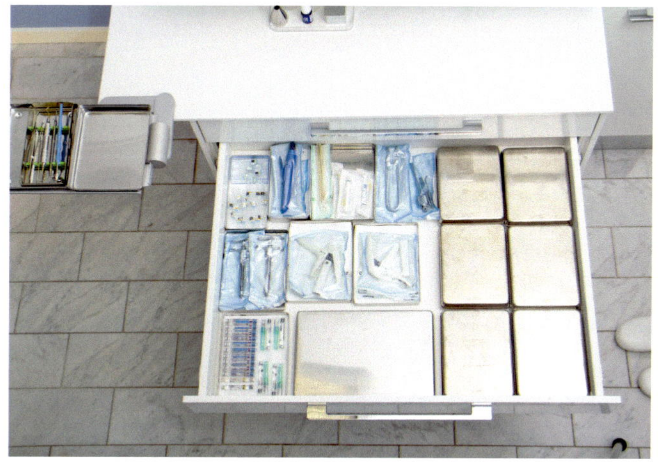

Fig 9–17 Cassettes stored in drawer. There is two of each type: when one is used, it is replaced by another.

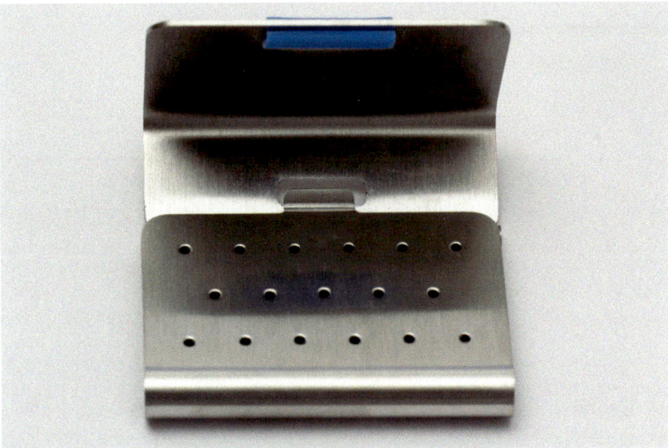

Fig 9–18 A bur stand in stainless steel.

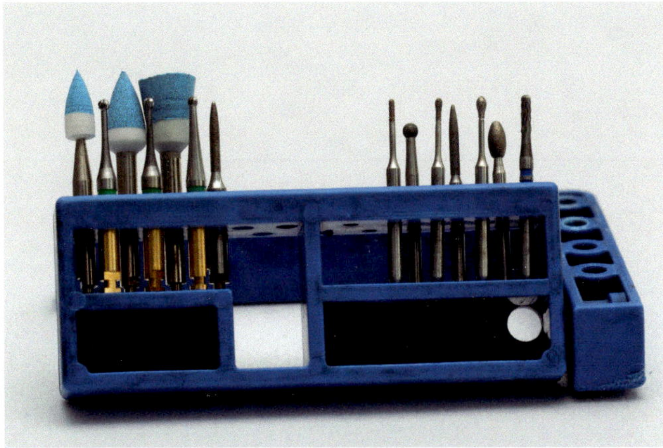

Fig 9–19 An example of a plastic bur stand, fitted out for composite.

ORGANIZING ROTATING INSTRUMENTS

Functional grouping

In many practices the rotating instruments, such as burs and diamonds, are placed in an open bur stand. If it is not protected by a cover or placed in a drawer, then airborne spray droplets will contaminate it. We also know that touching infected gingival margins may result in bacterioemia. This can happen even from eating, brushing teeth or using interproximal cleaning.

Rotating instruments will very often touch infected gingival areas, so contamination of instruments from airborne spray droplets may cause cross infection and the intrusion of bacteria into the patient's blood vessels. Combining this knowledge with the increased risk from multi-resistant bacteria, as well as viruses such as hepatitis and HIV, leads to the conclusion that the use of rotating instruments is potentially invasive. Therefore, the protective measures used for sterilization should be upheld.

The treatment-specific bur stand

Similarly to how hand instruments are grouped, the most used rotating instruments for a specific treatment are selected and placed in a treatment-specific bur stand (Figs 9–18 to 9–20). So, say in perhaps 90% or more of cases, no other rotating instruments are necessary. In about 10% or less of cases, a specified bur or diamond may be taken from a chairside supplementary bur stand.

The treatment-specific bur stand can be made of metal with holes for friction grip burs/diamonds (high speed contra-angle or turbine/air rotor) with a diameter of 1.60 mm, and for burs for normal contra-angles with a diameter of 2.35 mm.

Modification of the bur stand

If the holes for friction grip burs/diamonds need to be enlarged for use with 2.35 mm burs, it is easy and quick to enlarge the holes using a drill with a precise 2.40 mm diameter.

Refill bur stand

After the rotating instruments are used chairside, they are placed back in the bur stand. When the treatment is finished, the content of the stand is checked. If a bur or diamond is lacking because it is lost or disposed, then a new bur is taken at a chairside refill bur stand, where extras of all rotating instruments from the treatment-specific bur stands are kept (Fig 9–21).

The refill bur stand is either placed protected in the inner part of the "most important drawer," or it is put under its cover. It should be placed at the dentist's side of the drawer, so they can take a bur or diamond too (with tweezers). The refill bur stand is refilled and sterilized once a day, from the refill drawer in the sterilization room (Fig 9–22).

The chairside assistant is responsible for ensuring that the bur stand already holds the rotating instruments, as described in the protocol for this treatment. (A photo of the different bur stands may be placed chairside in a visible place.) She provides the refill if necessary. This

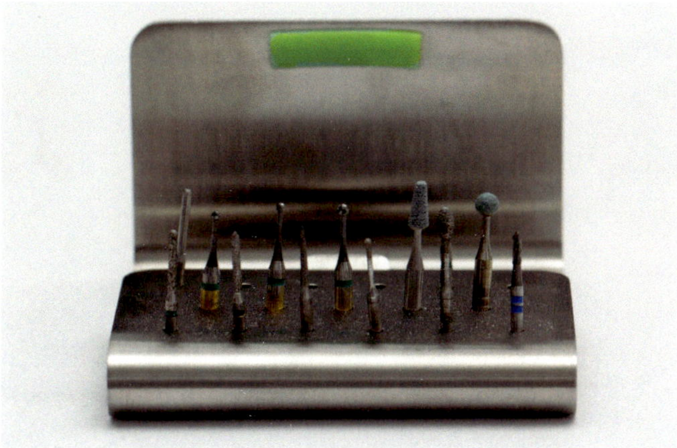

Fig 9–20 A stainless steel bur stand here fitted out for crown preparation.

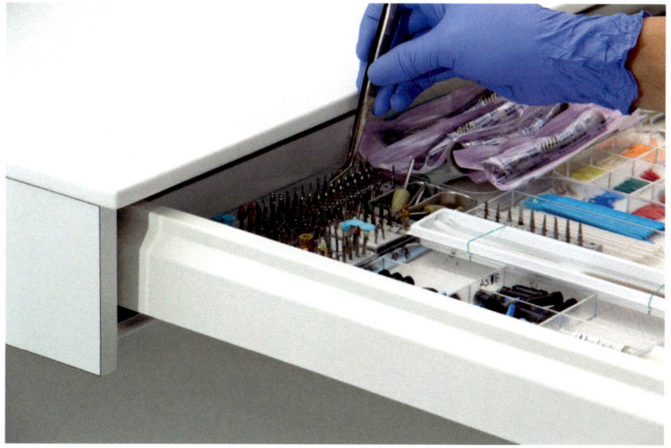

Fig 9–21 A supplementing and refill bur stand with extra burs and diamonds, which are picked up using tweezers. Both dentist and assistant are able to reach them.

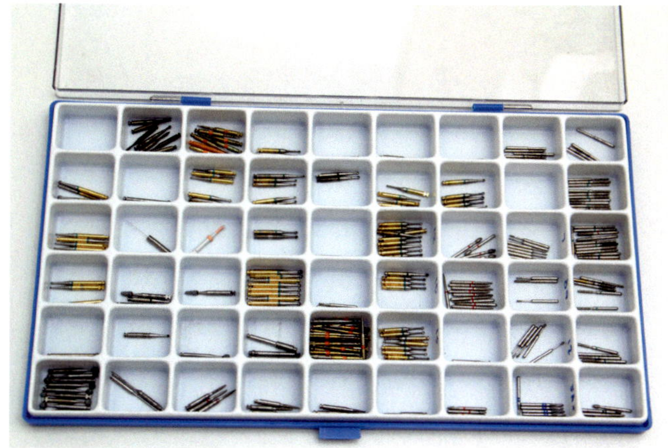

Fig 9–22 Refill bur stand replenished by the refill drawer in sterilization.

procedure is much faster to perform chairside than later on in the sterilization room, because the assistant is already giving her full attention to the bur stand.

After the patient's appointment, the bur stand is closed and placed in an ultrasonic bath for cleaning and disinfection. Then afterwards it is packed (in a paper bag or treatment cassette) and sterilized in the autoclave. The refill bur stand is sterilized once a day, after refilling in the autoclave (the author's preference).

Storage

The treatment-specific bur stands are stored in closed sterile cassettes or in sterile paper bags (Figs 9–23 to 9–25).

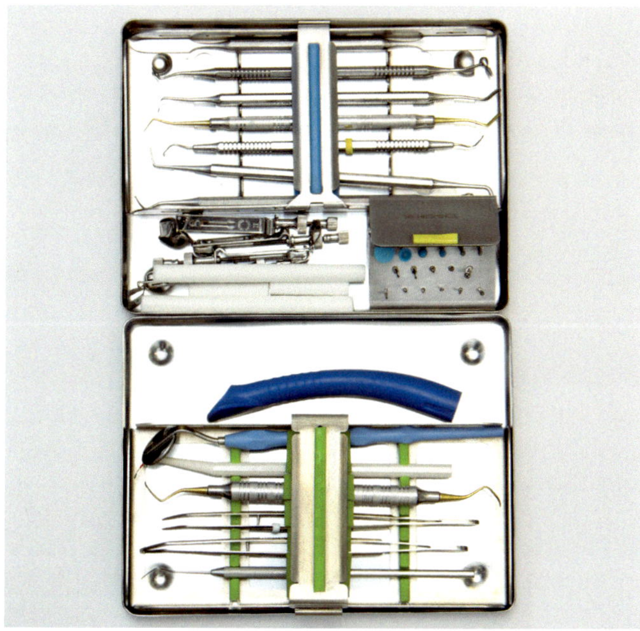

Fig 9–23 A bur stand in a cassette.

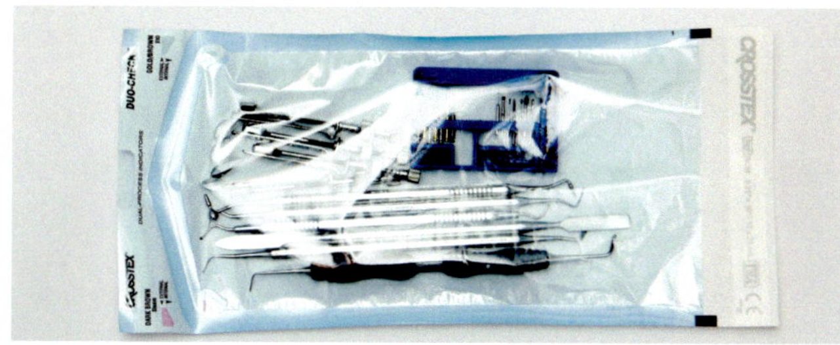

Fig 9–24 The bur stand in sterile paper bags, together with hand instruments.

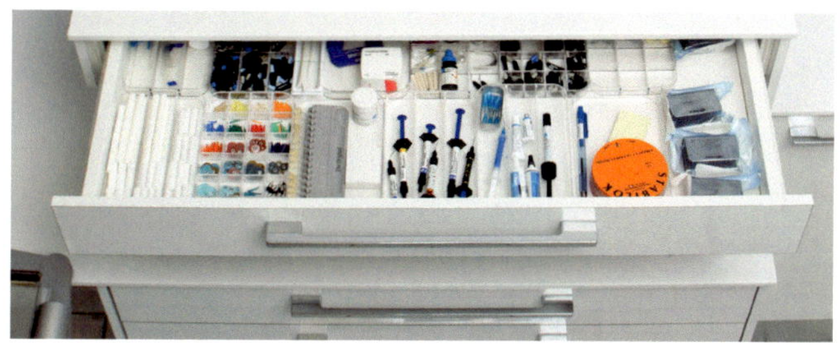

Fig 9–25 The "most important drawer" with bur stands in sterile paper bags at the right side of the drawer.

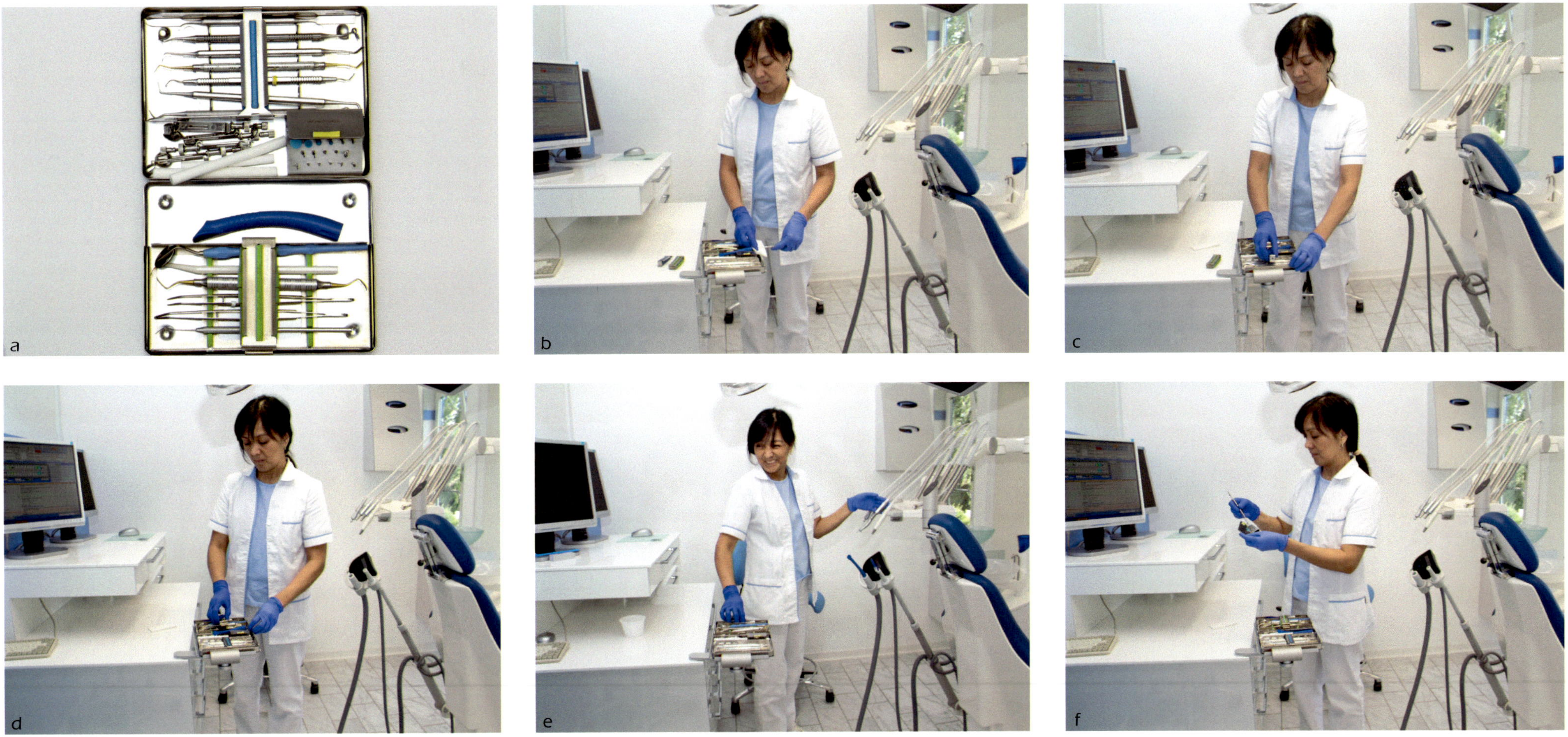

Fig 9–26 (a) A basic cassette with hand instruments ready for examination, and composite cassette ready for use. (b) The hand instruments used for composite, liner, cement etc, are cleaned with a wipe. (c) The treatment is finished and the assistant checks that all hand instruments are present and are lying in the clip in the correct position and sequence, according to the protocol. (d) Both clips are closed. (e) "Parking position" of unit instruments close to the tray: contra-angles, the tip of a 3-in-1 syringe, inserts, and suction are dismounted from the dental unit and placed on the tray. Used burs are dismounted from the contra-angles and placed in the bur stand. (f) The assistant checks that all burs and diamonds are present and placed in the correct position, according to the protocol.

Cycles for the use of instruments and burs

The instrument washing machine is run shortly after each consultation, to wash the used instruments. If the instrument washing machine is not full, then a cold water rinse program may be run (Fig 9–26).

After washing, the contents are placed in the cassettes, while the contra-angles are also packed in sterile paper bags and sterilized in the pre- and

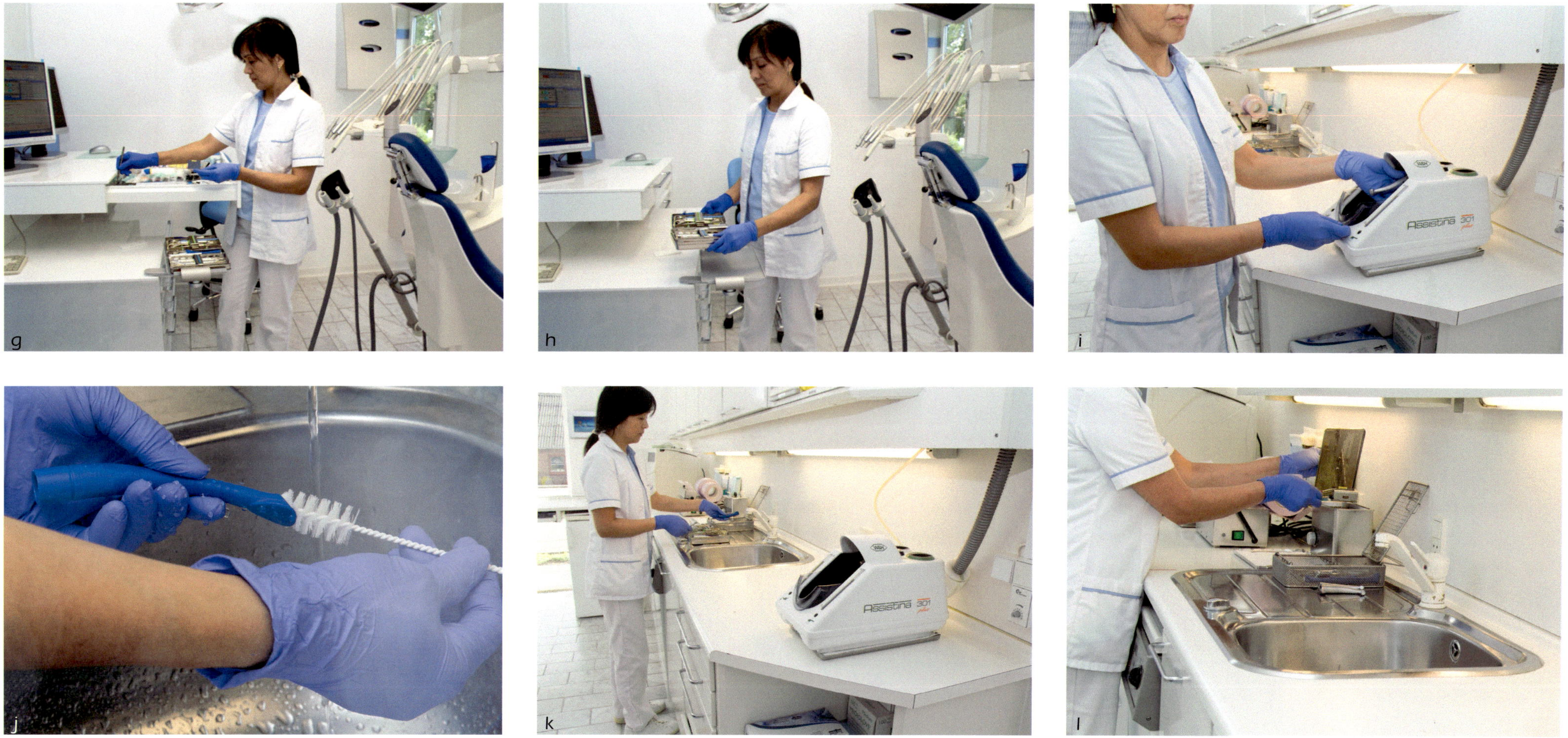

Fig 9–26 (cont) (g) A bur is taken from the refill stand. (h) Cassettes are carried to the sterilization room. (i) Contra-angles are placed in the lubrication and surface disinfection apparatus. (j) The large suction tubes are rinsed and cleaned from the inside out with a manual brush. (k) Suction tubes, the tip of the 3-in-1 syringe and the matrix system etc, are placed in the next box for the instrument washing machine. (l) The closed bur stand is placed in an ultrasonic cleaning bath.

post vacuum autoclave. No separate hand instruments, burs or diamonds are touched or handled in the sterilization room. This and the rinsing/running program of the instrument washing machine makes the pre-disinfection bath unnecessary. Only the occasional use of a supplementary instrument or bur/diamonds needs to be handled individually. Using this procedure can save much of the assistant's time.

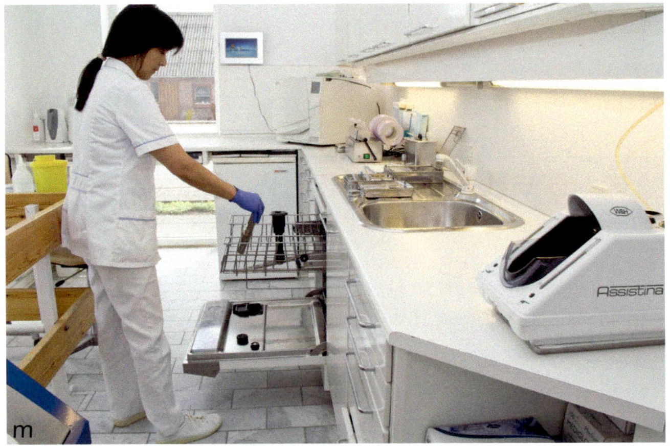

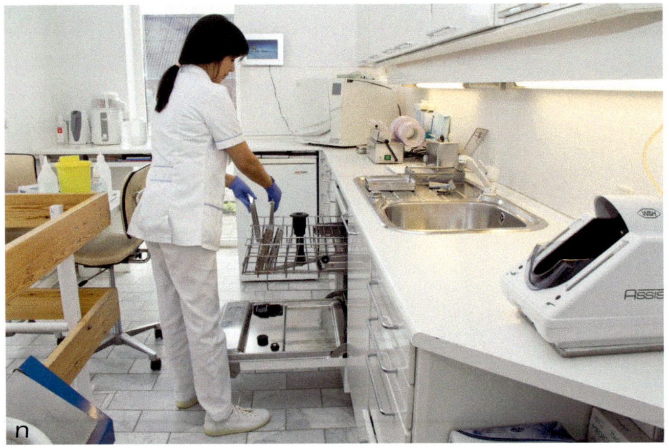

Fig 9–26 (cont) (m) The instrument clips are placed in the instrument washing machine. (n) Cassettes in the instrument washing machine.

DISINFECTION AND STERILIZATION

The standards and regulations for hygiene, disinfection and sterilization vary accordingly from country to country. They differ even more when regarding the standards in individual dental practices. The "opinions" for what is optimal or acceptable vary much. Standards are also always changing, so what may be acceptable one year, may not be so in a few years.

Changes in the widespread opinions held by dentists can take a very long time. For example, the sterilizing of contra-angles began with the spread of hepatitis in the late 1980s, but in some countries 25 years later the sterilization of contra-angles is still a matter of debate. There is often a vigorous discussion between scientists and practitioners about standards of hygiene, because some programs lead to considerable costs. Every practitioner has to make their own choices, and there is always something that could be improved.

The author of this book follows and participates in this discussion in different countries, but has decided not to go into this discussion here. But it is fair to describe the author's **personal** reflections and protocol for hygiene circa 2012, because this influences in part the organization of instruments and materials in the previous chapters.

The author knows that in order to develop a protocol for hygiene, a lot of priorities and details may be discussed before reaching any conclusions; some may find the following information insufficient, while others may find it too much!

The author's point of view is as follows:

1. Some of our patients may be infected with the hepatitis virus, HIV virus or by multi-resistant bacteria, which in past years have spread rapidly. We do not know if our patients are infected, and the patient themselves may not know, but our hygiene programme should cope with the potential problem of transferring infectious viruses or bacteria between our patients.
2. When we work with spray, spray droplets are spread over the whole treatment room and even to neighboring rooms. So in the practice, it is effectively "raining" droplets of spray everywhere, with a possible saliva content of bacteria and viruses (airborne contamination).
3. Contact with an inflamed gingival margin often leads to bacteria being transferred to the blood circulation, known as bacteremia. This indicates that all instruments etc, which touch the gingival tissues, should be sterile.
4. We could possibly enter situations where by law we have to prove our standards of sterilization. (This can be documented with computer prints from the autoclave, with printed documentation for temperature and time noted, or scanned on the patient card.) Patients will have a right to demand documentation for our procedures.

A look at 2012 operative dentistry hygiene protocol

The author chose the year 2012.

- Hand instruments are cleaned in an effective instrument washing machine, and sterilized in closed instrument cassettes in a segmented pre- and post-vacuum autoclave.
- Rotating and endodontic instruments are cleaned in an ultrasonic bath while placed in a bur/file stand. After packing into trays or in sterile paper bags, they are sterilized in a pre- and post-vacuum autoclave and are then finally stored, maintaining sterility.
- An autoclave without a pre- and post-vacuum function will not be able to sterilize internal spaces in contra-angles, as well as the internal part of the spray channel. A few non-vacuum autoclaves can inject hot water vapor to sterilize spray channels, but not the internal cavities in the contra-angles.
- Contra-angles and hand pieces are washed under cold water, lubricated and disinfected in an apparatus, packed in sterilized paper bags, sterilized in a pre- and post-vacuum autoclave, and then stored, maintaining sterility. To do this, the practice must have sufficient contra-angles.
- An autoclave sterilization cycle takes place in a pre- and post-vacuum autoclave for about 40 minutes plus cooling time, for contra-angles. If the assistant is not ready to start the autoclave again immediately, a half hour or more may pass because the contra-angles can also be placed in the lubrication and disinfection apparatus unit before starting the autoclave again.
- Single supplementary hand instruments are sterilized and then stored in small sterilization paper bags. These bags are stored in compartmentalized drawers.

Unit instruments

Unit instruments are disinfected with an alcohol/chlorhexidine mix.

The 3-in-1 syringe

The tip is sterilized pre- and post-autoclave, and the rest of the syringe is covered by a narrow and pointed protective plastic bag permitting only the syringe tip to pass through. The plastic bag is held in place above the syringe by a small orthodontic elastic band. The protective cover is replaced when changing patients.

Ultrasonic scaler

The insert of the scaler is sterilized in a pre- and post-vacuum autoclave, and the handpiece protected with a protective plastic bag as it is positioned by the multifunction syringe.

The suction tubes for retraction and aspiration are cleaned internally with a mini-bottle cleaning brush, cleaned in the instrument washing machine, packed, and then stored either in the tray for examinations or in a sterile paper bag for sterilization in a pre- and post-autoclave.

ORGANIZATION OF MATERIALS

The most important drawer and large material trays

Materials

For some treatments, quite a lot of materials are used, eg, procedures for crowns or bridges may use up to 60 different materials. For endodontics, if using both manual starting files and rotating files, then the number of materials will be very high as well.

The problem

When the materials for a specific treatment are prepared, the assistant collects the materials from the different storage places. The number of storage places can be astonishingly high, seldom under 12, often more than 20, and sometimes more than 30.

The assistant may take a considerable time "running around" to collect materials. And when the treatment specified above is finished – everything is replaced at all these places again. This "ritual" may be performed every day, year in, year out. It is very rewarding to improve the organization of materials, as the assistant can save much time and energy every day.

The solution

The solution is to organize the materials in groups according to their use. The materials can be organized in trays, small tubs, boxes or the like. The author has seen many variations of this used in different dental practices. Some were made many

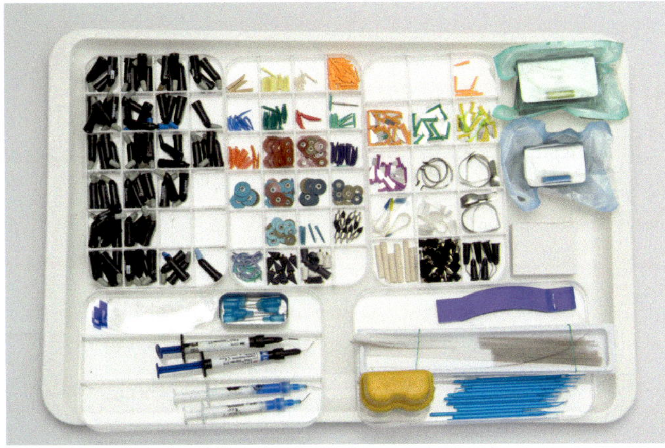

Fig 9–27 Large material tray for composite, with all the materials required.

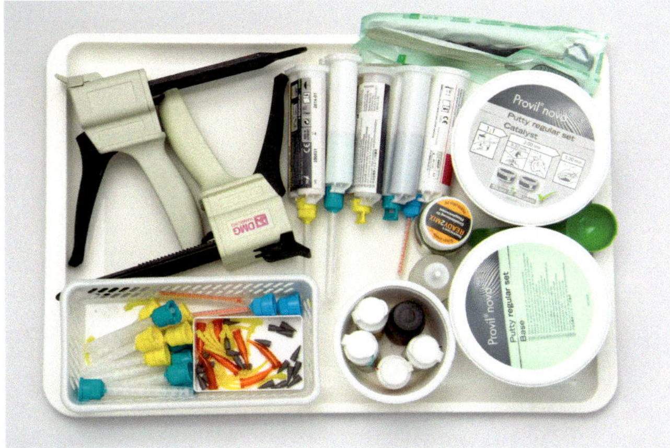

Fig 9–28 A large material tray for crown and bridge procedures.

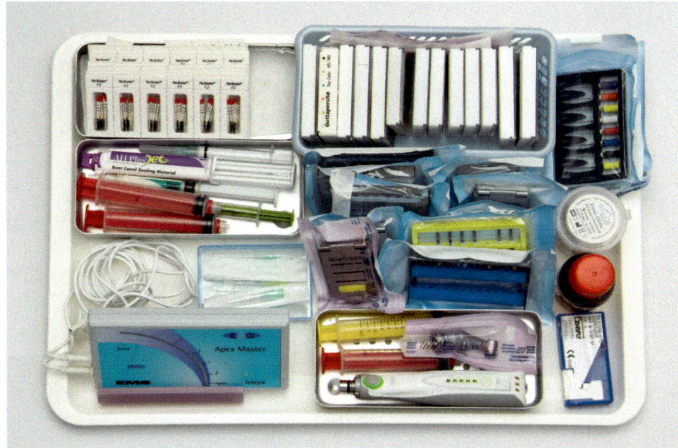

Fig 9–29 A large materials tray for endodontic treatment.

years ago when the number, volume and complexity of dental materials were small. If the materials are placed in one layer and if the border around the "storage unit" is low, the materials can be seen and grasped directly.

The best and cheapest solution is shown here. A large cafeteria-style tray, eg, measuring 45 × 30 cm is excellent. There is sufficient space, it is easy to see everything, and the space is fully used (Fig 9–27). And it is easy to pick up materials because the border is very low, so there is no reason for picking the materials out of the tray when they are going to be used.

The material tray for a temporary crown procedure, including temporary cement, can supplement this (Figs 9–28 and 9–29). Cassettes may be used for smaller groups of materials as well.

Examples of cassettes with materials:

- Post systems for crown build-up.
- Cementing cassette.
- The materials may be stored in a cupboard, either in each treatment room, or in a cupboard in a central place in the practice (Fig 9–30).

This means that instead of collecting individual materials for a certain treatment, you simply take the actual material tray from the storage drawer or storage shelf, and place it on the working table top close to the patient. In this way, the preparation of materials before and the replacement of materials after the treatment is finished, is greatly simplified. The time gained per day may easily be more than 1 hour.

Large restaurant-style trays have a good functionality, especially when combined with a well-designed workstation, where all the frequently used small materials are quick and easy to take for the assistant.

The use of large material trays is integrated in the MEGASPACE workstation (Figs 9–31 and 9–32). It is a workplace with immediate access, and incorporates "the most important drawer" in your practice. When working with spray, the material trays are covered with a protective serviette.

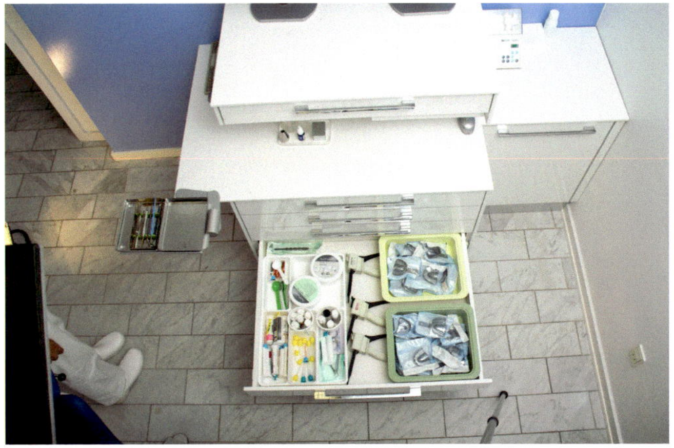

Fig 9–30 The large material trays are stored in a lower drawer on the left side.

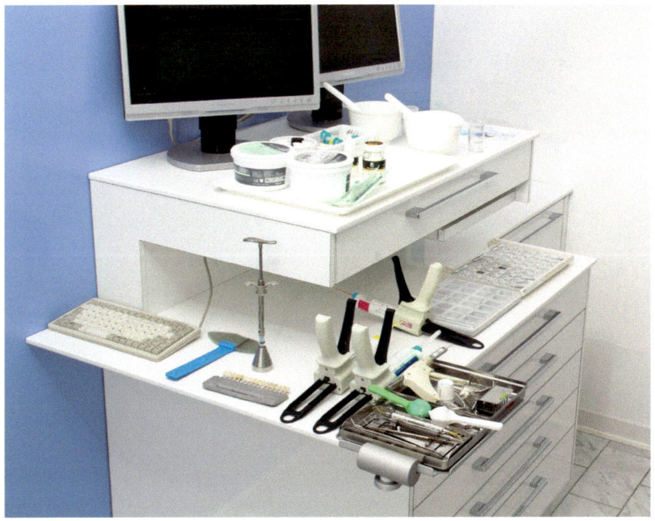

Fig 9–32 The material tray on the workstation's top work surface. Everything that is needed for crown and bridge procedures is placed here.

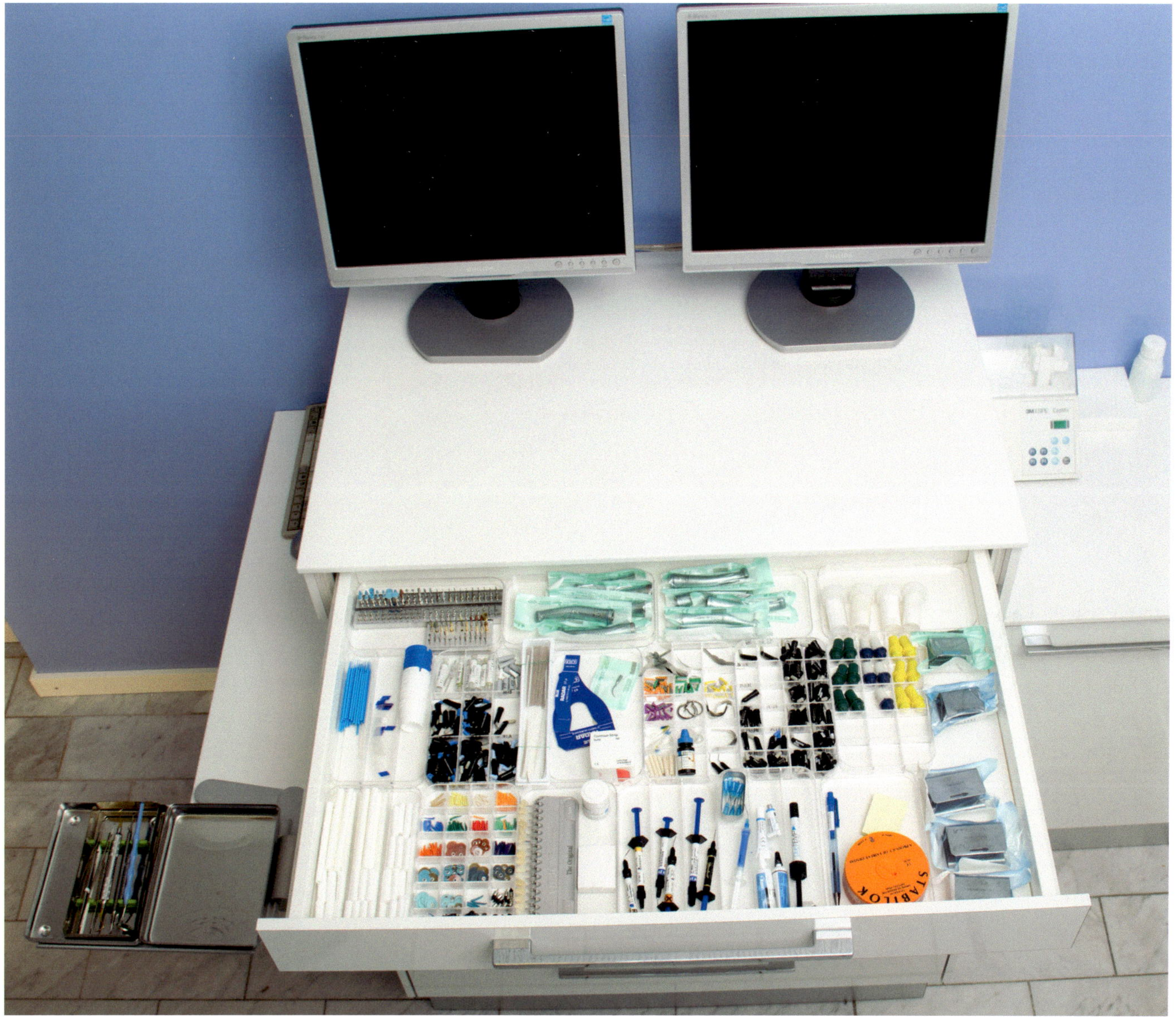

Fig 9–31 The most important drawer in the practice, on the MEGASPACE workspace. It is easy to reach, placed above the worktop. Over 100 small materials are stored here, including all materials for cavity preparation, filling and polishing. This drawer also includes the content of the large material tray for composite.

Chapter 10

ASSISTANCE AT TREATMENTS

ASSISTANCE WITH COMPOSITE FILLINGS

In the case of a workstation such as MEGASPACE or WORKSTATION 2, the materials for composites may be organized in the "most important drawer" (Fig 10–1) placed above the worktable, so it can be opened easily during the treatment procedures. In workplaces without this drawer, materials may be placed on a large material tray (Fig 10–2) with low edges so the content is easy to see and to grasp with an extra pair of tweezers from the basic instrument cassette.

Preparations

A basic instrument cassette and composite instrument cassette are placed on the hand instrument table (Fig 10–3).

The red contra-angle is mounted with a diamond according to protocol, and placed on the micromotor closest to dentist. The blue contra-angle is mounted with a round bur according to protocol and placed on the micromotor closest to the assistant (because burs on the blue contra-angle are changed more frequently than diamonds on the red contra-angle).

Then the etch and bonding system is prepared, and the color shade selected.

Assistance

Figures 10–4a to 10–4g show some examples of the teamwork for composite that demonstrate these principles.

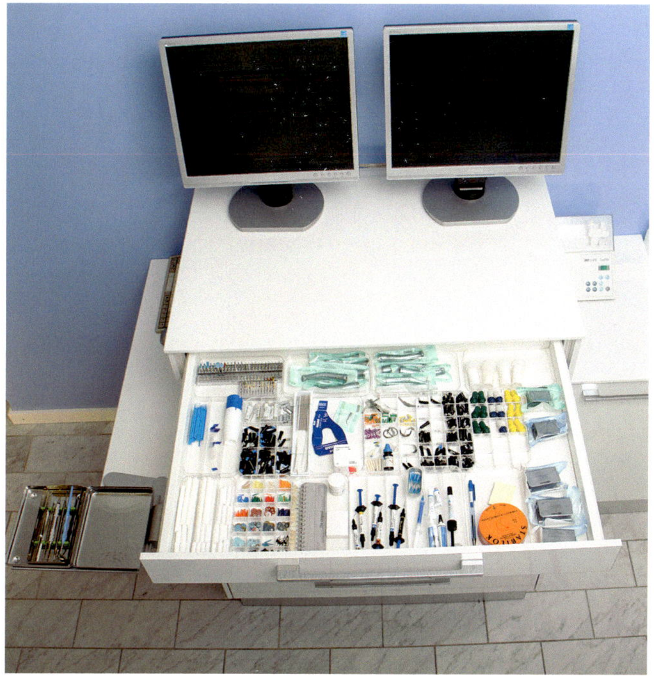

Fig 10–1 The most important drawer.

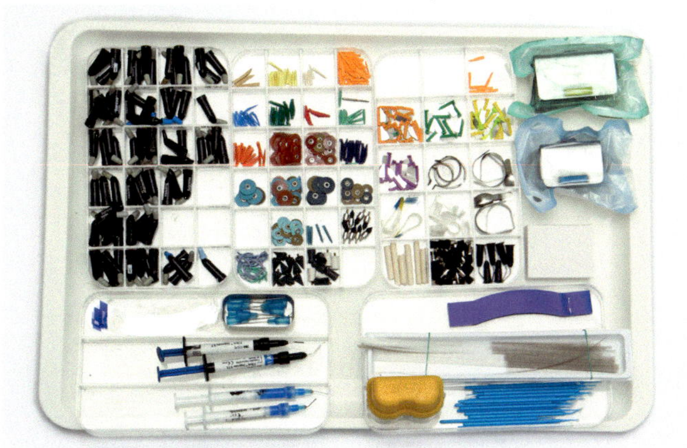

Fig 10–2 Composite material tray, the contents include: cotton rolls; liner; mixing pad; etching gel; primer and bonding system; microbrushes; color shade guide; fender protection of neighboring teeth; matrix systems; pincer for placing rings; plastic strip; contour strips of different shapes; corner matrixes; short retraction cords; interdental wedges, composite pistols; composite of the 10 most-used colors and types flow; high power LED composite polymerization lamp (wireless) if not placed on recharger; articulation paper.

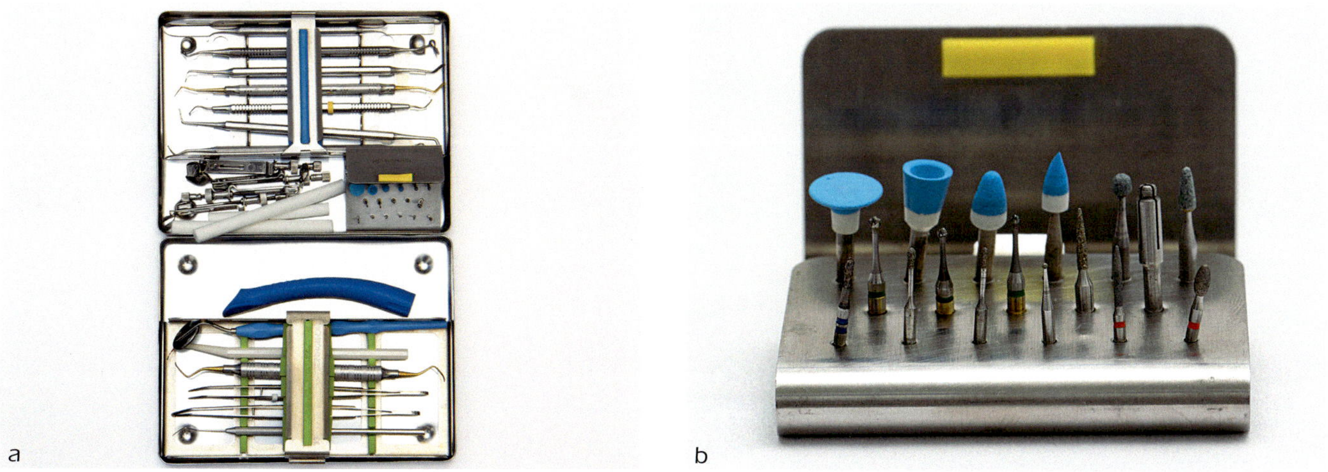

a b

Fig 10–3 (a) Composite instrument tray with hand instruments and bur stand. (b) Composite bur stand.

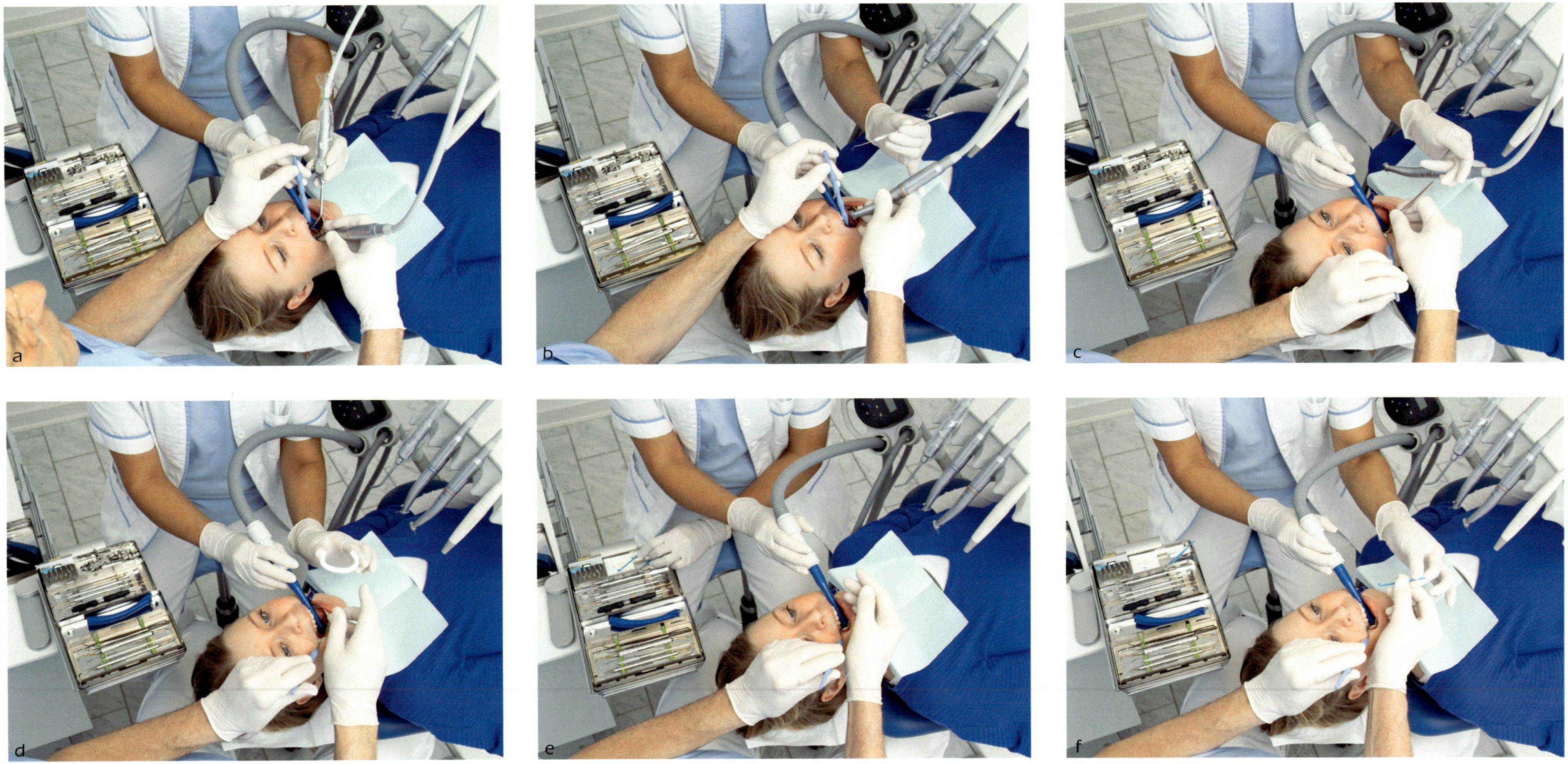

Fig 10–4 (a) Preparation. Mirror used and dried by assistant. (b) Assistant takes micromotor with high-speed contra-angle and (c) transfers the probe. (d) Cotton rolls placed vestibular for retraction and for drying. The assistant retracts the tongue. (e) The microbrush picks up the etching gel. (f) The microbrush is predirected towards the cavity and transferred. (g) Etching.

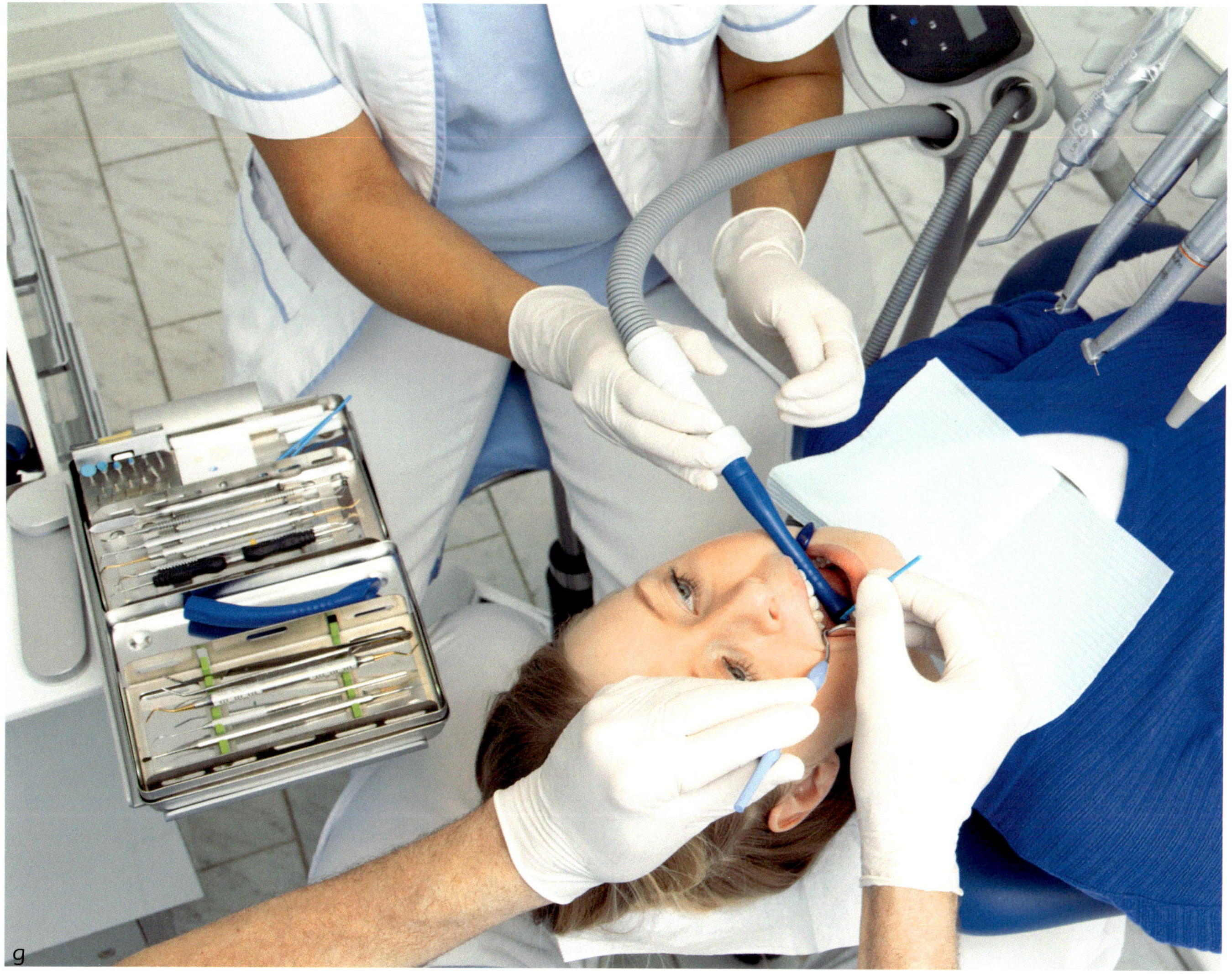
g

Basic four-handed assistance techniques are shown in Chapter 6. These are:

- preparation
- retraction
- keeping the mirror dry
- drying the cavity
- transfer of hand instruments
- transfer of different unit instruments with different methods, and transfer of materials.

Figures 10–5 to 10–7 show specific examples for composite, eg, the mandibular right molar. A few of the photos here have been shown before and are presented here within the context of a workflow.

Multilayer technique

There is a repeated shift using the multilayer technique, between the composite pistol (a hand instrument for adapting composite) and a polymerization lamp.

Repeated use of articulation paper and diamonds for adjustment of occlusion and articulation

In this situation, change from using a micromotor with a high-speed contra-angle to a micromotor with a blue 1:1 contra-angle and polishing point, discs and cups.

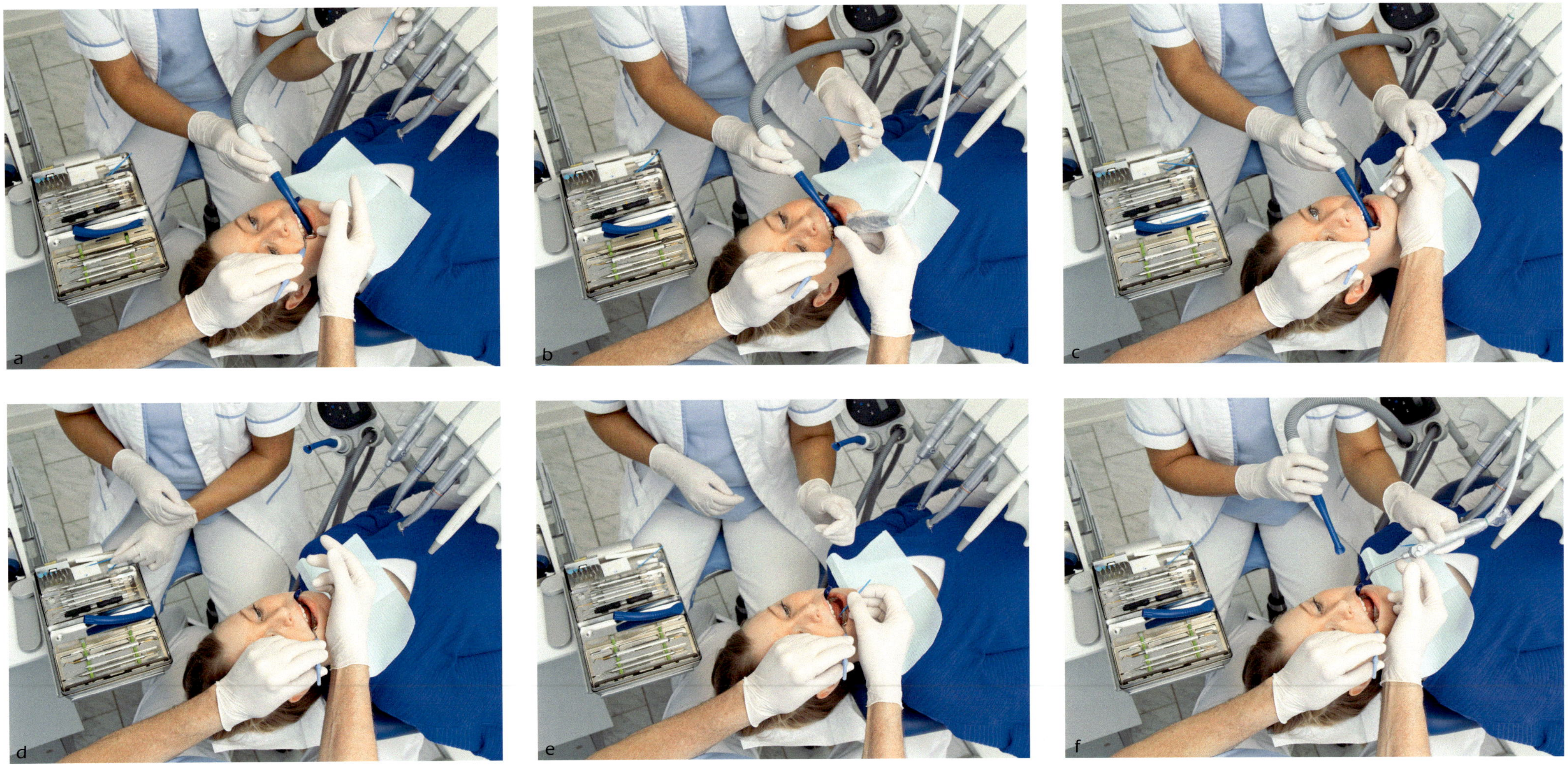

Fig 10–5 (a) The assistant has taken the microbrush, and takes the 3-in-1 syringe and transfers it to the dentist. (b) Rinsing and soft drying. (c) Transferring the cotton roll with tweezers, the dentist takes both and places the cotton wool lingual to the actual tooth. (d) The assistant takes the dentin primer, while the dentist is waiting. (e) Hydrophile primer on cavity. (f) Transfer of syringe.

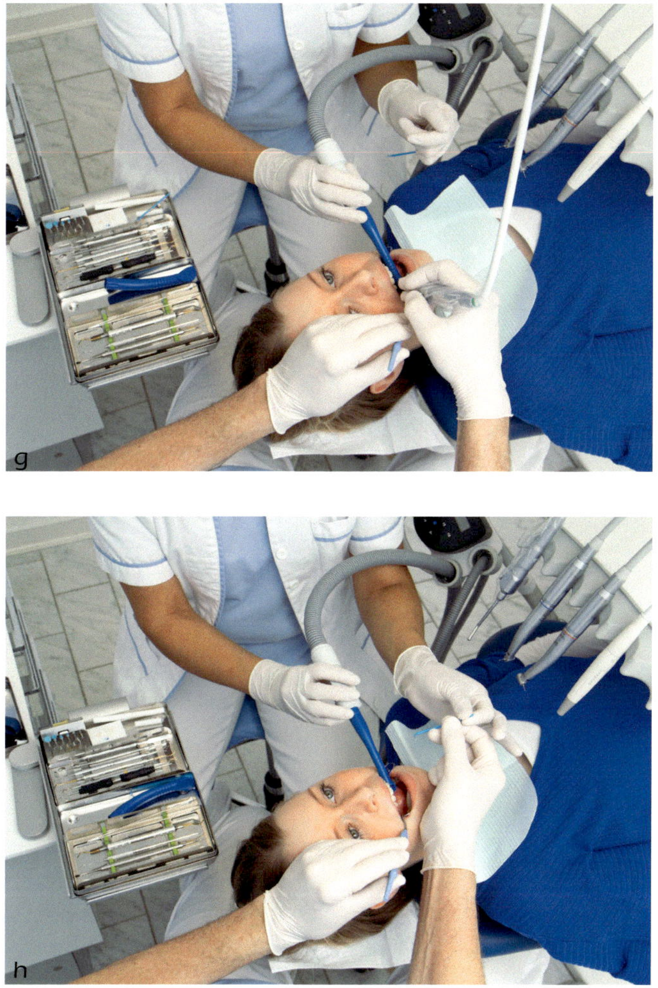

Fig 10–5 (cont) (g) Drying: the aspiration tube is close to the tooth in order to evacuate droplets of primer (allergy protection). (h) Transfer of predirected (bent and directed to cavity) microbrush with bonding.

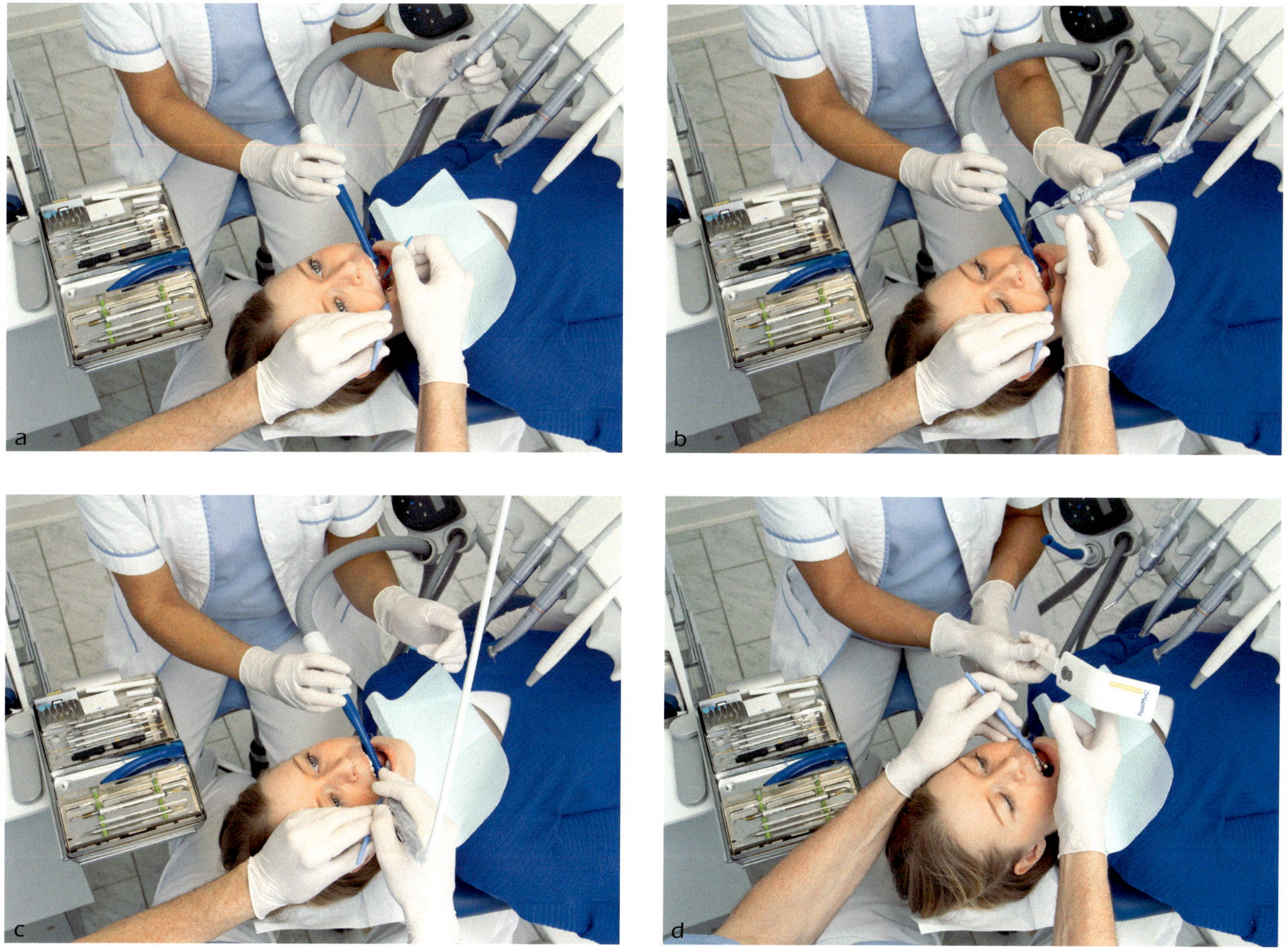

Fig 10–6 (a) Bonding. (b) Transfer of 3-in-1 syringe. (c) Soft air for even distribution of the layer. Aspiration collects potential droplets. (d) Transfer of battery powered rechargeable ultra high intensity 4W LED composite polymerization lamp. The polymerization time is about 3 s for 2 mm, but used for a maximum of 0.5 to 0.8 mm.

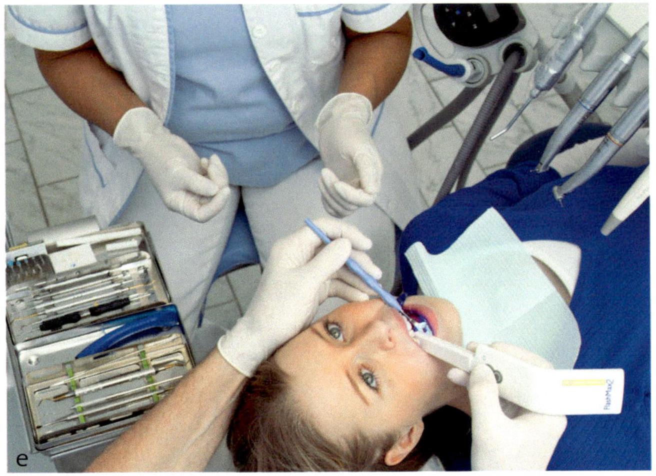
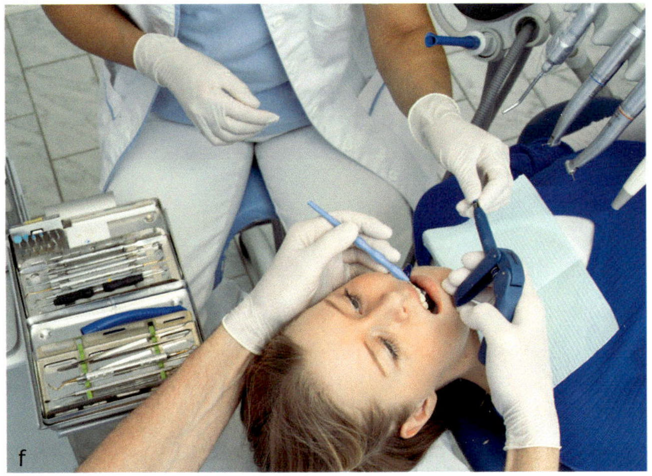
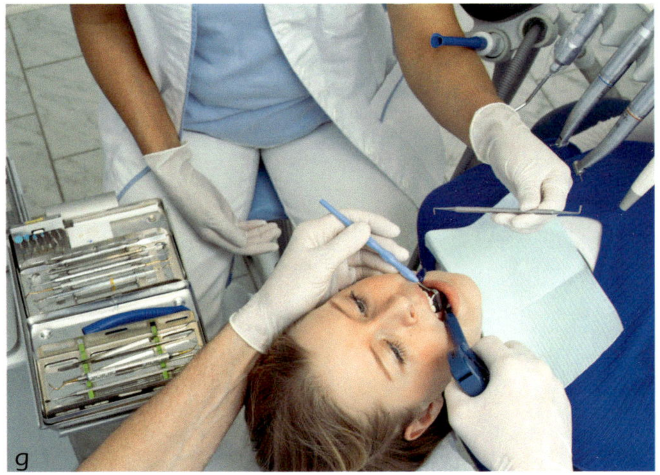
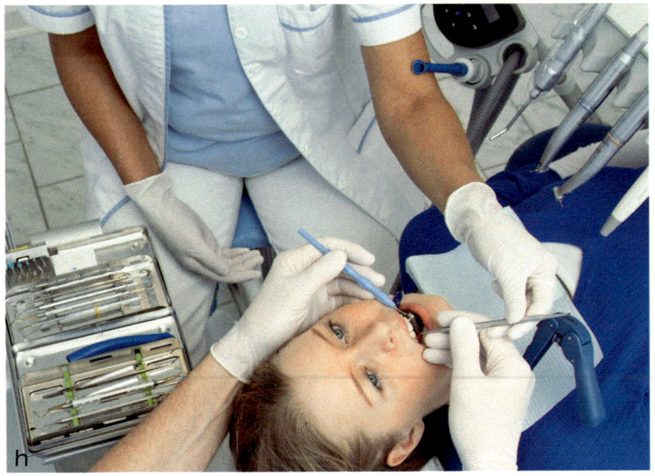
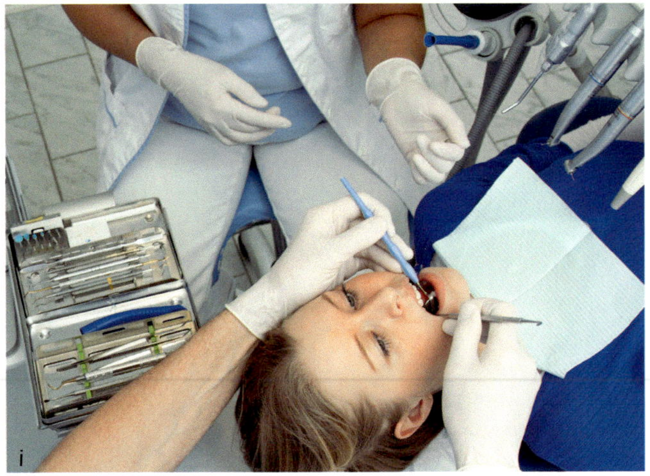

Fig 10–6 (cont) (e) Polymerization. (f) Transfer of composite pistol. (g) Applying composite – the hand instrument for adapting the composite stands by. (h) The assistant takes the pistol with the little finger and transfers the hand instrument. (i) Use of composite adaptation instrument.

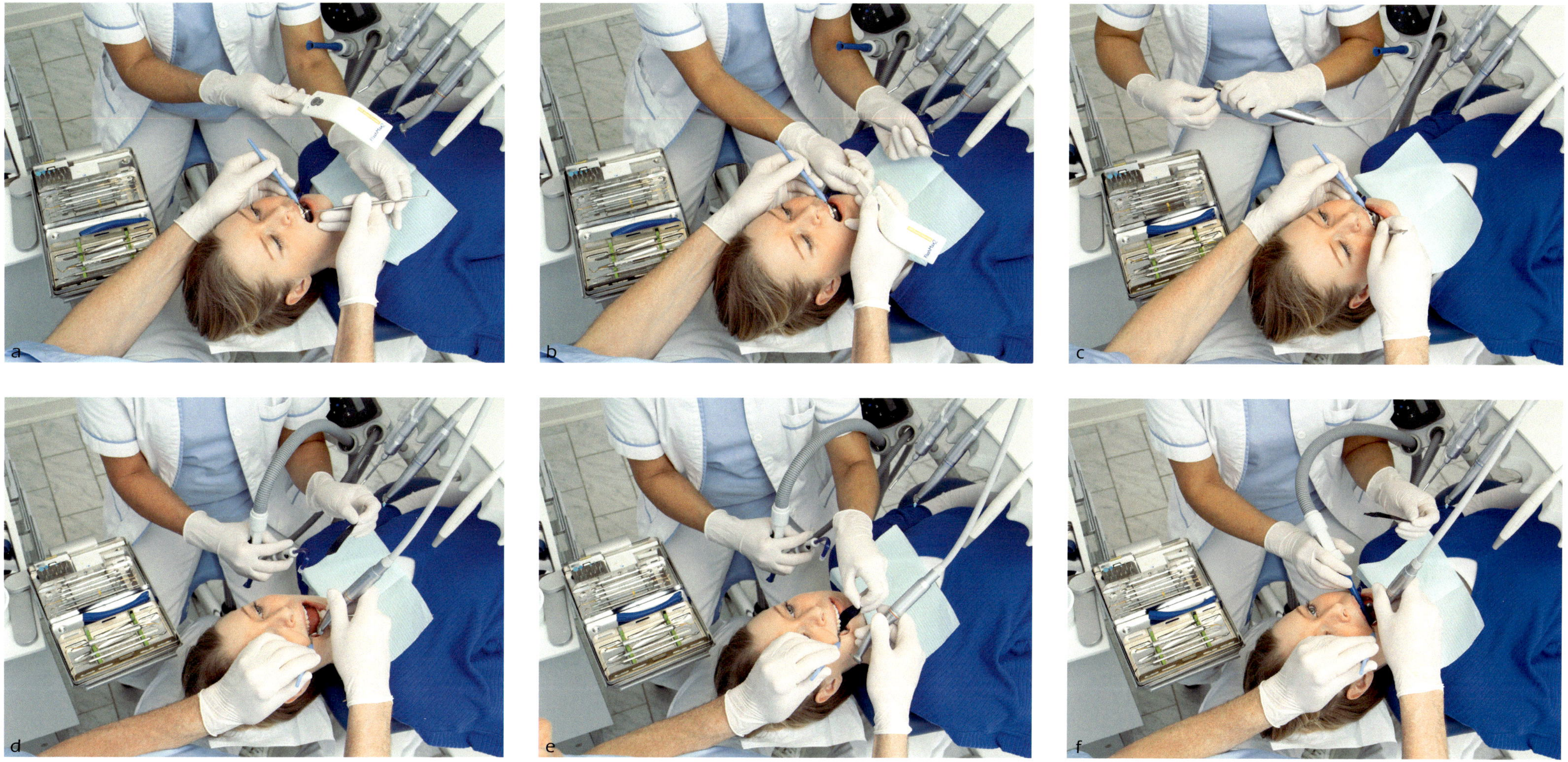

Fig 10–7 (a) The assistant picks up a hand instrument ready for the transfer of the polymerization lamp. (b) The polymerization lamp is transferred. (c) The assistant shifts the rotating instrument to be ready for polishing. (d) The small suction is removed and ready for the articulation paper (e) to be used. (f) Correction of occlusion and articulation.

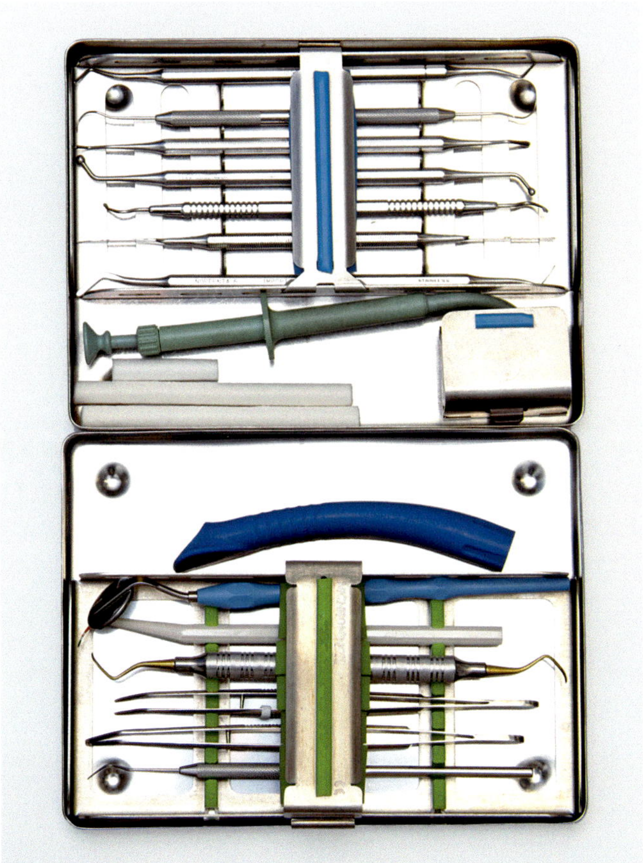

Fig 10–8 Basic instrument cassette and amalgam instrument cassette.

ASSISTANCE BY AMALGAM FILLINGS

Amalgam usage differs. In some countries, the use of mercury and mercury alloys are not used, allowed or only allowed on strict limitations. In other countries, amalgam is generally used.

The amalgam material tray is used if the treatment room does not have the "most important drawer." The content might be:

- cotton rolls
- matrix bands and matrix holders
- wedges
- liner
- mixing pad
- amalgam capsules – single, double, and triple
- articulation paper.

The basic hand instrument cassette

This is used for examinations and in combination with the amalgam treatment tray (Fig 10–8).

The amalgam instrument cassette, with hand instruments, amalgam carrier and bur stand

This may include:

- two matrix holders (right and left) premounted with large flat matrix bands for molars
- two matrix holders (right and left) premounted with small, flat matrix bands for premolars.

The material tweezers (from the basic hand instrument tray) are used for materials from "the most important drawer." Here the assistant takes the approximal wedges in the size the dentist asks for. Articulation paper is also taken from here. If an articulation paper holder is used, it may be placed in a sterile paper bag in the first drawer, and mounted with articulation paper before the treatment. A capsule mixer is used for the lowest risk of mercury spill.

When the capsule is opened, the amalgam is picked up with an amalgam carrier directly from the capsule (Fig 10–9). Training is necessary to fill the carrier with fewest possible movements. The amalgam carrier may be passed by the assistant's RIGHT hand to the dentist in two different methods, illustrated in Figs 10–10 to 10–14.

The assistant fills amalgam directly into the cavity

For medium to large fillings, the assistant fills the amalgam directly in the cavity, so the dentist can concentrate undisturbed on condensing the amalgam. The assistant fills amalgam into the cavity with precise and trained movements, eg, first the distal part of the cavity, later the mesial, and then finally the occlusal part.

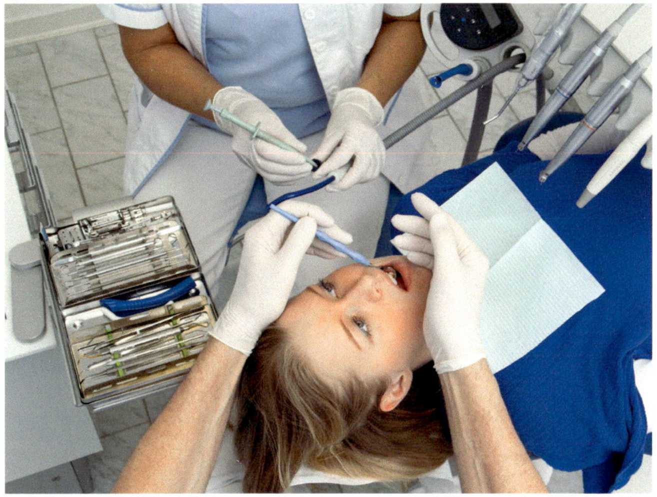

Fig 10–9 The assistant uses an amalgam carrier to pick up amalgam from the bottom part of the amalgam capsule (held in the left hand), together with the small suction tube used to pick up particles of amalgam in the patient's mouth. The small aspiration tube is held by the left hand's index and middle fingers.

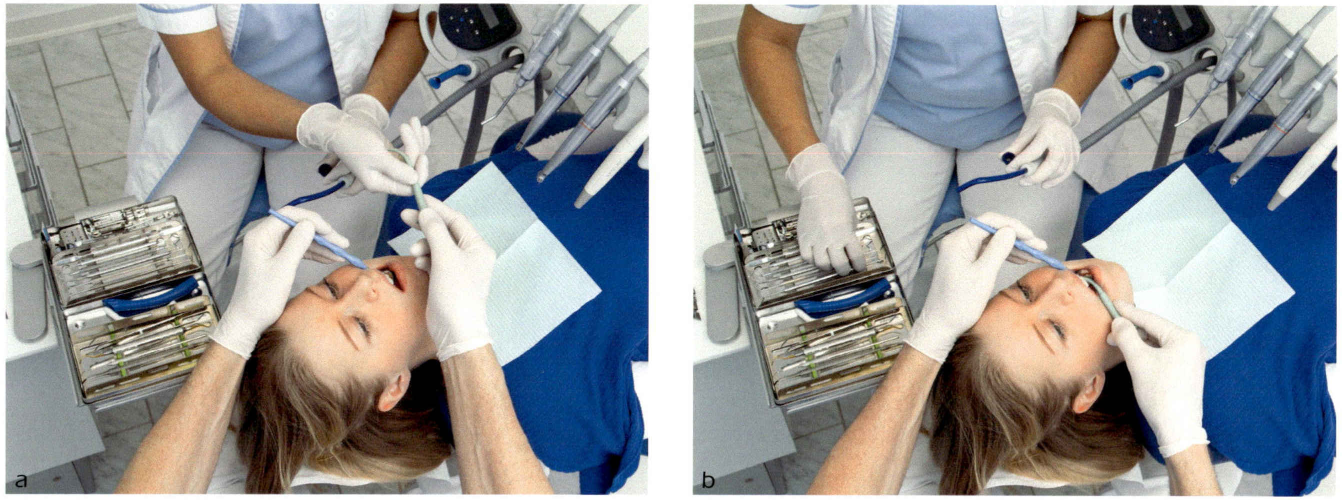

Fig 10–10 (a) The transfer of amalgam to the dentist. The amalgam carrier is in "contact to palm" grip. The assistant has a small suction in the left hand. (b) The assistant picks up the amalgam condensing instrument with the right hand.

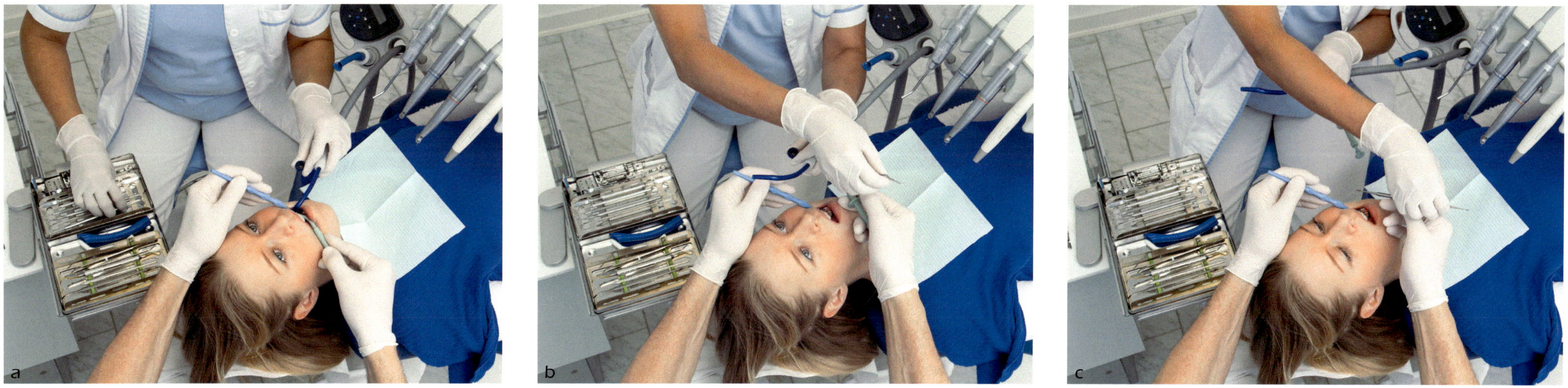

Fig 10–11 (a) The assistant uses a small aspiration tip when needed, held with the left hand. (b) She transfers the condensing instrument to the dentist using her right hand, while taking the used carrier with the little finger of her left hand. (c) Transfer of the condenser.

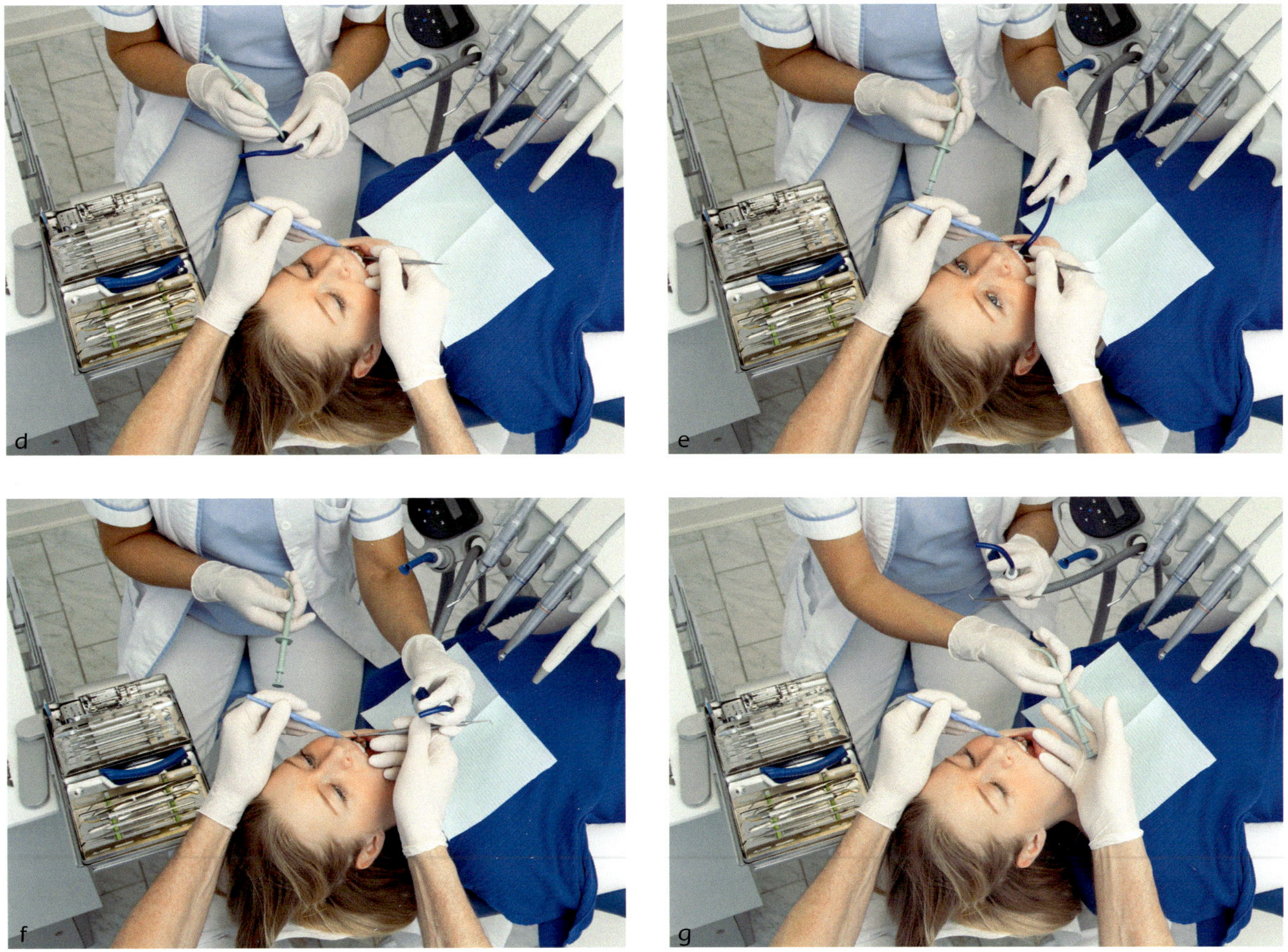

Fig 10–11 (cont) (d) The dentist is condensing amalgam while the assistant fills the carrier. (e) The dentist continues condensing while the assistant picks up any amalgam outside the preparation. (f) The assistant takes the condenser, and (g) transfers the carrier.

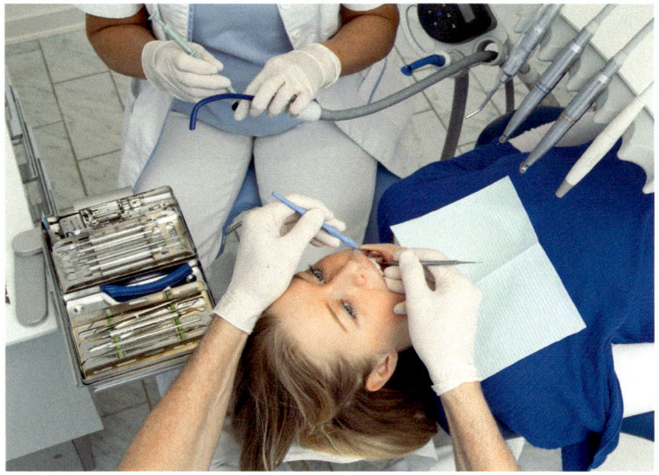

Fig 10–12 Filling the amalgam carrier again.

Alternative grip of amalgam carrier

If the assistant is well trained (and fast), and the cavity is large, the dentist may use a mechanical amalgam condenser – a special contra-angle mounted on a micromotor for very efficient condensation of amalgam.

For cavities that are small and deep and/or difficult to look into, the dentist fills amalgam into the cavity himself. Assistance for amalgam fillings is characterized by the transfer of a lot of hand instruments, for sculpturing, burnishing, carving and correcting the amalgam (Figs 10–11 and 10–12).

Four-handed instrument transfers are performed by the basic protocols shown on page 124.

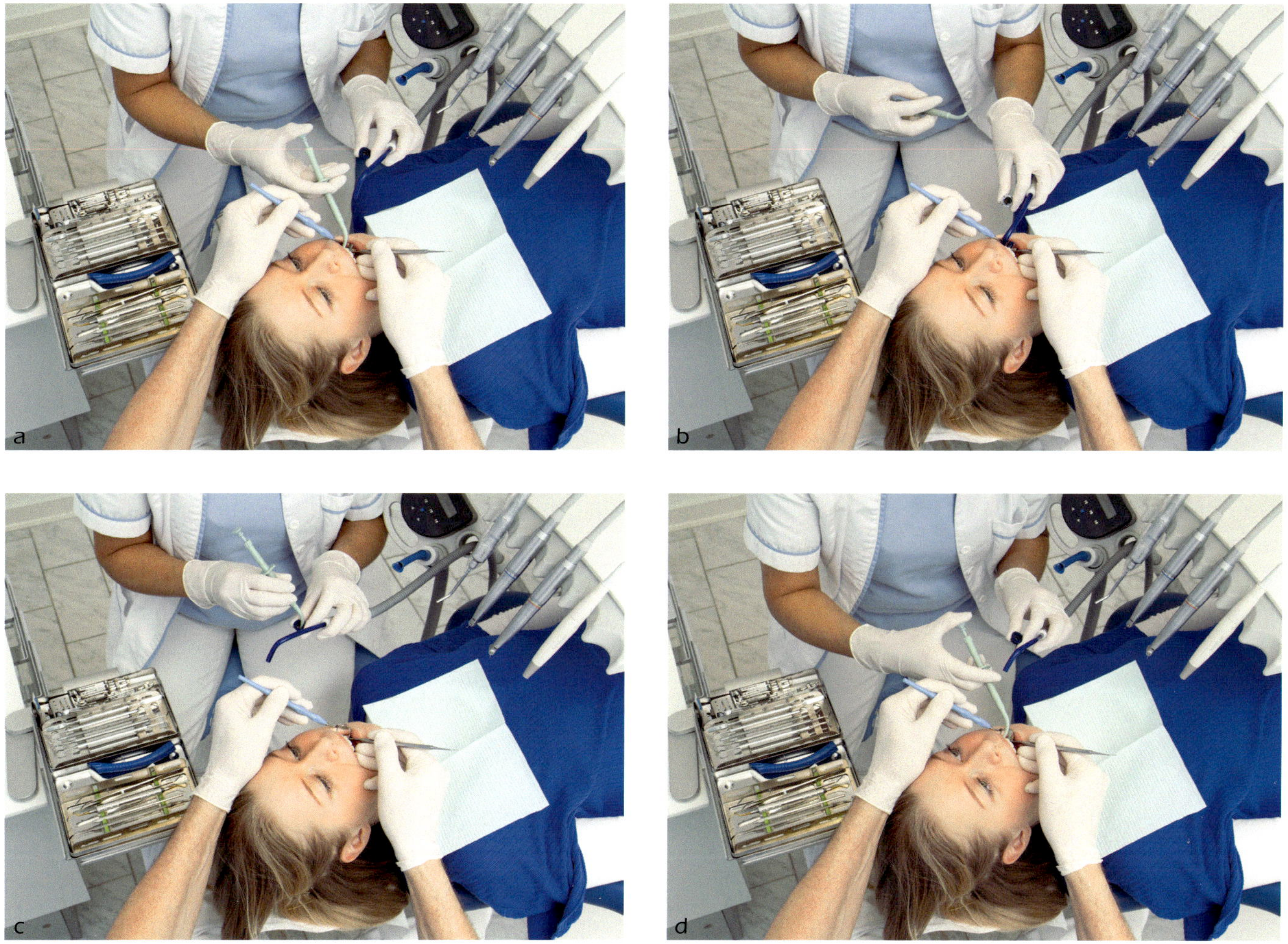

Fig 10–13 (a to c) The dentist tells the assistant where the amalgam should be placed in the cavity. The filling steps are as follows: The carrier is placed within the periphery of the matrix band (if there is one). The carrier is moved mesially or distally until contact is made with the matrix band. The carrier is moved to the bottom of the cavity and completely or partially emptied (the dentist advises). (d) The assistant fills amalgam carrier directly into the cavity as the dentist continuously condenses the remaining amalgam.

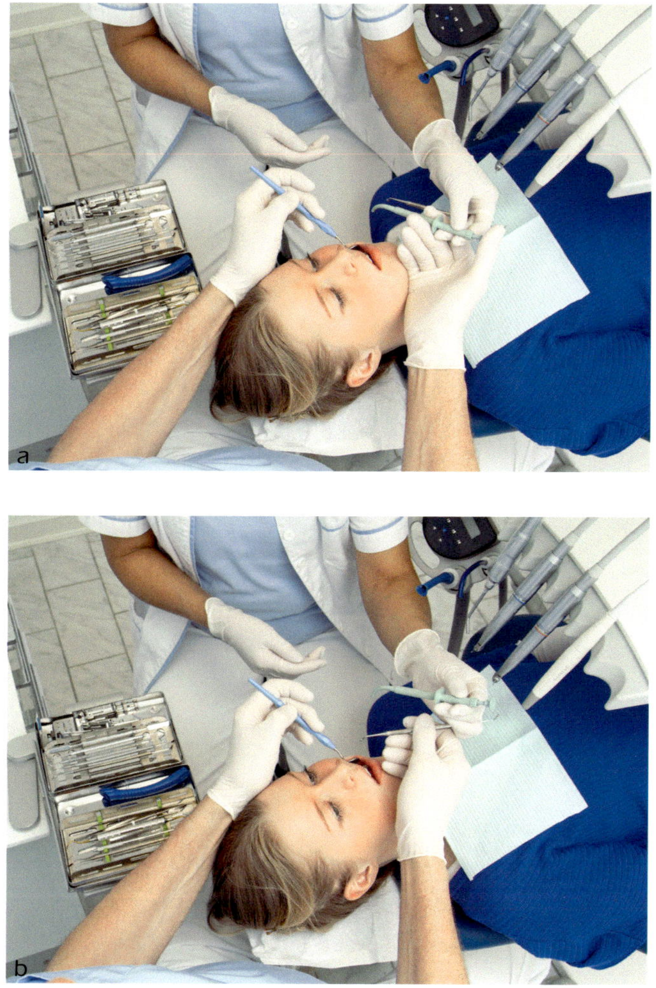

Fig 10–14 (a) A syringe grip. (b) When carving, the hand instruments are transferred with the standard method, described in Chapter 6. Some dentists prefer a syringe grip on the carrier.

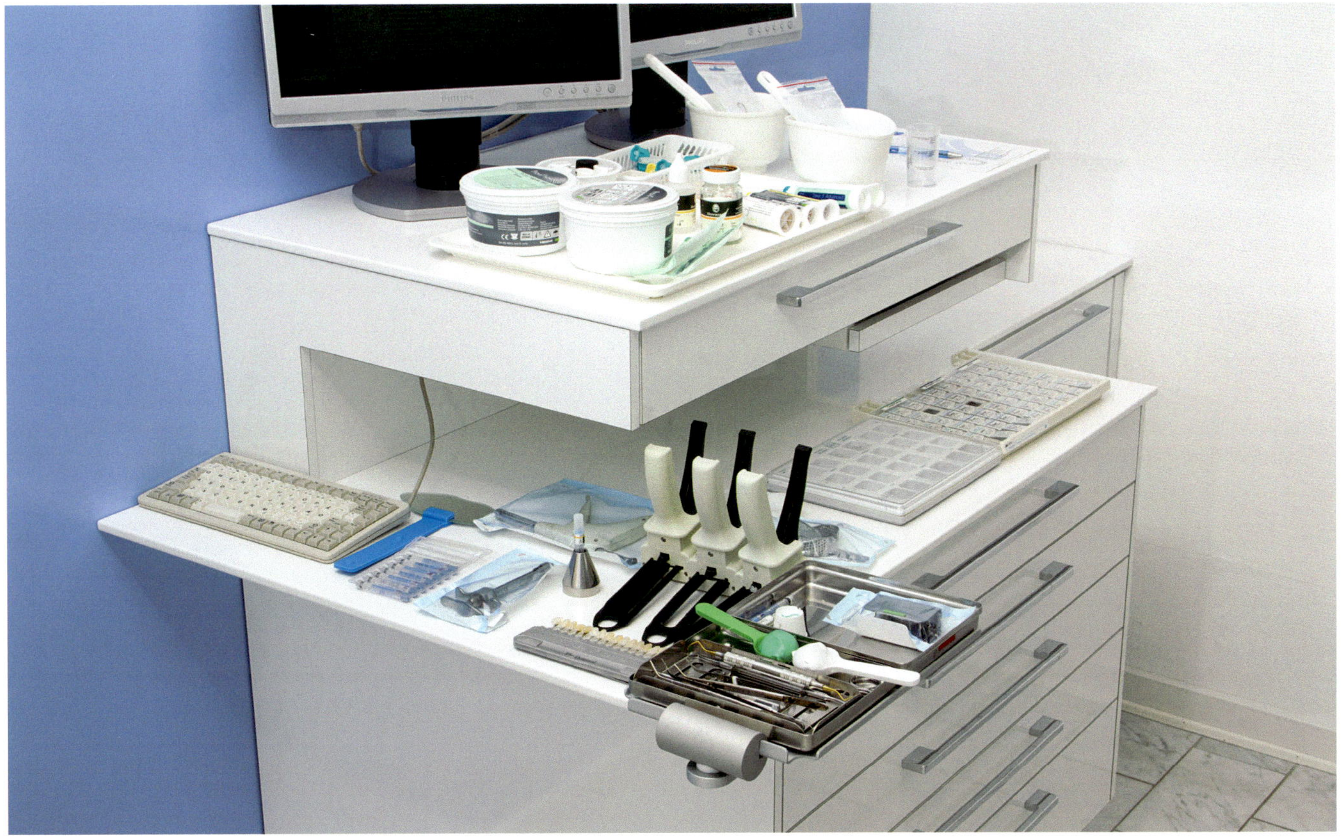

Fig 10–15 The MEGASPACE ready for a crown and bridge procedure. Note that the almost 2 m two storey workplate is full with materials. This is a test for the workstation's quality.

FIXED PROSTHODONTICS

Crown and bridge procedures, and inlays and laminates

Preparations for the treatment will be very dependent on protocol, and will depend on whether "digital impressions" or traditional impressions are used. Here are some examples of how to organize materials using "large material trays" and traditional impression methods. The MEGASPACE workstation is used as an example (Fig 10–15).

The assistant uses this photo as an example for the protocol for preparation of instruments and materials for fixed prosthodontics.

Crown and bridge material tray (large)

The contents of this could be:

- color shade guides
- alginate premeasured in small sealed plastic bags
- alginate mixing bowls, water measure and spatula
- bur stands (if not in a prosthodontic instrument cassette)
- retraction cords of different thicknesses
- gel or liquid for retraction cords
- dappen glass
- pair of scissors
- automix plastic model material for small models for evaluating parallelism and possible undercuts,
- impression materials, eg, putty, and measuring spoons
- impression material automix in cartridges
- automix tips with small injection tips
- cartridges with bite registration paste with automix tips
- scalpel for adjustment of alginate impression for temporary crown
- cartridges with Protemp (3M ESPE) and temporary crown material and tips
- correcting hand piece cutter for temporary crowns
- non eugenol temporary crown cement
- "pistols" for automix impression and bite registration materials, as well for temporary crowns are placed beside (Figs 10–16 to 10–19).

Boxes with premade "shapes" or "molds" for temporary crown in a drawer close to the workplace

In the MEGASPACE crown and bridge drawer, the crown and bridge bur stand is stored in a sterile paper bag.

The teamwork and assistance follow the same principles as described by other treatments. All materials and all instruments are transferred to the dentist's hand predirected towards the "object of action." So the dentist can take it and use it, without having to change the grip with fingers and hand. Protocol for the workflow is of course very important here too, because they enable the assistant to foresee each step in the treatment.

For more information concerning micromovements, biomechanics, perception, feed forward training and examples of tools, diamonds, etc, see Chapter 4. All the general principles of assistance and teamwork are applied. To read further on the positioning of the patient's head, chair, type of vision, dentists position, retraction by assistant, retraction by dentist, instrument grip (including modified grips), and hand/finger support – specified for tooth surface and type of action – please see Chapter 10.

The author will leave the detailed protocols to specialists in prostodontics. However you may wish to have a look at www.netergonomie.com for further information.

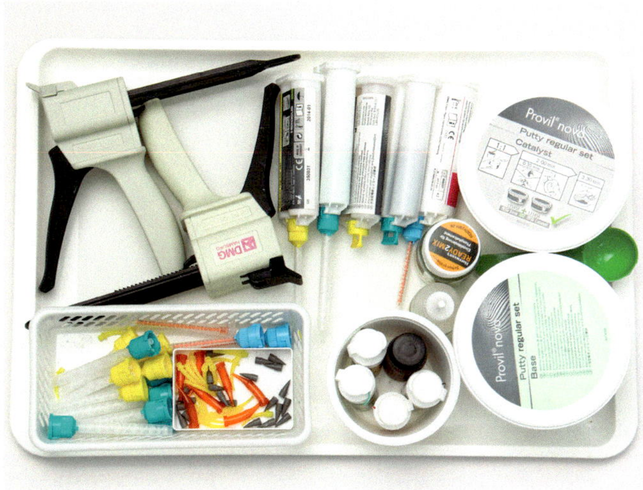

Fig 10–16 A crown and bridge material tray.

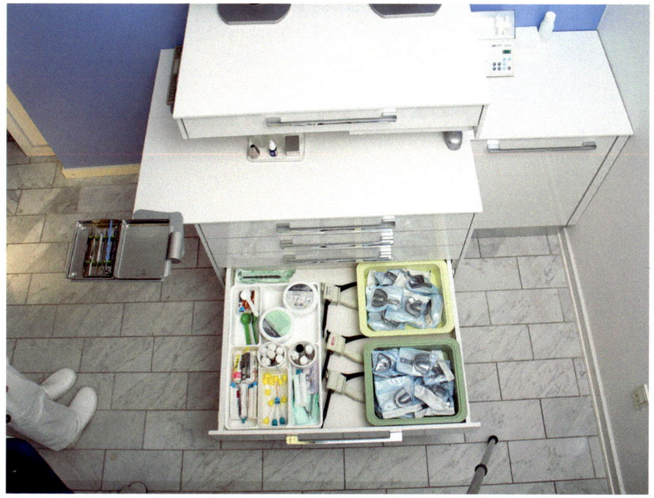

Fig 10–17 The crown and bridge drawer in the MEGASPACE (including the crown and bridge tray).

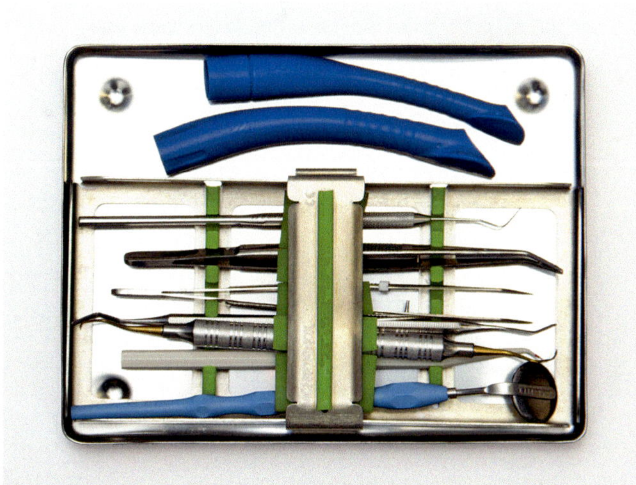

Fig 10–18 A basic hand instrument tray with open cover.

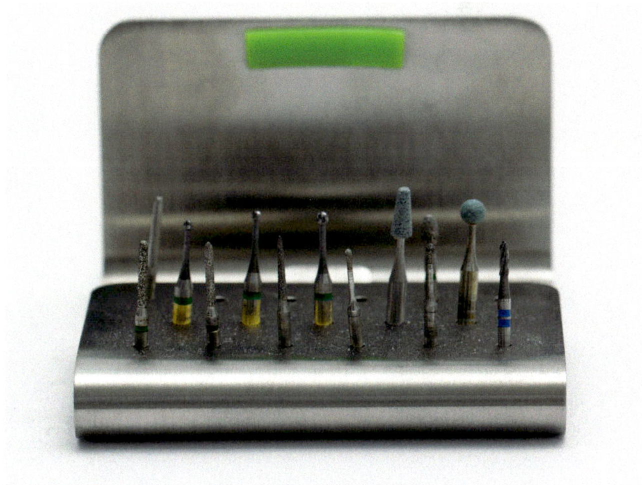

Fig 10–19 A bur stand for crowns and bridges.

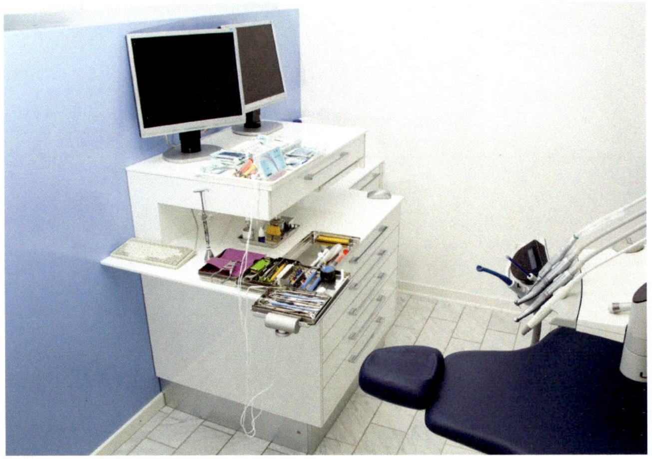

Fig 10–20 The MEGASPACE prepared for an endodontic treatment. Notice how a large workspace is necessary. The material tray for endodontic treatment is placed above the most important drawer.

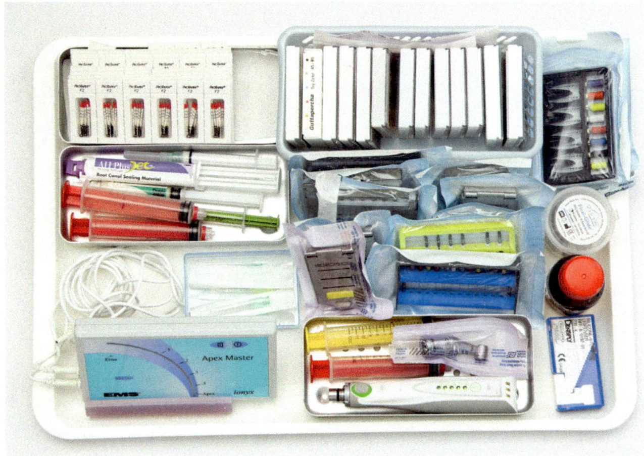

Fig 10–21 A material tray for endodontic treatment.

ASSISTANCE BY ENDODONTICS

There are a number of different concepts for endodontic treatments available. To follow the descriptions and illustrations in this book, the standards described in short here are applied with the ProTaper concept (Dentsply). When using other concepts, probably only smaller adaptions should be made.

The description is based on the following standards:

- The rubber dam is established.
- After opening of the dental cavity (cavum pulpae) with long 1.2 mm microprep diamonds and long burs, the root canal orifices are identified using loupes fitted with an LED light to enable visual inspection simultaneously as the burs are used.
- Caries detection liquid may also be used for coloring the orifices.
- The magnifying mirror may also be used for a total of 4 to 6x magnification.
- Hand files 0.10 or smaller are used. When a depth of say 5 to 6 mm is reached, a rotating file with very small point and large taper is used 3 to 4 mm into the superficial part of the canals to widen up the orifice, with the objective that repetitive use of files make them easier to place in the canals.
- The hand files are used until apex and length is monitored by an apex locator and followed up by radiographic verification.
- Then rotary flexible nickel titanium files are used, according to the system used with rinsing with 0.30 mm canules.
- After drying with calibrated paper points, the root canals are filled temporarily with CaOH, or with permanent filler according to the type of endodontic treatment.

Organization

Instead of collecting the materials and instruments for endodontic treatments, material trays are used. The material trays are large and have low edges, which allow direct vision to materials on the tray and make it easy to take materials from the side.

The material tray is placed on plate on top of "most important drawer" in workplaces like MEGASPACE or WORKPLACE 2, or constructions similar to these (Figs 10–20 to 10–22). The surface height where the material trays are placed is in both cases about 95 cm, so this is why the edges of the material trays have to be low, otherwise the assistant cannot see or take the content while sitting.

The following sections detail the materials used for the most frequent endodontic treatments are placed. A second large endo tray may be used for the seldom cases where the rotary file systems cannot be used because the canals are too large, too long or too curved.

Endo material tray – standard

- rubber dam fluid for sealing the rubber dam
- apex localizer

- endo motor if not in stand for recharging
- contra-angle for endo motor
- reciprocating contra-angle for hand files
- small box with many extra K-files in small sizes, eg, 0.08 mm, 0.10 mm, 0.15 mm and 0.20 mm
- syringes and micro canules for rinsing
- rinsing liquid, such as stabilized NaClO, EDTAC or alike in low bottles
- bottle with chlorhexidine
- file stand with extra rotating files
- file stand with hand held versions of the rotary files may be taken into use if the root canals are very curved
- file stand with standard Nitiflex hand files (Dentsply)
- abundant paper points calibrated to the rotary file system
- gutta-percha points calibrated to the rotary file system
- gutta-percha points calibrated for use after use of spreaders
- CaOH paste in syringes
- canules to CaOH paste
- root canal filling paste.

Endo material tray – special

- a file stand with rotary endo files
- a file stand with K-files from size 0.45 mm and "all the way up" –that could be two file stands (if the root canals are very thick)
- a file stand with K-files, width from 0.08 up to 0.45 mm, length 35 mm, if the root canals are very long

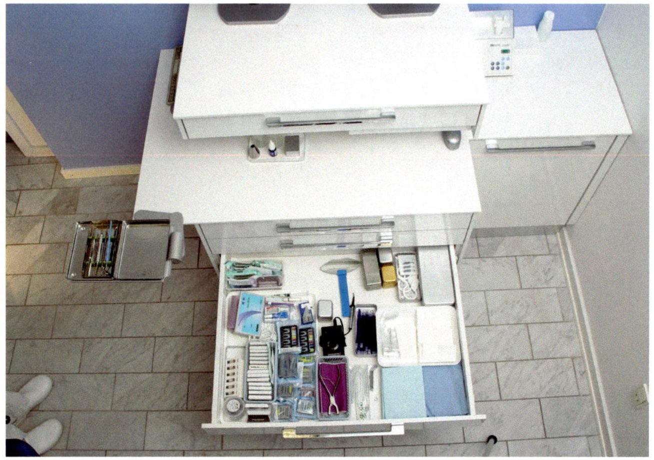

Fig 10–22 The MEGASPACE drawer for endodontics. The material tray is stored on the left side.

- a file stand with K-files width 0.50 mm and up to length 35 mm, if the root canals are very long and thick
- calibrated K paper points and gutta-percha points, for the rare cases where width and or length makes it necessary to finish the root canal instrumentation with K-files.

Other file stands

The endo material trays may be stored in a closed cabinet with shelves or in a lower drawer in MEGASPACE. This can store:

- rubber dam cassette with rubber dam
- clamps
- rubber dam perforator
- pliers for clamps
- mounting frame.

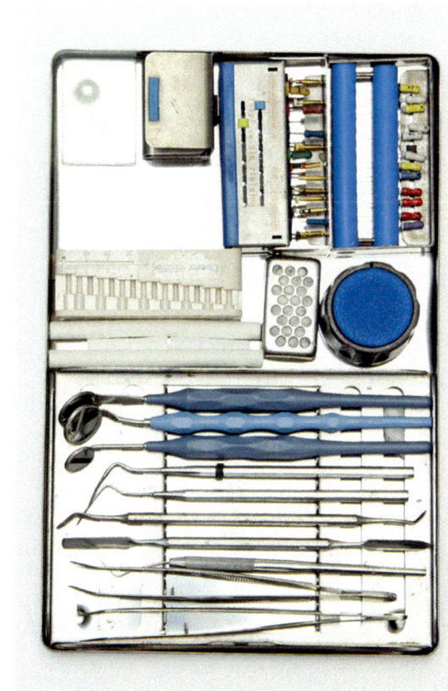

Fig 10–23 The endo instrument cassette, containing: hand instruments (including front surface mirror and concave magnifying mirror); file stand with thin K-files and an extirpation needle; file stand for the rotating files, and spreaders; file measuring block; endo bur stand; glass pad for mixing; file "carrier" with foam, cotton pellets and cotton rolls.

Preparing for endodontic treatment

- Anesthetic is prepared.
- A standard endo instrument cassette is placed on the hand instrument table (Fig 10–23).
- A standard endo material tray is placed on the working area.
- A rubber dam cassette is placed besides opened and prepared rubber dam clamp (with wings), mounted with the rubber dam, and placed on pliers.
- The standard endo material tray is placed on the working area.

Assistance where "everything" is transferred to the dentist

When using loupes, see the special endo transfer technique on page 214.

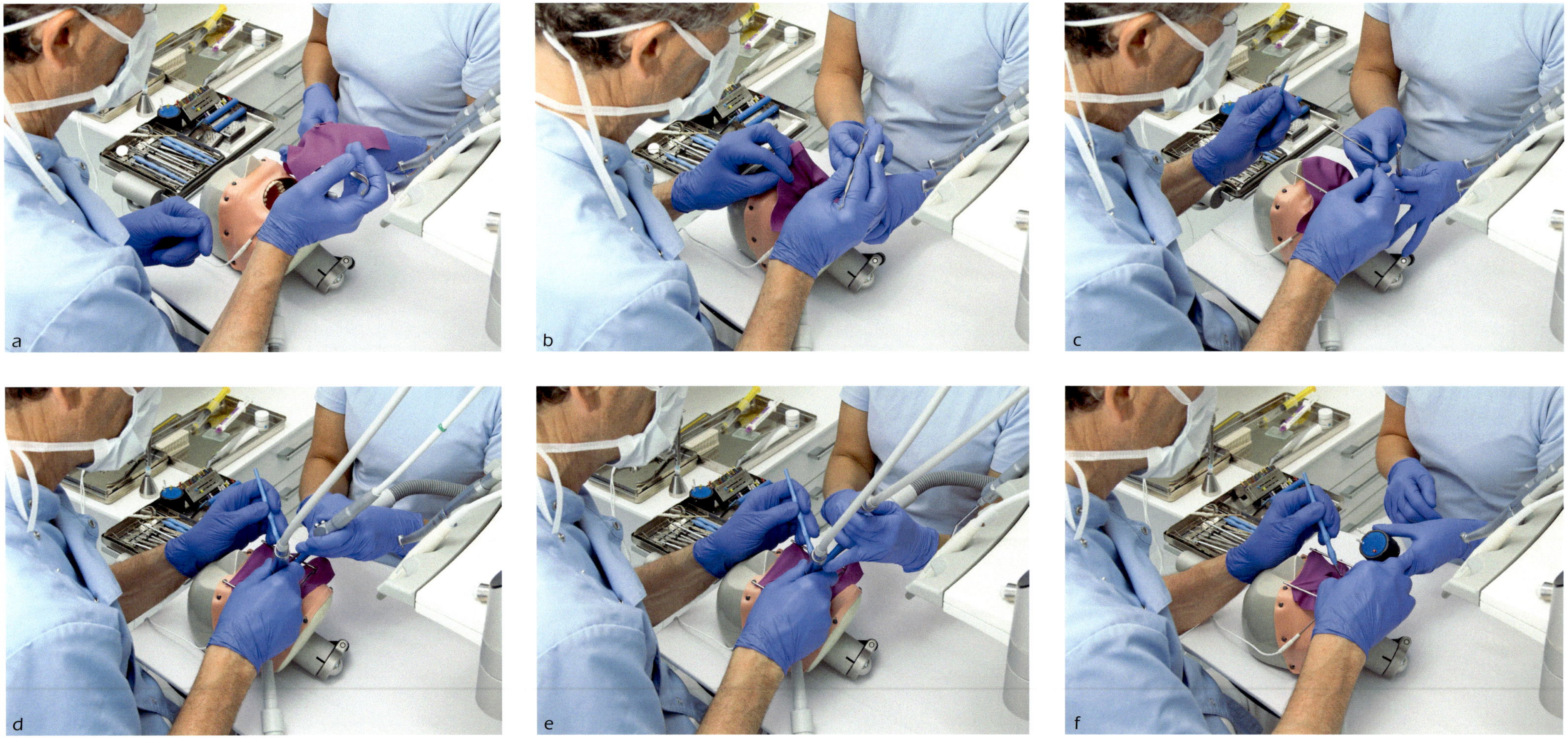

Fig 10–24 (a) The rubber dam is mounted on wing clamps on the clamp forceps, transferred to the dentist and then placed on the actual tooth. Here is the maxillary left molar. (b) The hand instrument is transferred and used for lifting off the rubber dam off the wings of the clamp. (c) The frame is transferred and the rubber dam mounted. (d) Opening the pulpal cavity with a diamond. The mirror is kept dry by the assistant using the 3-in-1 syringe. (e) The assistant takes the unit instrument and is ready to transfer the 3-in-1 syringe to the dentist. (f) The hand files are transferred in a file holder with polyester foam dampened with chlorhexidine.

Some examples of endodontic treatment assistance are shown here in Fig 10–24. (Notice how the small aspiration tube is placed opposite the operation field, with the tip placed behind the last molar. The "ground electrode" for the apex localizer is also placed.)

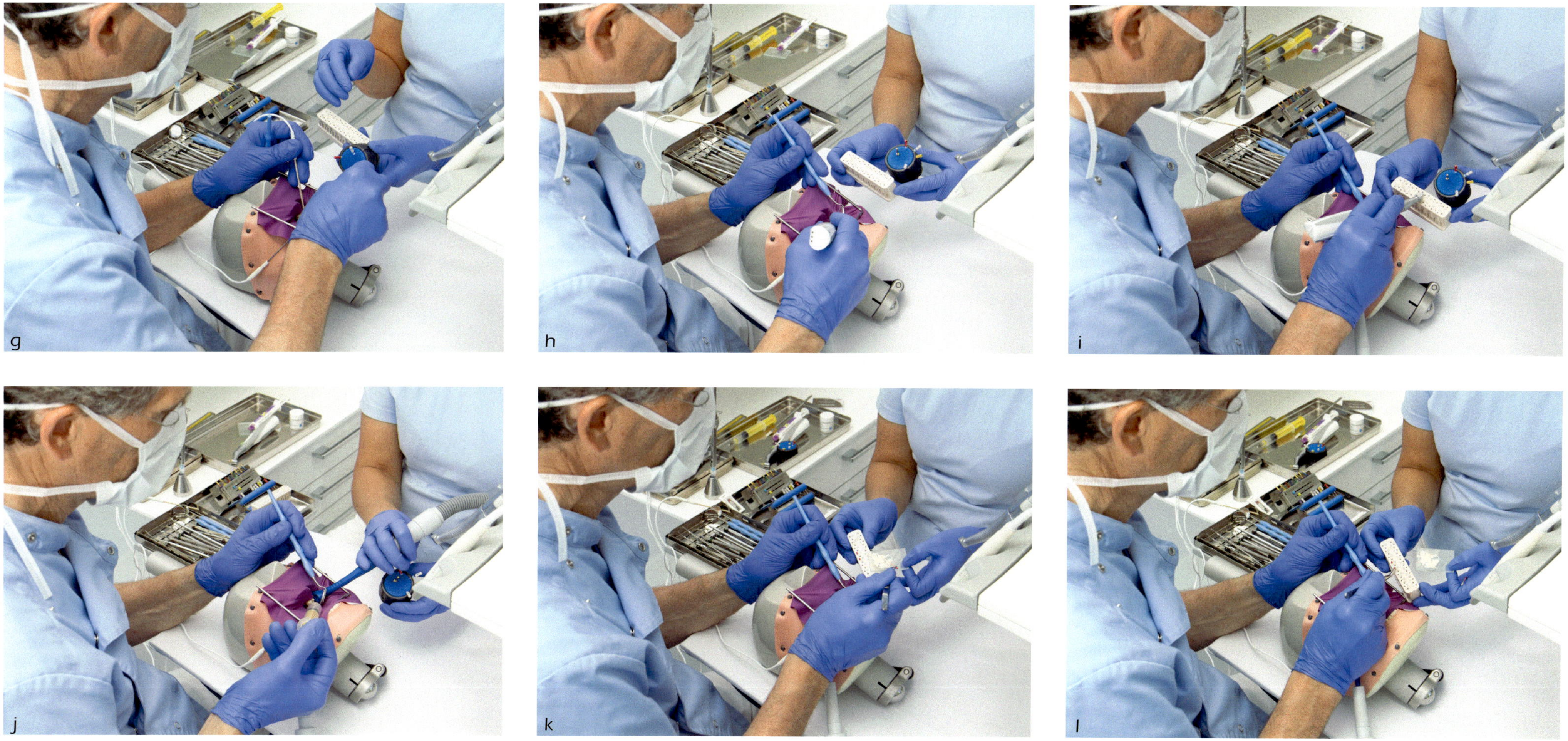

Fig 10–24 (cont) (g) An apex localizer, used for measuring root length. The assistant mounts rubber rings according to the root length measurements. (h) The assistant mounts rotating files on a torque-regulated endo motor, with the rubber rings in position for the shortest root length. She has already passed the endo motor to the dentist who is now using it. (i) The assistant presents the file measure. When the shortest root is instrumented, the file – while mounted on the endo motor – is placed in the root measure block according to the second shortest canal. So the rubber ring is placed in position according to the length of this canal, which is then instrumented, and so on for other root canals, one by one. Then the next file is mounted on the endo motor and the instrumentation continued, as shown above. (j) The syringe with NaClO is transferred to the dentist, who is now using it for rinsing. (k) The paper point is presented to the dentist, who then takes them with tweezers. (l) Gutta-percha points are presented in the file measuring block for correct measurement of root length.

ASSISTANCE WHEN WORKING WITH LOUPES

When the loupes are (correctly) inclined 45 degrees downwards, the dentist can easily look over the loupes to look at unit instruments or the assistant.

The size of the loupes's visual field will depend on distance between the eyes of the dentist, magnification of the loupes, and on the ocular. The shorter the distance, the larger the visual field.

The blind field

A ring-shaped area around the field seen in the loupes is not visible for the dentist (it is covered by the enlarged visual field seen through the loupes).

When the assistant transfers instruments, unit instruments or materials to the dentist, this happens in the blind field. The transfer is not visible for the dentist. Therefore, the transfer must be highly trained by both parties. The method is the same as described earlier.

The assistant places takes the used hand instrument and places the next hand instrument, unit instrument or material in the hand, prepositioned for immediate action. The assistant marks the moment of delivery with a small firm movement, indicating to the dentist that now the next instrument is in his hand.

Endodontic file transfer in blind field

For endodontic procedures, the file transfer can be made using a "file carrier" made with polyester foam dampened with chlorhexidine. (This is described in the chapter on endodontics, page 214.) The file carrier is approached by the dentist's right hand, with the ring finger stretched forward slightly.

When the file carrier touches the ring finger, the thumb and ring finger are closed on the hand file. The assistant must turn the file carrier, so the file shaft is exactly where the two fingers are closing.

USING A MICROSCOPE – A FEW CONSIDERATIONS

You don't work with a microscope, you use the microscope while working

For some procedures, magnification is important. The use of a microscope gives a sharp and perfect picture, which is important for some procedures. A microscope provides a larger magnification than loupes. It has built-in light and provides a super sharp vision with magnifications from 5× and up.

For endodontic use and for microsurgery, a magnification of 10 to 12× is used. This magnification creates a visual field a little bigger than a molar. It is important that the microscope has an objective (lens closest to object)-to-object distance of about 25 cm in order to avoid disturbing the work with unit instruments and hand instruments, as well as the assistant's transfer of these to the dentist.

The arm system supporting the microscope may be mounted on the wall behind the chair of the patient. If this is to be possible, it will depend on the geometry of the arm system and must be tested properly. If the microscope is mobile, the base of the supporting "system" may be placed on to right side of the patient chair. The eyepiece of the microscope may also be adjusted, so if the dentist has a comfortable head position, and is slightly inclined forward, then the working position can be fine.

When using the microscope, the eye-to-ocular distance must be very precise too. This means that although the work position of the dentist is fine, the position is completely fixed. To comply with this, frequent compensatory exercises are proposed. In the near future, this may be solved by connecting a high definition camera to the microscope, and using a high definition retina projection of the image.

Using a microscope can cause complications. It cannot be placed so you are able to look into the mouth of the patients in the same directions as by the unprotected eye. Positioning microscope according to the direction of vision is often not possible difficult to achieve depending on the geometry or the supporting "arm system."

When the microscope cannot be placed in a position that enables a vision into a specific exterior surface or an interior surface in a cavity, then the mirror must be used.

Training to work with microscope is largely a question of:

1. Learning to adjust the microscope, and learning when and where the microscope cannot be used using direct vision.
2. Learning to work in a mirror also at surfaces, where a dentist without a microscope will work directly.

How to learn to work with a mirror

In some positions, the use of a mirror leads to unusual optical phenomenon, with the result that the dentist must train intensively to learn new eye-to-hand relations (if the are not learned already). The patient is lying horizontal as always for sit down dentistry. The following three examples are the same as for working without a mirror.

Example 1

Working with a mirror in the occlusal maxillary jaw (or MOD) cavity:

- Up (which is mesial) is seen as up and down is seen as down.
- Left is seen as left and right seen as right.

Example 2

Working with mirror in the occlusal mandibular jaw (or MOD):

- Up and down is reversed 180 degrees.
- Up (which is mesial) is seen as down, and down seen as up.

Example 3

Working with a mirror in lingual mandibular jaw at incisors:

- Up and down is still reversed 180 degrees.
- Up, which is here in labial direction (eg, approximally) is seen as down, and down is seen as up.

The following examples are more tricky:

Example 4

Looking through a mirror at a line on a buccal surface of a mandibular right molar "drawn" from the disto-occlusal "corner" to the mesiolingual "corner."

This will be reversed 90 degrees as seen through the mirror placed distobuccal from the tooth, but will not be reversed seen with a mirror in a mesiobuccal positioning.

Example 5

Looking through the mirror at the buccal side of a mandibular left molar, a movement from the distal to mesial part will be seen as a movement to the left side.

New training program for microscope users

The examples reveal the major problem of learning to use a microscope while working. That is, to identify, learn and train hand-eye co-ordination in some new situations. This training can be structured to be more systematic and with a faster learning effect without the microscope, which reduces the visual 3D perception.

The training program tasks (details are not covered in this book however!) contain many repetitions for the trainee. The training involves mental 3D animations, and intensive biomechanic and proprioceptive training. A mix of practical exercises and mental movement animation is advantageous.

Assistance when working using microscope

Blind dentist – invisible hands

Everything outside the small working area is invisible, which means that high-end, four-handed teamwork is a condition for work. Every inclusive unit instrument has to be placed in the hand of the

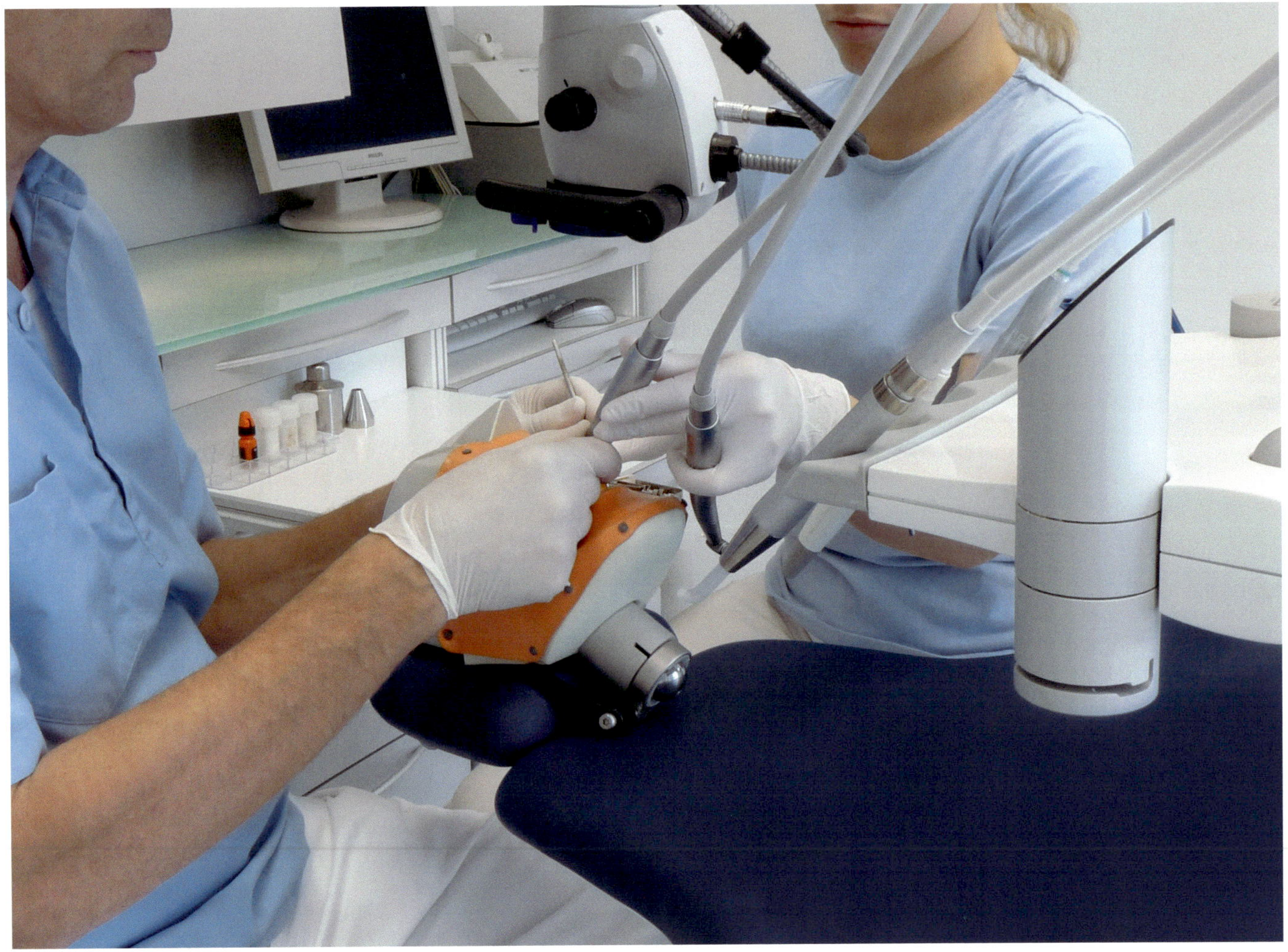

Fig 10–25 The assistant guides the instrument transfer until the working part of the instrument is visible in microscope (often just a few mm from the tooth).

dentist. So for working with a microscope, a centrally placed unit is an important factor, so that the assistant can transfer the unit instruments to the dentist (Fig 10–25).

The assistant guides the blind dentist

Instrument transfer is made as for dentists using loupes. But compared to using loupes, the visual field using a microscope is much smaller, so the assistant guides the instrument in the hand of the dentist until the working part is visible in the microscope.

When the instrument transfer is completed, the assistant does not leave her grip on the instrument but maintains the grip a short while after the dentist has the "new" instrument in his hand. Doing this, she also guides the dentist in holding the instrument until the working part of the instrument is visible in the microscope. Dentists using a microscope require absolutely excellent assistance.

SUPRAGINGIVAL SCALING AND POLISHING

Instruments and methods

Microergonomic considerations for the use of hand instrument and ultrasonic scaler for supragingival scaling and polishing

In some countries, a large part of or even large majorities of dental patients are educated to and have an established habit of regular preventive and interceptive recall. The interval between the recalls are individualized, perhaps every 3 months for high risk patients, and 6 months for average patients, with longer intervals for low risk patients. In connection with the recall examination and hygiene control, there is also a supragingival scaling.

The recalls can be performed by the dentist SOLO, by a hygienist SOLO or DUO by a dentist with assistance.

Supragingival scaling of recall patients

Without periodontal disease and a maximum of 3 mm periodontal pockets

Diagnosis of dental calculus may be done visually, if visible over the gingiva, or tactile in case of dental calculus, which is not visible like approximal calculus or calculus in gingival pockets.

Diagnosis and scaling by use of hand instruments

For tactile diagnosis, a probe may be used or it may be done with a hand instrument for scaling into pockets up to 2 to 3 mm. To look for and to remove calculus hidden deeply in narrow approximal spaces, the instrument has to be thin and pointed, and the working part so long that you can reach a bit over the middle of the approximal space between large teeth, such as the first and second molar (Fig 10–26). Three movements are now carried out:

1. The use of the hand instrument is now carefully planned, so the working part is used step-by-step with light-touch scraping movements over the surface of the tooth from – if indicated – the bottom of the pocket.
2. This first "strike" is a light movement as the scaler removes biofilm (plaque) from the surface. The movement with the instrument is light in touch, in order not to harm the surface of tooth or risk to remove cementum. The first movement done with the scaler has a second objective, which is that the scaler functions as a probe for identifying the presence of dental calculus. If no roughness caused by calculus can be felt, then move on to the next instrumentation position. If there is a resistance, more power is used in order to smooth the surface.
3. Then a second probing and scraping movement at same position is made. If the surface is smooth, then proceed. If not smooth, then the scraping is repeated until the surface is smooth.

There are three purposes as explained with each movement:

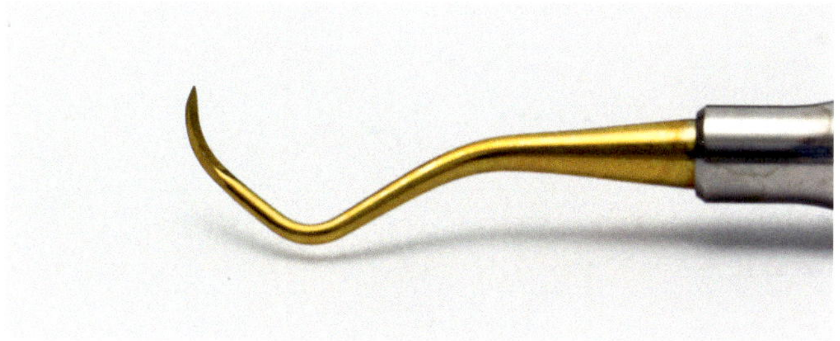

Fig 10–26 Scaling instruments.

- to remove biofilm
- to diagnose dental calculus
- to remove dental calculus.

This could be called: "feel, remove, and control scaling." The planning of the movements is done with each stroke slightly overlapping the previous. When movements are consciously trained, each movement may take less than 1 second. The sharper the hand instrument, the less power used, and the less tired the hand of the user will be.

Where traditional hand instruments have to be sharpened frequently, there are now hand instruments that are very sharp and which do not need to be (or can be) sharpened. This is because of a very hard surface (eg, American Eagle AE C M 13-14 S XPX – for the same reason they cannot be sharpened and after a very long time of use, the instruments are replaced by new instruments).

As the scaling instrument is so sharp, they are much easier to use. The force required for its application is considerably lower than that needed for

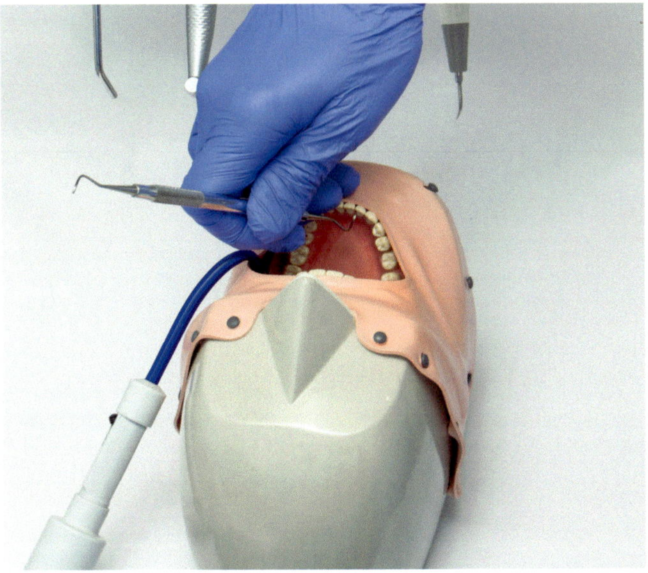

Fig 10–27 Scaling lingually at mandibular teeth. If the sideways inclination of the working part of the hand scaler is less than 45 degrees, it is difficult to use with the dentist in an 11 o'clock position, for example, and leads to a poor work posture. (See Fig 1–7, page 5.)

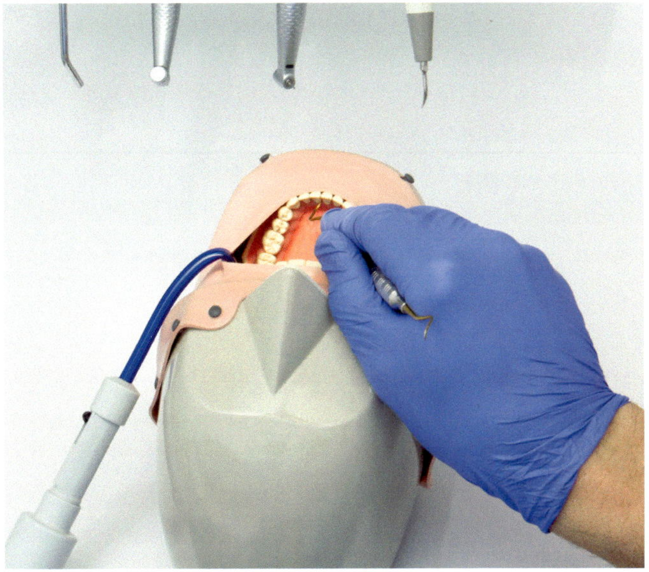

Fig 10–28 This scaler is bent sideways 45 degrees to the side. The grip of the scaler is so much to the right side of the patient's nose that there is room for the dentist's thumb. The dentist or hygienist can perform the scaling relaxed in 11 o'clock position using direct vision or mirror.

traditional instruments, and is less tiring for the hand of the user.

Supersharp hand scalers are in most cases much faster to use on recall patients with limited and rather "fresh" calculus, than the ultrasonic scaler. The reason is that the ultrasonic scaler provides almost no tactile feedback, and where subgingival and approximal visual examination is not possible, one is working "blind." The advanced "feel and remove/control" method used with the supersharp hand scaler is not present.

In the case of abundant dental calculus and hard dental calculus, the ultrasonic scaler is used initially and is followed by hand scaling for refinement. In cases of prolonged clinical crowns of the teeth, the ultrasonic scaler is more easy to use than hand instruments. A hand scaler is used lingually at the mandibular front teeths (Fig 10–27).

Often dentists or hygienists perform the scaling at the front of the lingual mandibular teeth with this instrument grip leading to an elevated right arm and a twisted back working in about an 8 o'clock position. There seems to be two reasons for this:

1. The working part of the scaler is not sufficiently bent to the side to allow scaling when dentist sits in an 11 o'clock position. The shaft will touch or be so close to the patient's nose that there is no room for the dentist's thumb between the shaft and the nose. If the sideway angle of working part of the scaler is 45 degrees, then this problem is not present.
2. The dentist is not trained to work with a mirror in the mandibular jaw, with the mirror behind the mandibular incisors and the dentist in an 11 o'clock position with a horizontal patient (here a labial movement is seen as a lingual movement, and vice versa – a labial–lingual direction reversed 180 degrees). Try it for yourself and see. The intuitive solution is to work with a half-sitting patient and the dentist at an 8 o'clock position twisted over the patient with an elevated right arm. Looking in the mirror in this position does not show the 180-degree reverse vision.

The solution to this common problem is:

- a 45-degree sideways-angled working part of the scaler (Fig 10–28)
- horizontal patient, dentist 11 o'clock with direct vision
- working with a mirror when direct vision is not possible, and
- brain/hand training to manage the 180-degree reverse vision.

How to move the hand scaler

In order to improve tactility "through the instrument," one can reduce or avoid using finger movements.

- Hold the instrument with your fingers, and feel with your fingers.
- Move your hand to move the instrument with flexible support of the ring finger or extraorally on the patient's skin.
- The fingers grip the instrument shaft in order to place the working part correctly on the part of the surface where the instrument is used, and than the fingers and the wrist are – as far as possible – no longer moved.
- This is the simplified biomechanics technique described earlier in Chapter 4.

The movements are done mostly by the upper arm and forearm. The fingers, hand and wrist are only supporting the instrument.

The hands and fingers hold your instrument and the movements are made by your arm (for the most part).

The author is aware that this working method is different to traditional scaling techniques based on active finger movements. The truth is that active finger movements are very tiring to perform, hard for the fingers to do, and the tactile feedback is reduced. The variety of instrument grips shown in Figs 10–29 to 10–31 secure good working postures, which are difficult to perform. When only the fingers are used to fix the grip and movements are performed with instrument/finger/hand/lower arm complex:

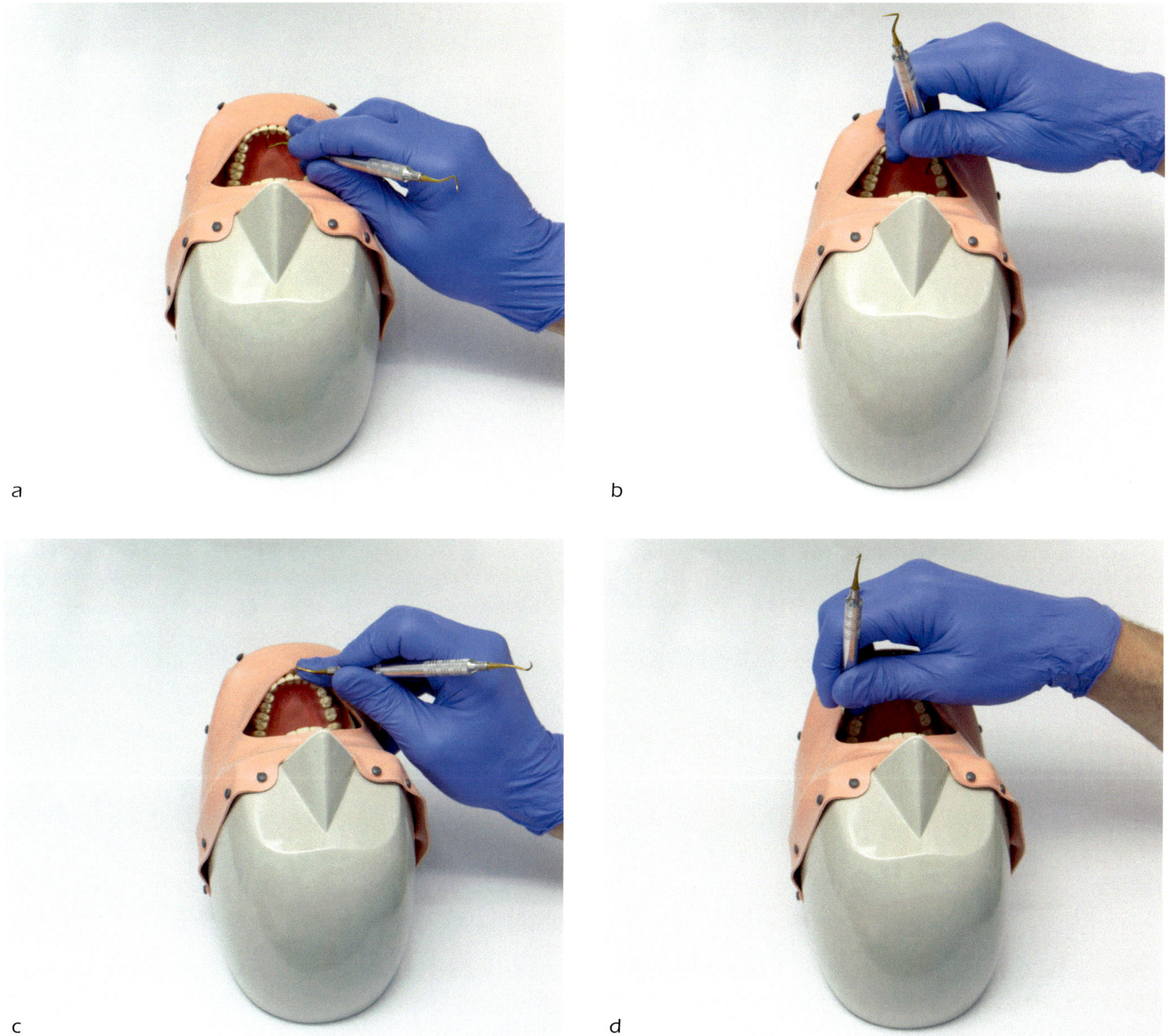

Fig 10–29 (a to d) The principles combining instrument grip and finger support are included in these further examples applied on different tooth and root surfaces in order to enable precise and relaxed scaling in good working positions.

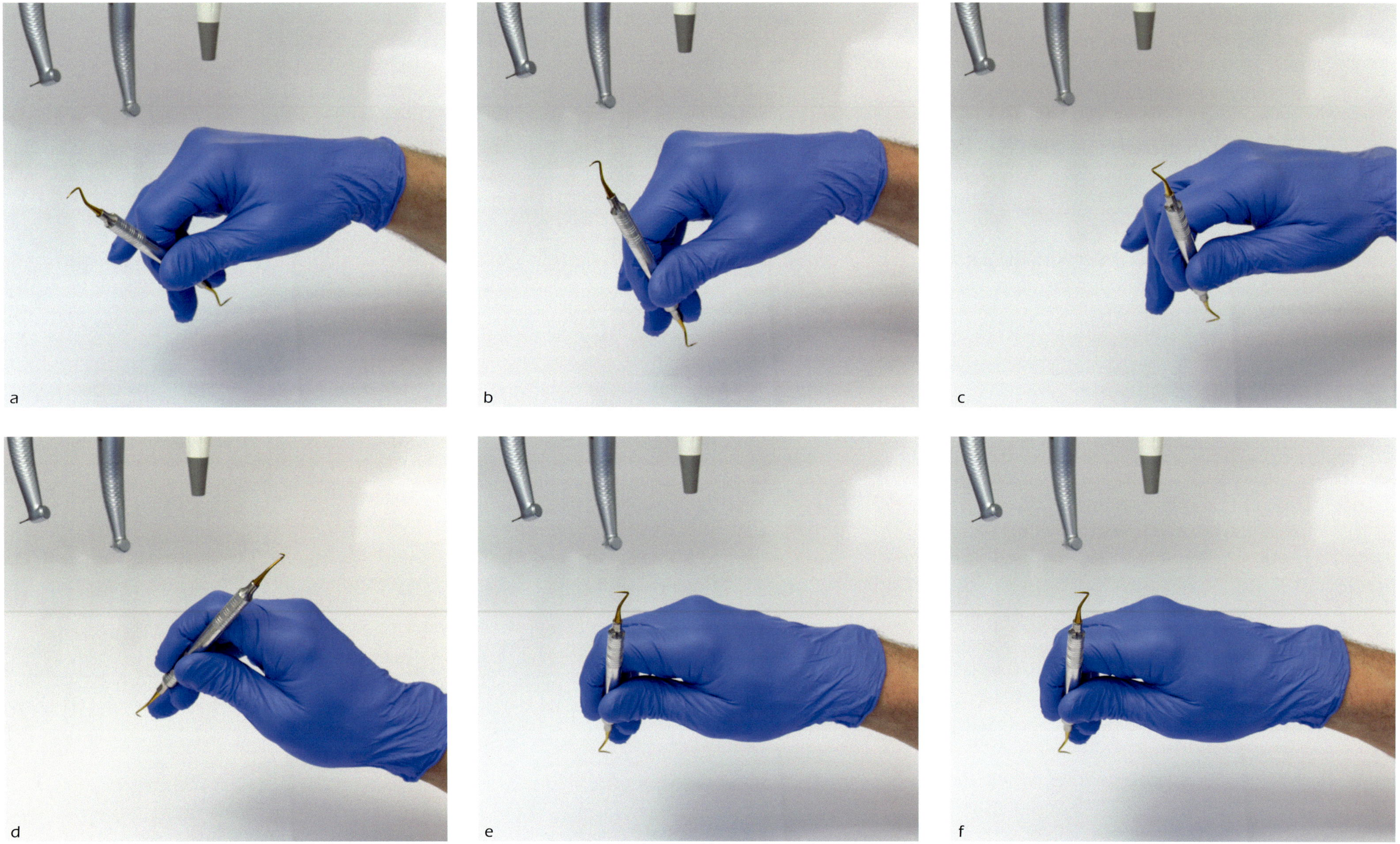

Fig 10–30 (a to f) Here are variations of finger support and instrument grips.

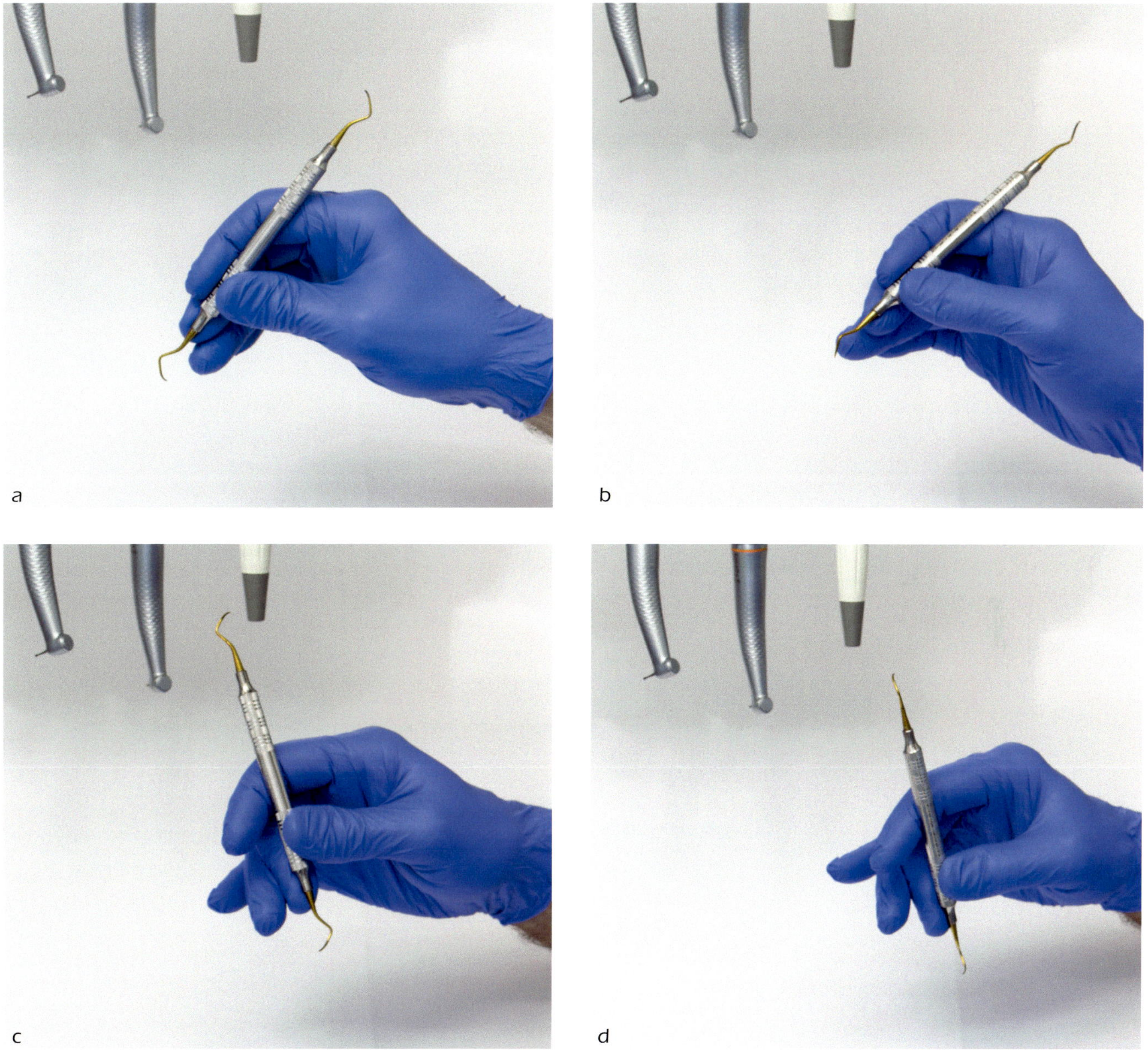

Fig 10–31 (a to g) Further examples of variations for finger support and instrument grips.

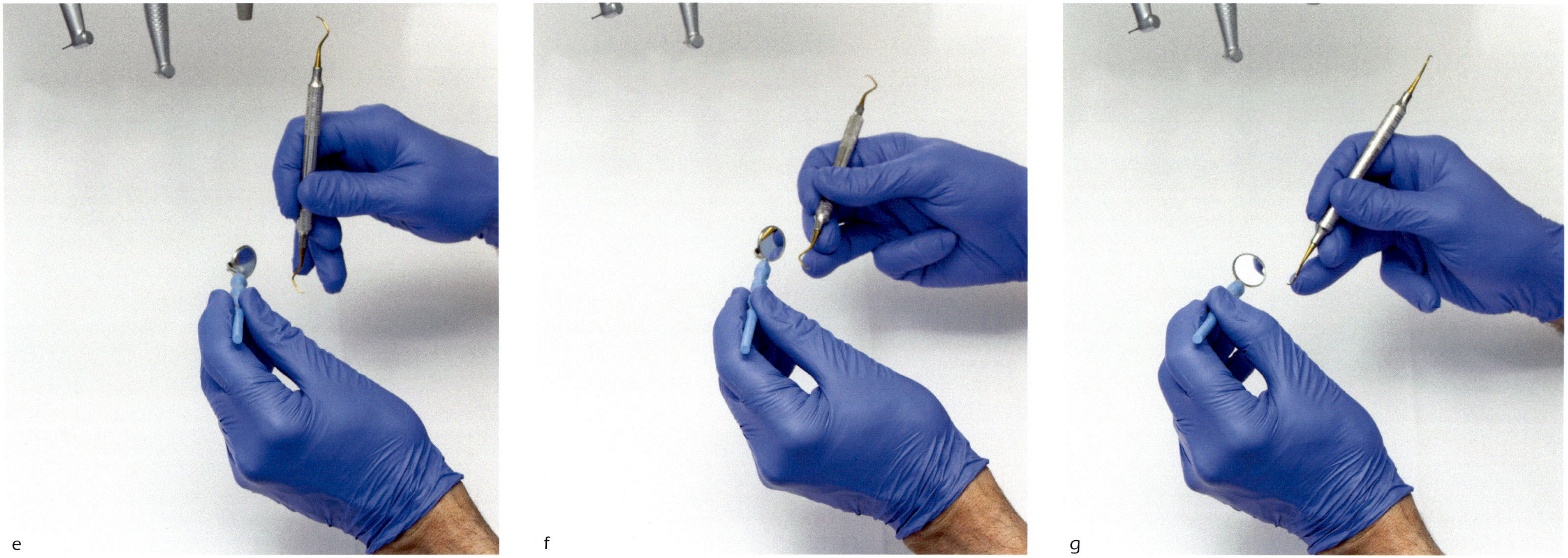

Fig 10–31 (cont) (a to g) Further examples of variations for finger support and instrument grips.

- ▲ The tactility is much better.
- ▲ Fine postures are easier to maintain.
- ▲ It is much less tiring.
- ▲ The skills are easier to train.
- ▲ The sitting position for precision vision in a fine posture is easier to reach, and:
  - – the scaler has to be bent sufficiently to the side.
  - – working with a mirror in the mandibular jaw has to be deliberately trained.

The movements are now guided by feed forward or movement planning, where each skill can be trained and later automatized. The instrument grip must ensure that the dentist can achieve an arm position that enables a good work posture.

The support is made on the ring and little finger to teeth or by parts of the user's hand, with extraoral support on the patients skin (Fig 10–32). Using supersharp hand scalers, with the correct angle and simplified biomechanics, scaling with a hand instrument is considerably easier to perform.

If dental calculus is abundant, and hard, and in cases of gingival retractions with surfaces difficult to reach with hand instruments, the ultrasonic scaler still is the choice. The ultrasonic scaler is efficient and requires little force for use.

The different instrument grips of scaler are similar as described by use of contra-angle and by hand instruments. The objective of the grip is to place the working part of the instrument correct AND work with precision vision in a fine posture. The support on teeth or extraoral on the patient's skin are the same.

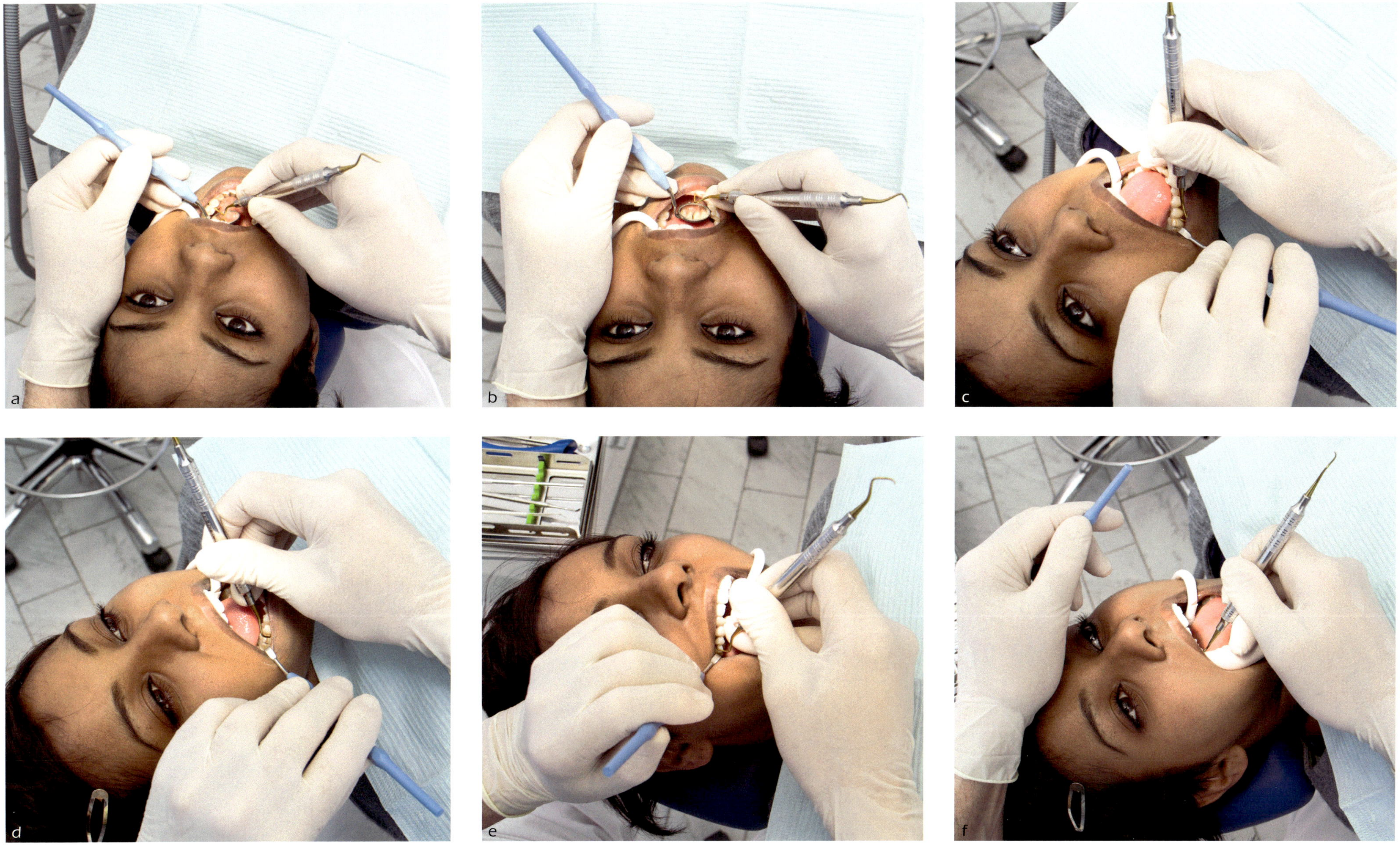

Fig 10–32 (a to f) More examples of finger support and instrument grips.

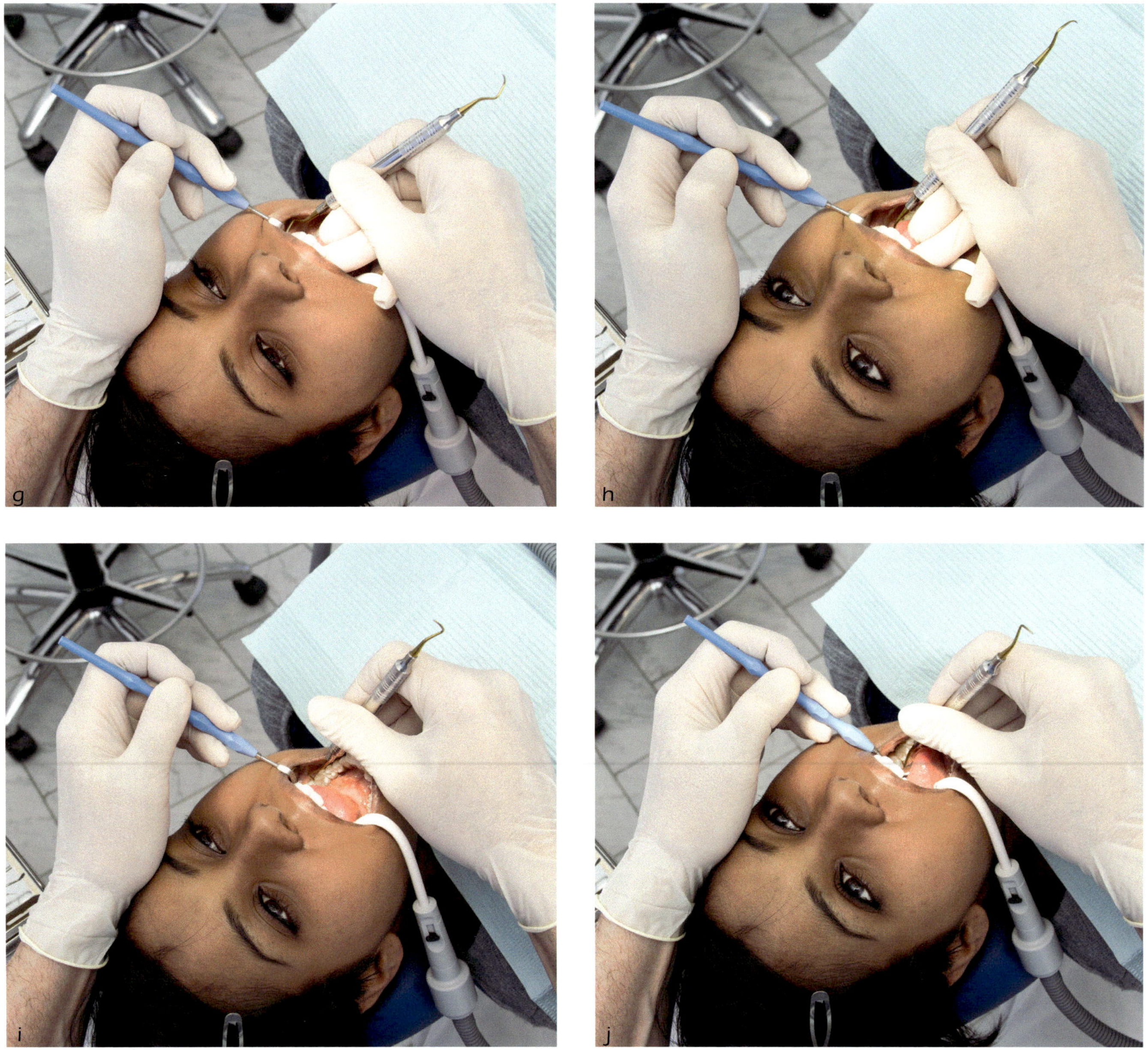

Fig 10–32 (cont) (g to j) More examples of finger support and instrument grips.

Ultrasonic scaler and mirror working

The spray from a scaler consists of water droplets larger than the droplets created by the mix of air and water from a contra-angle. When the water droplets cover the mirror, a finger may smoothen out the droplets to a thin film on surface of the mirror, which it is possible to see through with sufficient visual precision for the use of the scaler.

If a thinner water film is desired, one can make a solution of 1 drop of hand-dishwashing soap on 0.25 l of water. A bit of this solution is held in a dappen glass, a fingertip is dampened with the solution and afterwards spread on the surface of the mirror.

Use of an ultrasonic scaler hurts some patients

About 10 to 15% of patients feel unpleasant to strong pain if an ultrasonic scaler is used on their teeth.

An air scaler does not hurt

Where an ultrasonic scale move with say 40,000 oscillations/min, an air scaler is much slower, with oscillations around 6,000 to 8,000/min. Almost all patients who do not tolerate an ultrasonic scaler can tolerate an air scaler without problems (Fig 10–33).

The air scaler is a little less effective as an ultrasonic scaler, but because of the less rapid movements it gives a certain feedback to the hand of the user, also when it touches calculus.

One could therefore have an additional air scaler for use on sensitive patients (the air scaler is mounted on an air rotor/turbine coupling).

Brush for removing stains from tobacco or chlorhexidine

Tooth surfaces covered with tobacco or chlorhexidine stains may be removed with a "criss-cross" movement with an ultrasonic scaler but it is considerable faster to use a brush mounted on the prophy contra-angle (Fig 10–34). The brush must not touch any gingival areas, where it can make scratches.

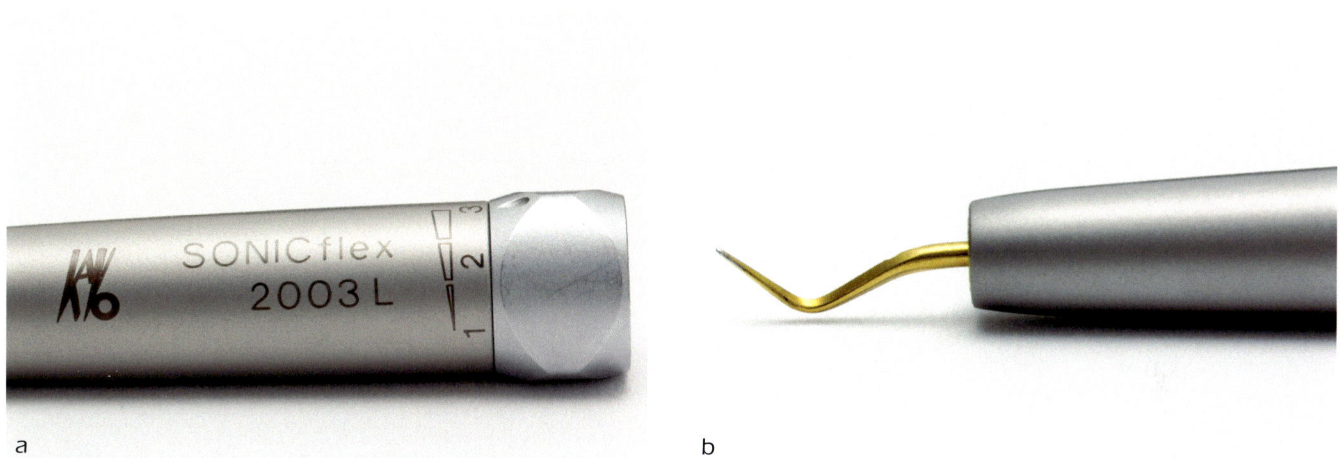

Fig 10–33 (a and b) Examples of air scalers.

Final polishing of tooth surfaces with rubber cup and polishing paste

Four-handed polishing

A rather thick polishing paste is used, like toothpaste, mixed manually with pumice to a thick consistency (Fig 10–35). The assistant transfers the micromotor with the rubber cup already filled with polishing paste to the dentist. The polishing starts on the lingual side of the mandibular left molars (where the assistant has difficulty placing polishing paste) (Fig 10–36).

The micromotor with the prophycontra-angle is then started and is not stopped before the polishing of all tooth surfaces is finished.

This is possible because the:

1. Polishing paste is thick
2. Surplus polishing paste on the exterior side of the rubber cup is aspired by the assistant using the small suction tube before it is thrown out in the air (and may hit the dentist's face!)

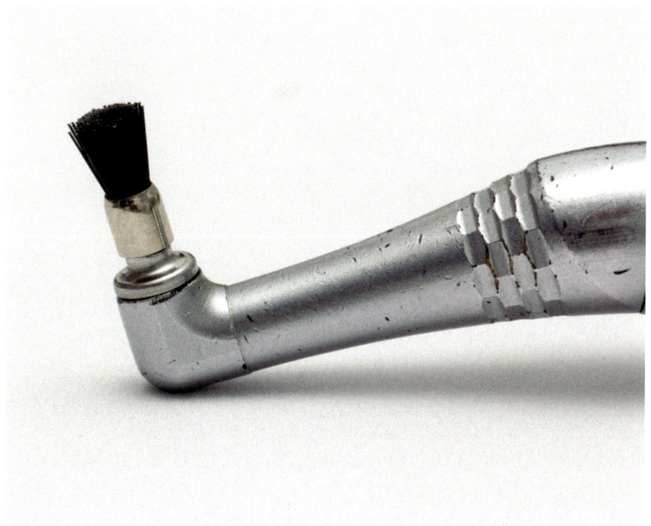

Fig 10–34 Brush-on prophy contra-angle. Effective for stains, but avoid contact with the gingiva.

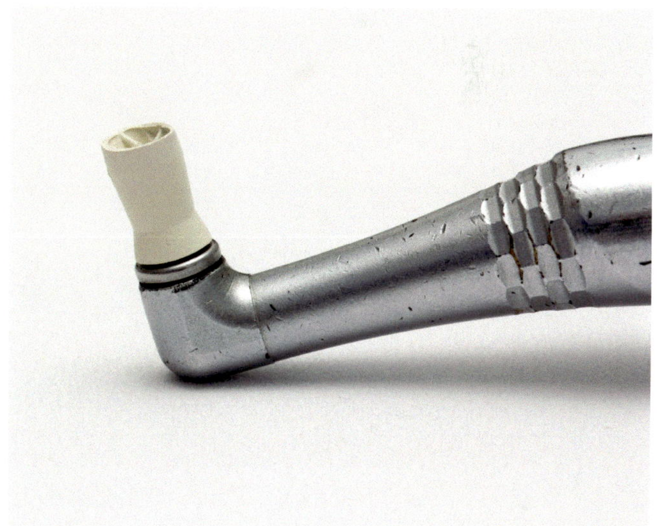

Fig 10–35 Final polishing with rubber cup and polishing paste.

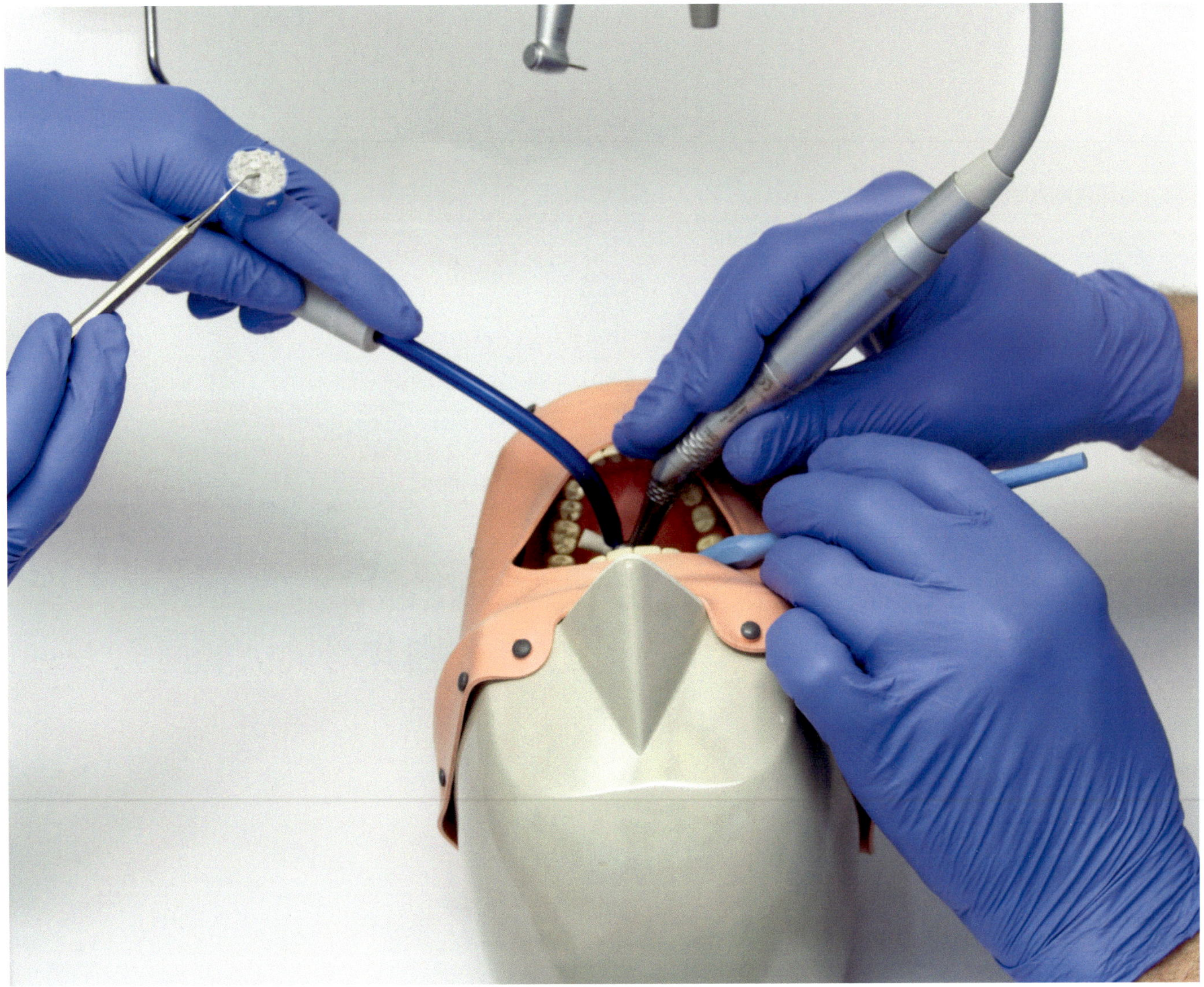

Fig 10–36 The assistant holds the polishing paste on a finger ring cup grip on the left index finger, while also holding the small suction tube without a tip, maintaining a slightly bent horizontal position with the left hand. In her right hand, she has a small metal spatula for picking up the polishing paste from the finger ring cup and placing it on the surface where the polishing is to be performed. The dentist takes the micromotor from the assistant, mounted with a prophy contra-angle with a rubber cup full of polishing paste.

3. A little polishing paste is placed by the assistant using the spatula on the surface of teeth 2–3 teeth ahead of the dentist.
4. If the dentist continues to polish on the same surface for more than 5 seconds, the assistant places more polishing paste on the same surface in order to avoid "dry polishing."

The whole polishing is performed in a sequence of movements without stopping, so the rubber cup is active by polishing 100% of the time. This means time for polishing compared to "what usually is done" is reduced to maybe 40% of the time used before (Fig 10–37).

The challenge for the assistant is always to place polishing paste on tooth surfaces before the dentist reaches them by the polishing cup, so there is no waiting time. The second challenge is to do this and, at the same time, use the small aspiration tip to:

- Aspirate the side of the rubber cup.
- Aspirate the bottom of the mouth of the patient when needed.
- Aspirate for saliva and too much polishing paste in the working area.
- AND to do this without "covering" the direction of vision.

This must be learned by using a variety of grip positions as shown in Fig 10–38.

It is important to note that it is a challenge for the assistant and much less tiring for the dentist,

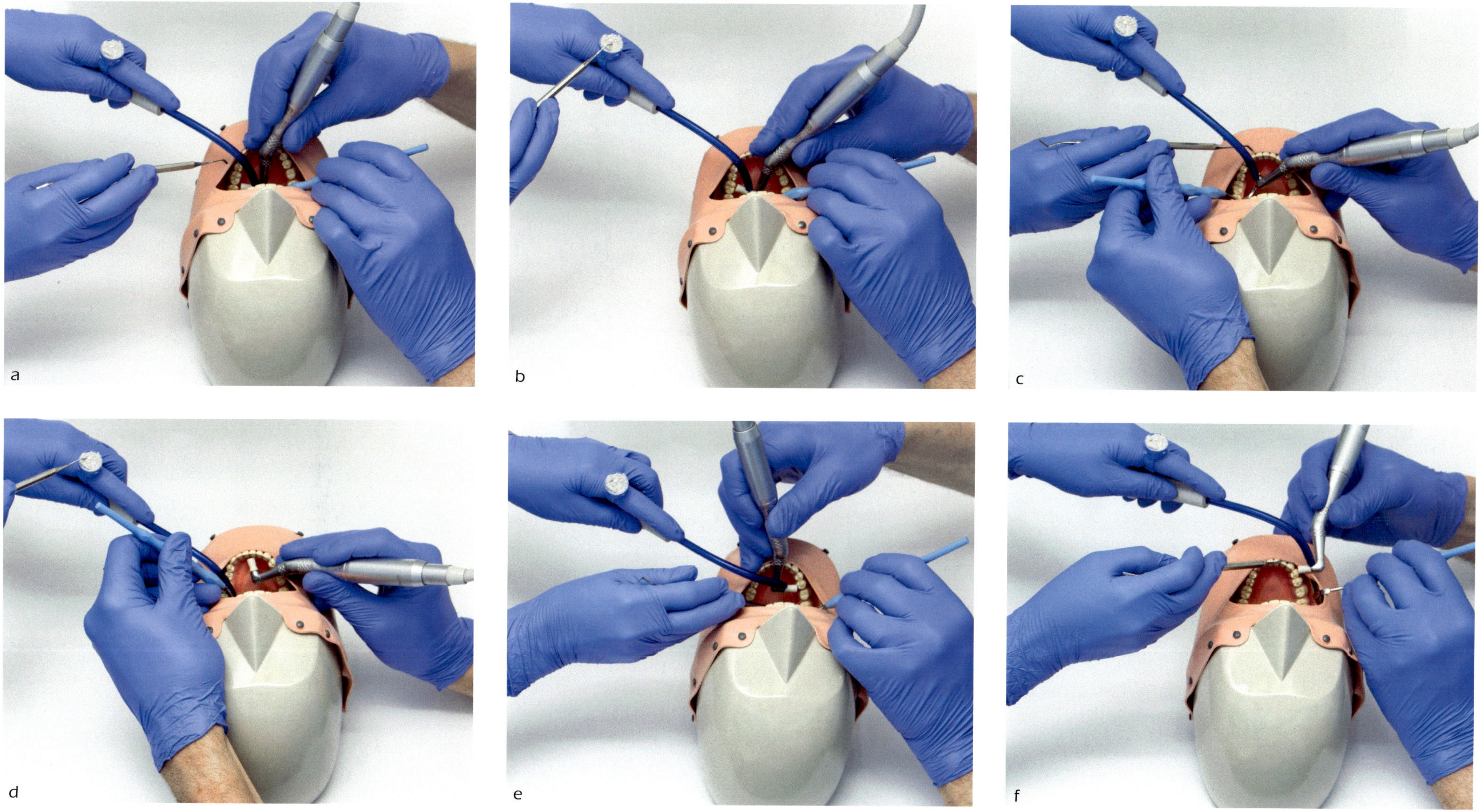

Fig 10–37 (a) Polishing the lingual mandibular left side. The assistant has already placed the polishing paste on the rubber cup. A small aspiration tube without the tip is ready for aspiring saliva on the side of the rubber cup, as well as excess polishing paste. (b) The assistant takes more polishing paste from the ring finger using a small spatula, and (c) places the polishing paste on the surface of three teeth, in front of the tooth that the dentist for the moment is polishing. (d) More polishing paste is picked up, and (e) is placed on the tooth surface. (f) Saliva on the side of the rubber cup is aspired before it can be thrown out into the air (or the dentist's face).

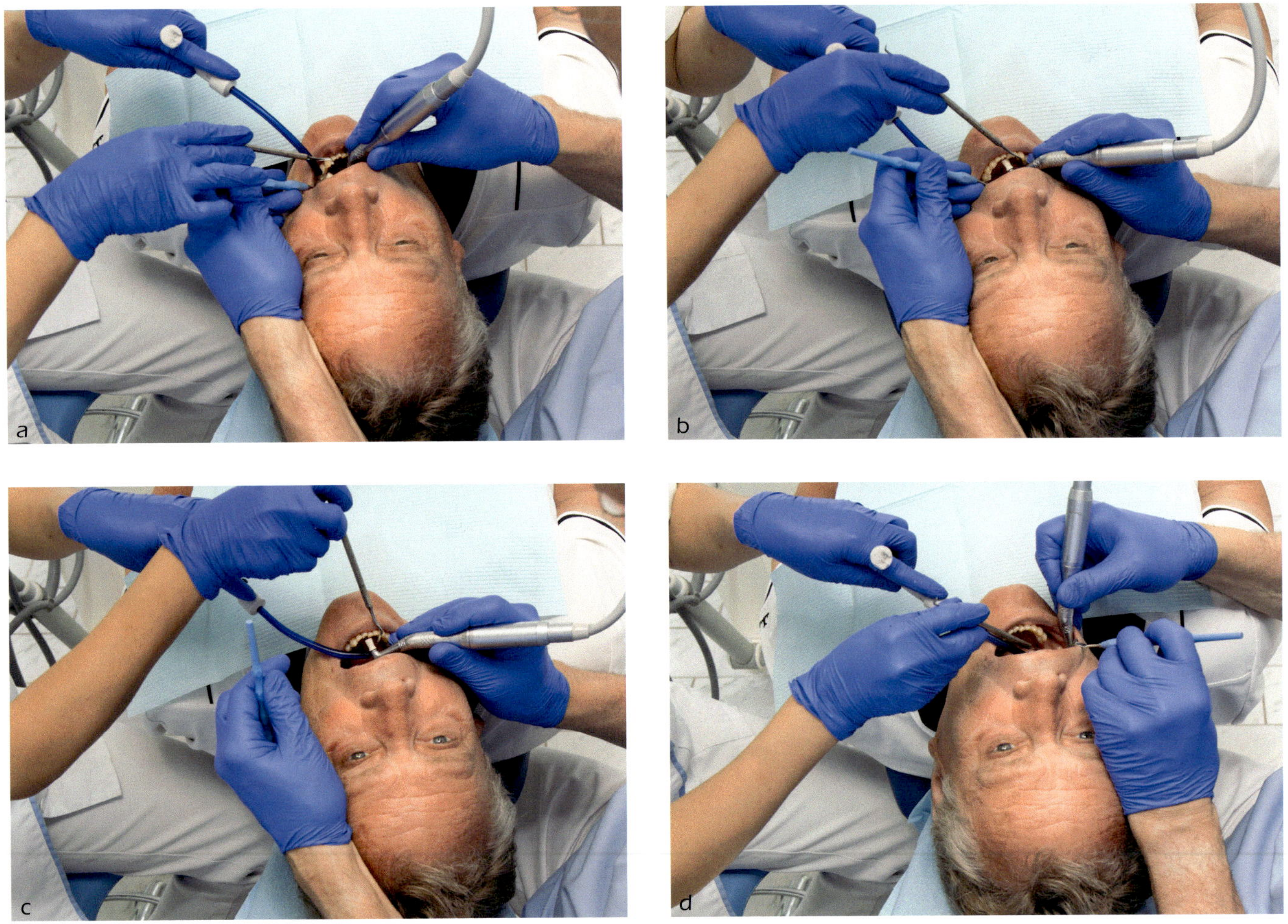

Fig 10–38 Polishing with polishing paste. Note the retraction done by the dentist. Note the different instrument grips the assistant is using in order to avoid disturbing the dentist's line of vision.

who no longer needs to stop the micromotor again and again to pick up polishing paste, then restart the micromotor having to again find the "right" speed. The dentist can instead concentrate on performing the best movements.

Recall patients – scaling and polishing

If the patient visits the dentist for regular recalls, the amount of dental calculus may in most cases be moderate to small. In such cases, the use of a supersharp hand scaler is faster or much faster than an ultrasonic scaler.

For maybe 10 to 20% of the patients with hard and abundant dental calculus, an ultrasonic scaler is used, but only where there is much calculus (like the mandibular lingual incisors and maxillary buccal first molars).

In the few cases where general use of the ultrasonic scaler is useful because of the amount of calculus, one could consider having the patient use an electric toothbrush and have recall visits every 3 months, for optimal prevention for this patient and easier scaling.

Using the best instruments, best and well-trained manual method and best assistance, treatments are also made in a precise, fast and relaxed manner in this case.

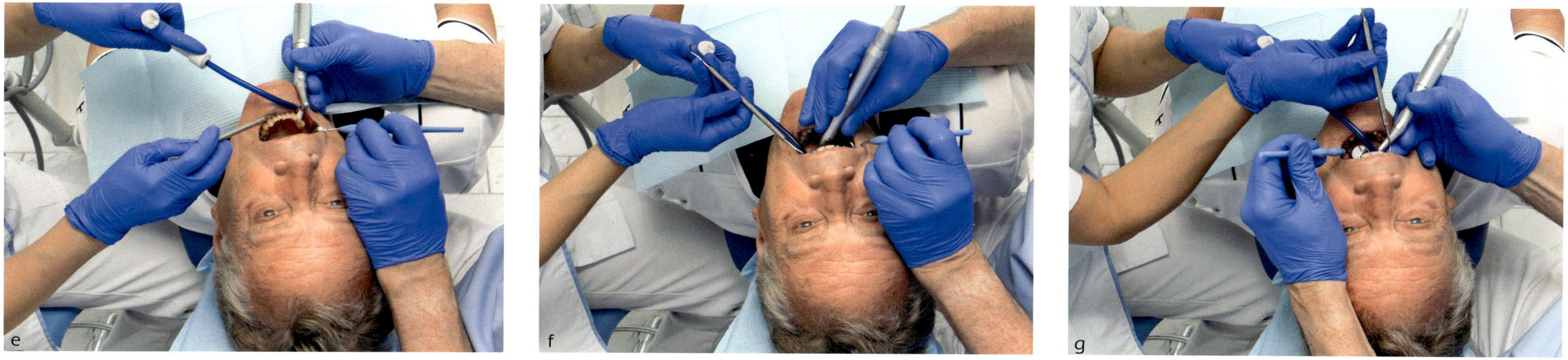

Fig 10–38 (cont) Polishing with polishing paste. Note the retraction done by the dentist. Note the different instrument grips the assistant is using in order to avoid disturbing the dentists line of vision.

Scaling and polishing – working SOLO

If the dentist or hygienist is working SOLO, all the procedures are the same as described above, except for the assisted polishing.

Solo polishing

The dentist or hygienist has the finger ring cup with the polishing paste on the left index finger, which is also used for the mirror (Fig 10–39).

A small hole in the side of the small suction tube is cut about 1 cm from the tip. The small size means that the suction is effective on both the hole in the tip and the hole on the side (Fig 10–40).

The small suction tube is bent and placed in the left side of the patient's mouth, so that the tip slightly touches the trigonum retromolare behind the last molar, where the tip aspires at the deepest site in the horizontal patient's mouth.

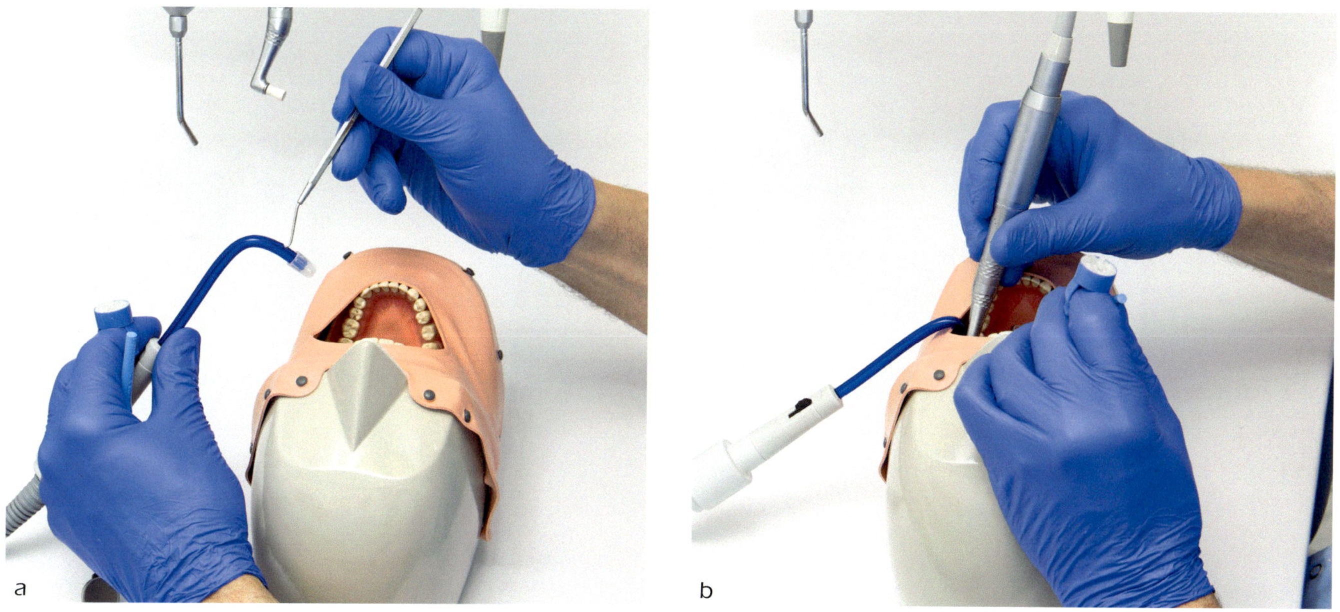

Fig 10–39 (a) A ring finger with polishing paste is placed on left index finger. (b) The small suction is placed behind the last mandibular molar on the left side. Here the lateral hole in the suction tube is easy to touch with the side of the rubber cup for cleaning when needed.

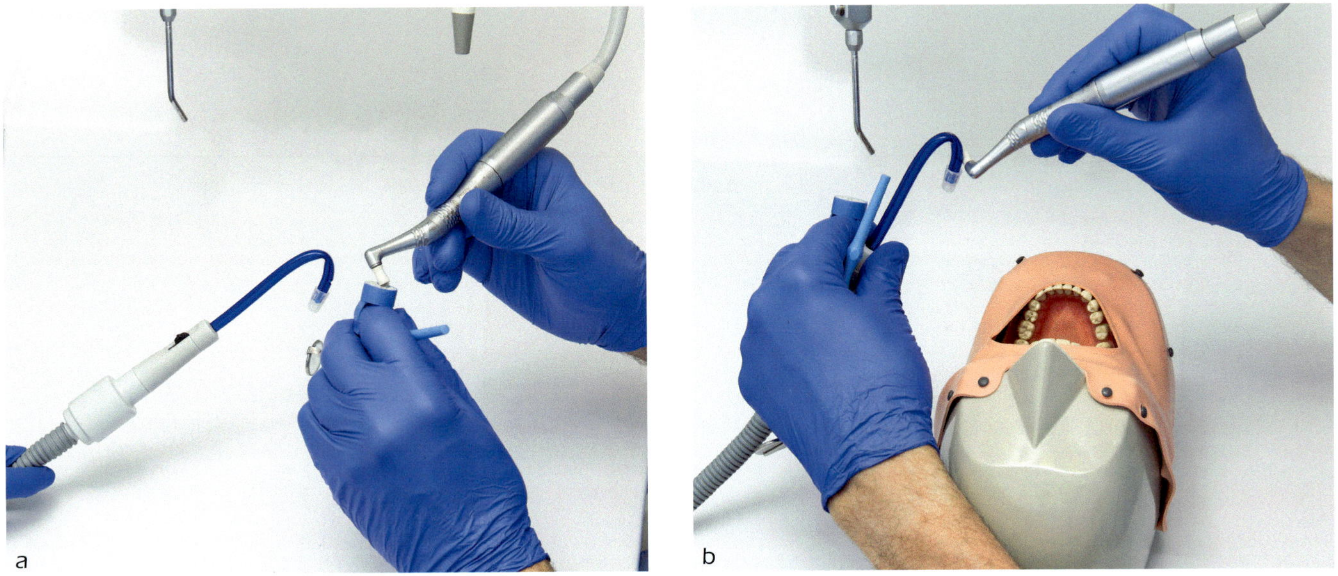

Fig 10–40 (a) Polishing paste is picked up by the rotating rubber cup. (b) The lateral hole used for aspiration of saliva. Possible polishing paste is at the side of the rubber cup, as demonstrated here with a small aspiration tube. Here it is shown how the lateral little hole in the aspiration tube is used for cleaning the rubber cup for saliva and polishing paste. But the small aspiration tube – of course – rests in its position behind the last left mandibular molar.

The dentist/hygienist picks up polishing paste with the rubber cup and starts to polish the surfaces. When saliva starts to move around the rubber cup, it is moved to touch the hole at the side of the small suction tube, and immediately the saliva (and polishing paste) is removed from the rubber cup. More polishing paste is picked up and polishing continued (Figs 10–41 and 10–42).

As the polishing paste is rather thick, it can be picked up by the revolving rubber cup. Therefore, the micromotor with the contra-angle is not stopped until all tooth surfaces are polished. An alternative is to use a spatula to place a deposit of polishing paste on the occlusal surfaces of the molars and premolars and "refill" the rotating rubber cup from here.

The time needed for supragingival scaling and polishing will vary. Many recall patients only need a very short time, and some need more. Scheduling recalls should therefore be based on the individual, and depending on the time needed for – among other procedures – scaling and polishing. It is fair to say that a reasonable time gain for 15 recalls a day will be more than 1 hour per day.

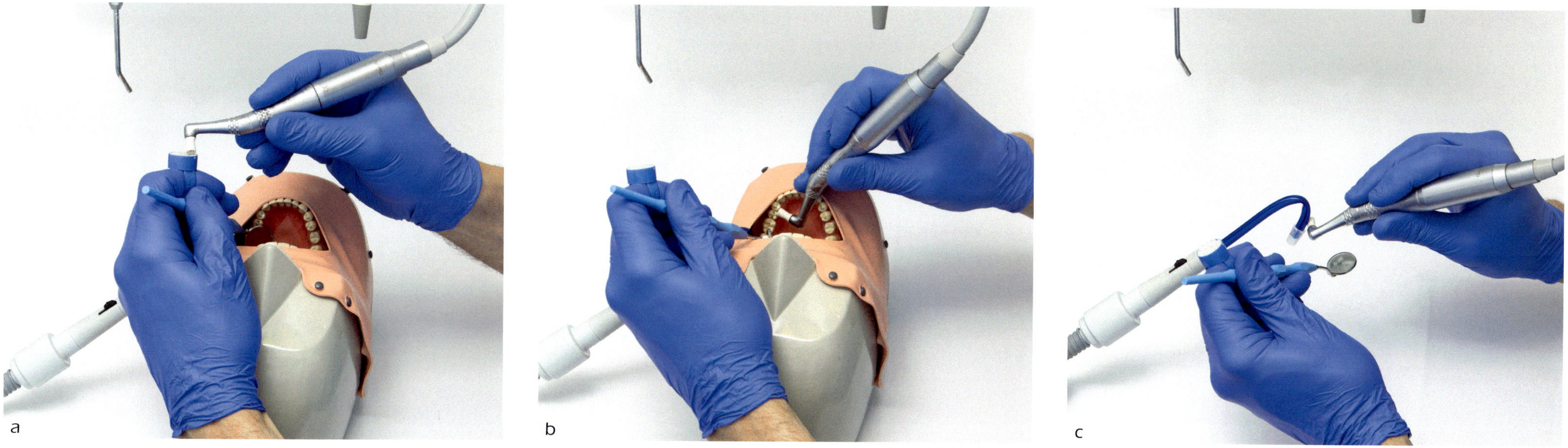

a b c

Fig 10–41 (a) Polishing paste is picked up from the ring finger, without stopping the rotation of the rubber cup. (b) Polishing. (c) When saliva and polishing paste rotates on the side of the rubber cup, it is cleaned by touching the hole in the side of the small aspiration tube – again without stopping the micromotor (shown here outside of the mouth). The aspiration tube remains in the patient's mouth.

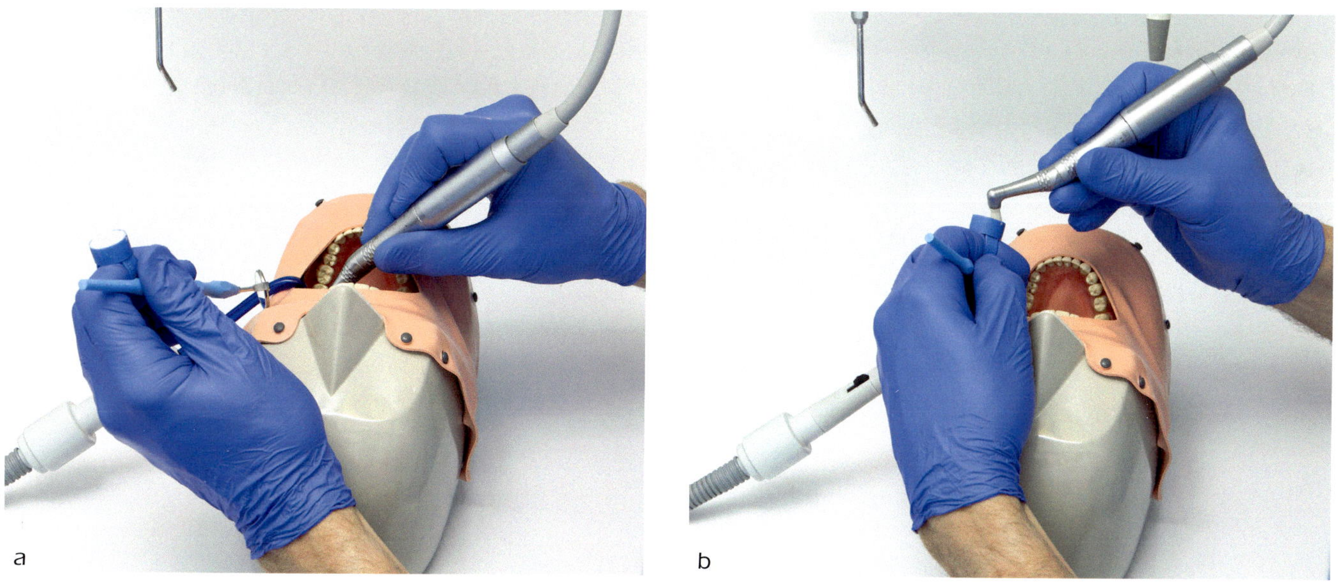

a b

Fig 10–42 (a) The rubber polishing cup in the patient's mouth. (b) Fresh polishing paste is picked up, and the polishing continues. Here the side is touching the lateral hole in the small aspiration tube for external cleaning of saliva/polishing paste.

SUBGINGIVAL SCALING AND ROOT PLANING BY PERIODONTAL TREATMENT

There are different schools of scaling methods, with a wide variation of hand instruments for scaling.

The author sees the task as follows:

- The working part of the hand instrument should have a size and form adapted to the surface of the tooth.
- The working part of the scaler must be longer for flat roots, like the mesial and distal mandibular first molars and mandibular incisors. The working part must be shorter for round roots and very short for round root surfaces of small diameter.

The angle of the working part (related to the instrument shaft) must allow access to all root surfaces and scaling movements in the direction of the axes of the roots.

The hand of the dentist/hygienist grips the shaft of the instrument in a direction and positioning that places the working part of the instrument in a position correct on the root surface and places the dentist's or assistant's arm in an ergonomically sound position.

For subgingival scaling, a supersharp hand instrument (as described on page 215) is excellent. Here an instrument grip, hand and arm position and support is provided for all surfaces using an American Eagle Gracey deep pocket AE G 15-16 DP XPX.

The scaling movements

If possible, avoid finger movements because they reduce tactility and are very tiring to make. The principles of simplified biomechanics are used here as well.

After the working part of the instrument is placed in the bottom of periodontal pocket, the axial movements are the same as described previously.

The fingers are used to create an instrument grip, so the working position of the instrument is correct and the dentist has a fine work posture. The support is made on the teeth by a flexible ring finger or extraoral area on the flexible skin of the patient. The movements are made by the arm (which has much more power than the fingers).

Ultrasonic scaling

The instrument grip is made by the dentist's fingers, while the support is made on the teeth by a flexible ring finger, or extraorally on the flexible skin of the patient.

The movements are performed with systematic, small and overlapping "zigzag movements," while moving the instrument in the direction of the tooth axis. Optimal scaling of deep subgingival pockets is a difficult task, which is the reason for open surgical scaling and root planing.

SURGICAL PROCEDURES

Here is an example of organization for surgical procedures in a general practice. For the surgical specialist, all these materials and instruments will already be present in the room specially designed and fitted for surgery.

Organization of disposable materials

This may be done in one or two large boxes (see Figs 10–43 to 10–46).

Organization of hand instruments

Hand instruments are organized in different sterilized cassettes (Fig 10–47).

Organization of implant systems

Implant systems are organized in a number of sterile boxes and cassettes.

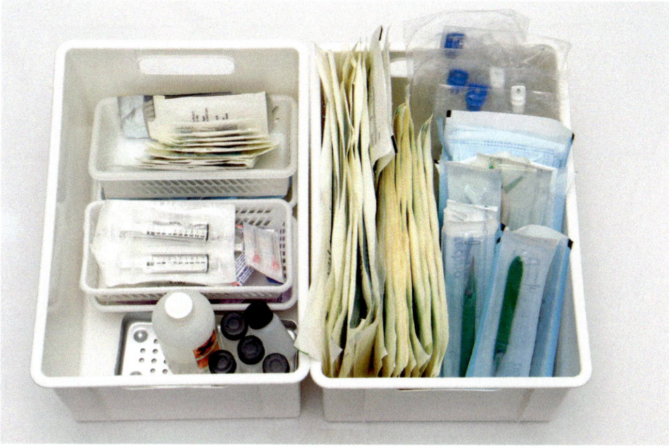

Fig 10–43 Surgical masks, hat, eyewear and protective clothing. The sterile gloves come in different sizes, alongside the sterile covers for the patient's head and surroundings. Scalpels, which are adjustable by angle and position for shaft; sutures; sterile gauze; sterile cotton rolls, sterile disposable surgical aspiration cannulas in two sizes; bottle with sterile isotonic NaCl solution for rinsing; syringes and cannulas for rinsing; glasses for biopsy with proper liquid; requisition block for histological examination.

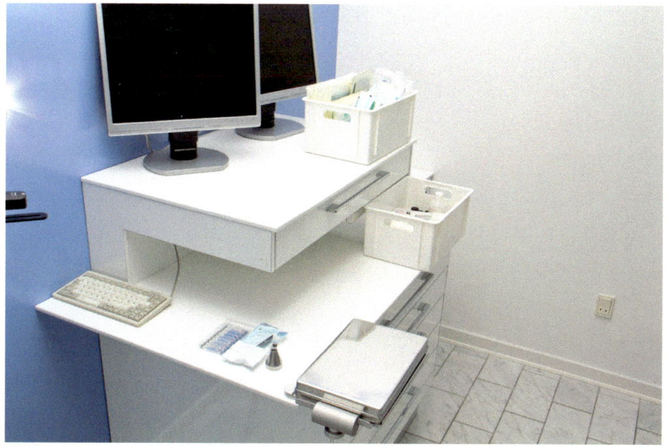

Fig 10–44 The two boxes on the MEGASPACE.

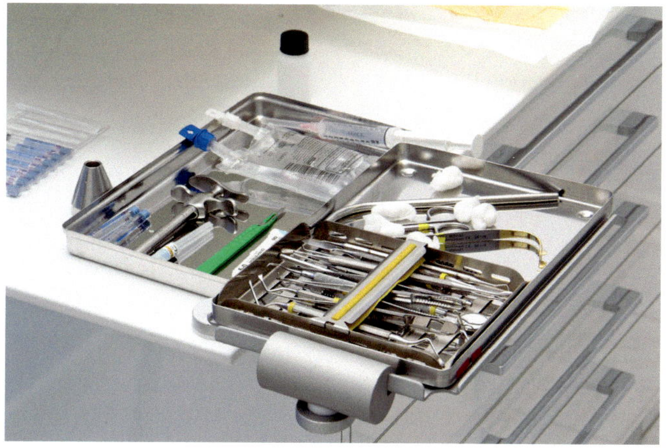

Fig 10–45 Hand instrument cassettes for surgery.

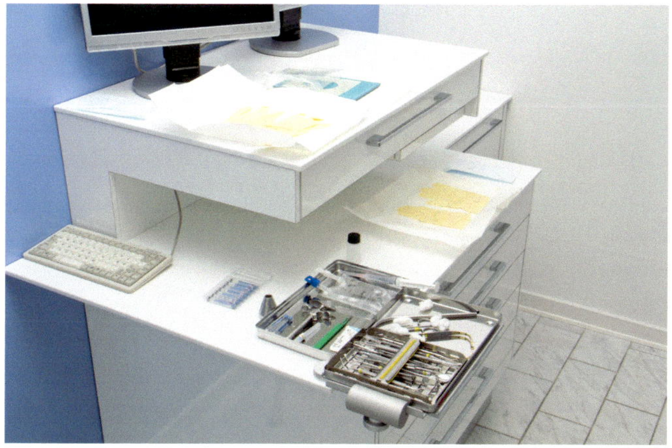

Fig 10–46 The opened sterile packings.

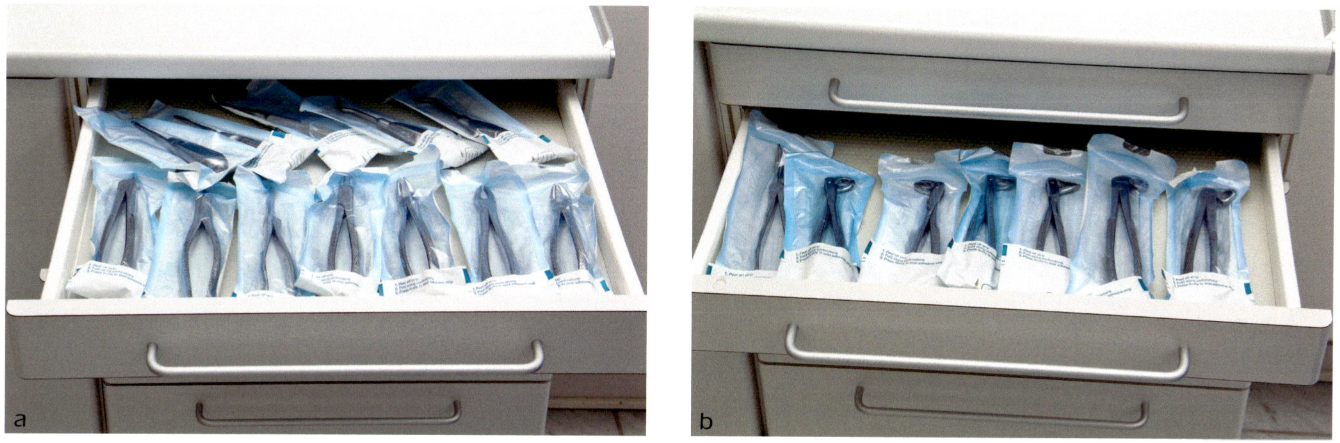

Fig 10–47 (a and b) Drawers with forceps.

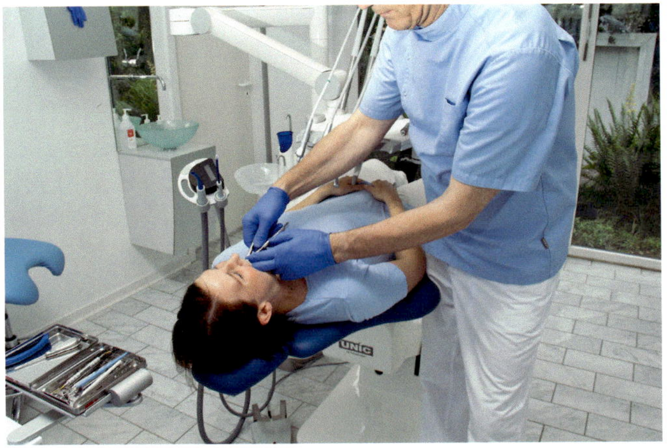

Fig 10–48 Maxillary extraction.

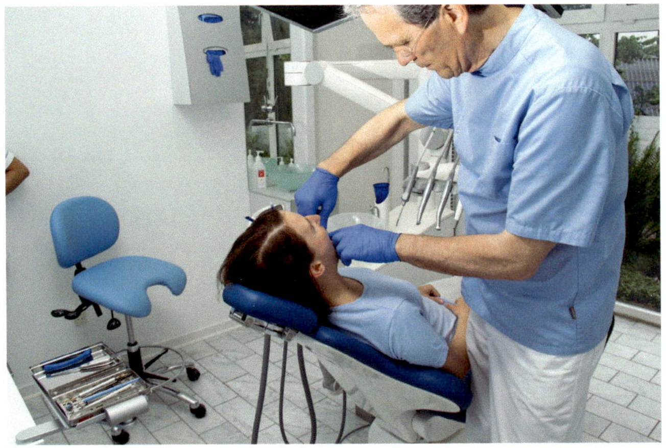

Fig 10–49 Mandibular extraction left side.

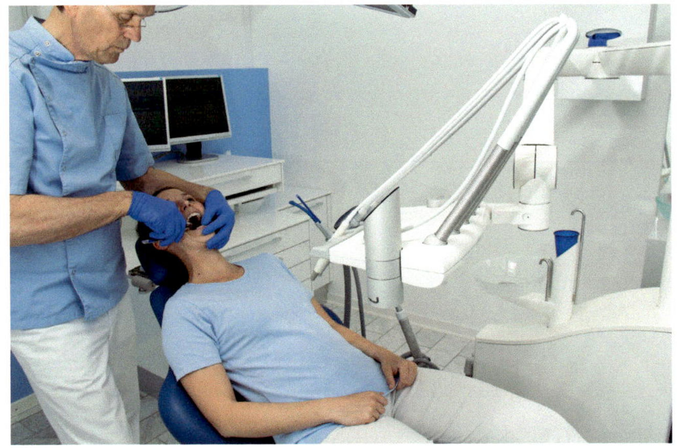

Fig 10–50 Mandibular extraction right side.

A FEW ERGONOMICAL CONSIDERATIONS

Working postures and positions for instrument grips

Wider details will be left for specialists in surgical procedures.

Extractions

In cases where luxation and extraction is a quick and easy task to perform, most dentists would probably accept the compromise of being in a bad working position for a couple of minutes. In cases with prolonged luxation, using some force (according to biomechanics and position) can be suggested.

Power extractions

To make luxations where power is necessary, one holds the forceps or elevator fixed in the hand while keeping the wrist still, in order to keep proprioceptive and tactile sensitivity in the hand and wrist (Fig 10–48).

Luxation movements are made in the lower arm, where the fingers, hand and wrist are – even in case of firm grip – used for sensitivity for the direction of luxation where the resistance is smallest. The left hand is used for a security check of mobility of the dental alveoli.

Extraction in the maxillary jaw

- The patient is lying, head turned to the right.
- The dentist is standing in a 7 o'clock position.
- The dentist is standing in order to have sufficient mobility of the lower arm for the luxation movements.
- It is important for the molar extraction that the left hand is in permanent contact with the alveolar process – buccal and palatal – for sensing mobility and risk of luxation in the maxillary tuberosity (tuber maxillae).

Extraction in the mandibular left jaw

The patient is sitting with the head turned to the right. The dentist is standing in a 7 o'clock position (Fig 10–49).

Extraction in the mandibular right jaw

The patient is sitting with the head turned a little to the right. The dentist is standing in an 11 o'clock position (Fig 10–50).

Use of elevators

In this situation, the author's advice is to not worry about work postures, and focus only on attaining a secure movement of the elevator. The grip on the elevator may be supported by the left hand to prevent the elevator slipping from the working position, risking damage to surrounding structures.

Use of scalpel for flap operations

This may lead to quite awkward and bad working positions.

Scalpel with adjustable angle

The disposable and sterile packed heads of the scalpel has a round "ball" shape. By "unscrewing" the shaft, the head of the scalpel may be directed in any position desired, allowing the dentist to use it in a good working position (Fig 10–51).

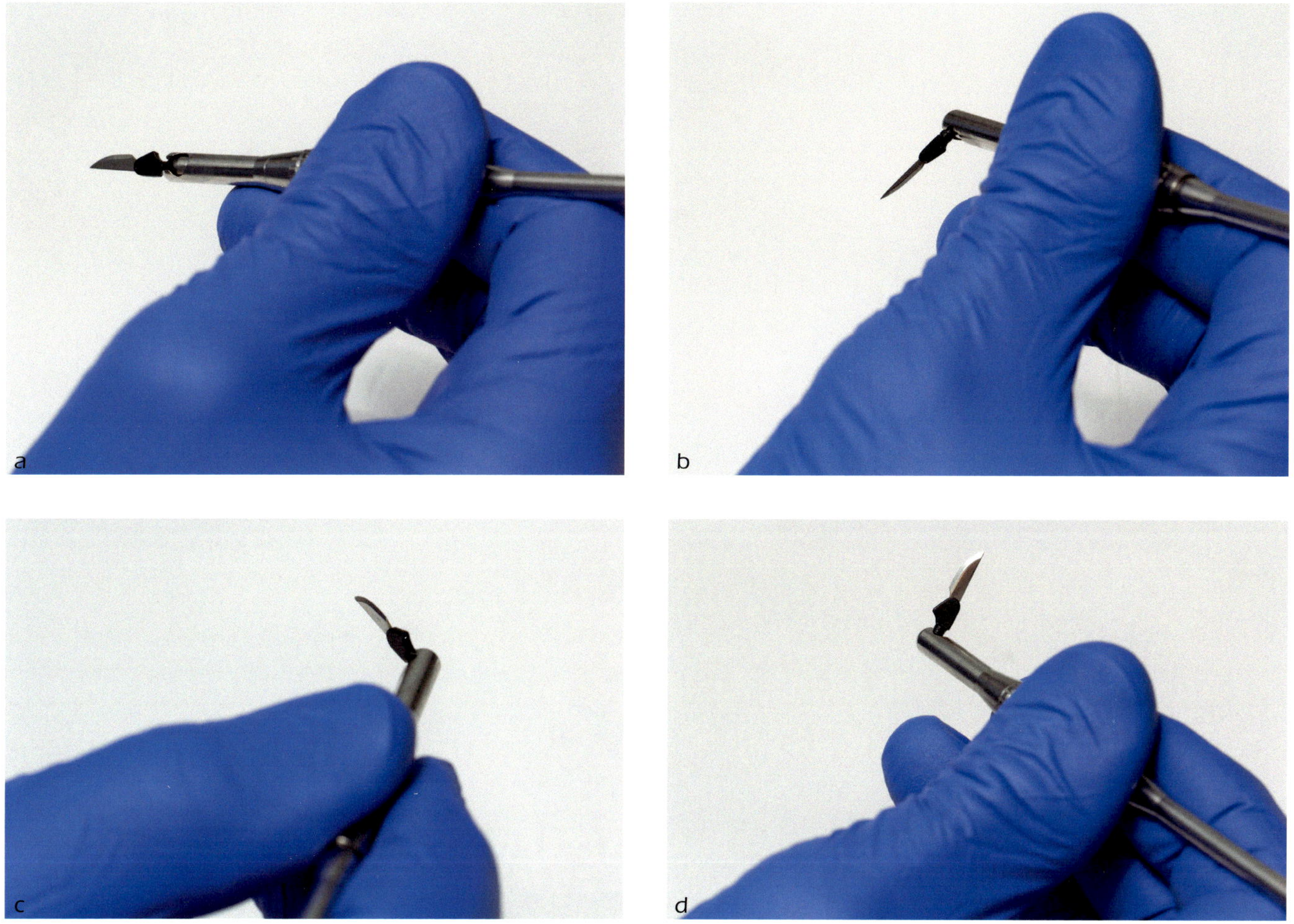

a b c d

Fig 10–51 (a to g) The blade of the scalpel can be adjusted in all directions, which together with the whole variation of instrument grips and hand supports enable the surgeon to use the scalpel in any position and maintaining a fine posture.

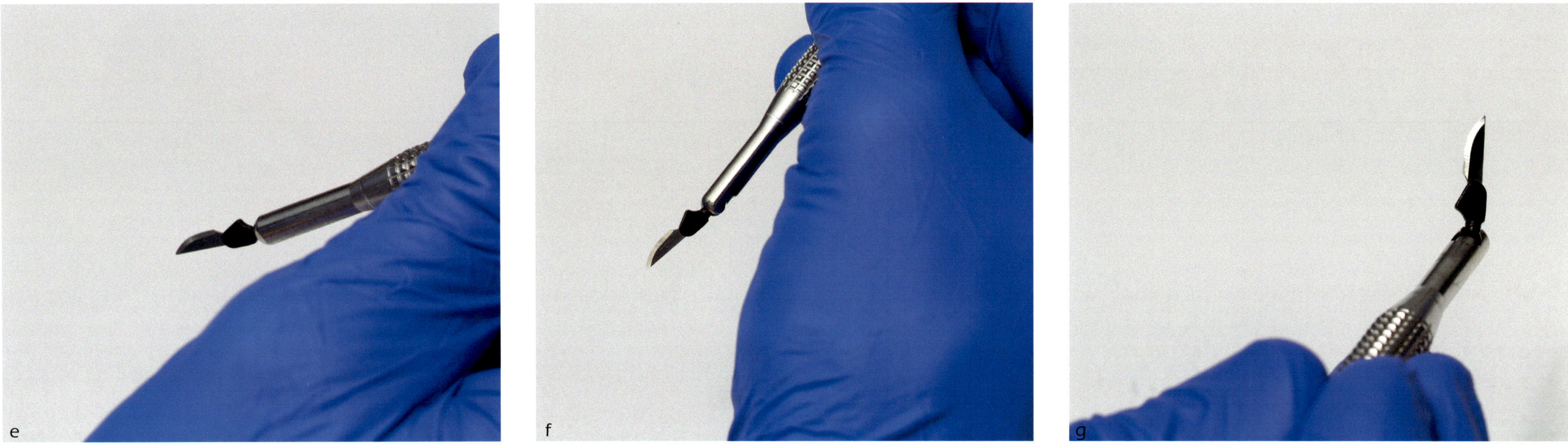

Fig 10–51 (cont) (a to g) The blade of the scalpel can be adjusted in all directions, which together with the whole variation of instrument grips and hand supports enable the surgeon to use the scalpel in any position and maintaining a fine posture.

Moving the contra-angle for fixture preparation when not using a bur guide

Making a preparation for a fixture while maintaining direction is difficult to do visually, because the continuous directing must be monitored from two directions, which differ by 90 degrees.

Instead one can train the biomechanics of parallel movement:

- The bur mounted in the contra-angle is placed at correct starting position and in right direction verified visually from direction, which differ 90 degrees.
- Then the hand grip is fixed and not to be changed.
- The wrist position is kept unchanged as well.
- That means that the bur, contra-angle, fingers, hand and lower arm are one fixed unit.
- The precise movement in longitudinal direction of the preparation bur is now a matter of a parallel motion by the dentist's lower arm.
- The fine motor movement is now transferred to a macro and visible movement.

HOW TO DO IT – GOOD WORKING POSTURE, PERFECT VISION AND INSTRUMENTAL ACCESS

The following pages will offer a tooth-specific guide for:

- working at specific tooth surfaces
- patient's head
- direction of vision
- dentist position
- instrument grip
- hand support
- retraction
- aspiration.

On a surface, one can work with cavity preparation and excavation more or less perpendicular to the surface, eg, for crown preparation or polishing, using the side of a polishing diamond or a polishing point.

Purpose of the positions

- All exterior or cavity-interior surfaces can be seen with precision either directly, or with a mirror. This is combined with the assistant's and dentist's retraction.
- The dentist's position and the patient's head position secures the necessary direction of vision working in balanced position without inclining or twisting head or spine.
- The instrument grip secures a fine working position with elbows in light contact with body.
- The hand support secures precision and mobility.
- The visual field down to 2 × 2 cm or down to 1 × 1 cm is sufficient. This means a "visual tunnel" of same size.

The patient in the following Figs 10–52 to 10–85 was chosen because the access to the mouth is limited-to-difficult, in order to demonstrate the principles of using these working methods under rather difficult conditions.

1	
TEETH	17,16
SURFACE	vestibular
HEAD OF PATIENT	back left
BACK OF PATIENT CHAIR	horizontal
VISION	direct
DENTIST POSITION	9
ACTION	cavity preparation
RETRACTION BY ASSISTANT	large suction tube
RETRACTION BY DENTIST	mirror
SMALL ASPIRATION TUBE	retromolar opposite side
INSTRUMENT GRIP	90 degree pen grip angle, modified until the dentist's right elbow is in slight contact with the body
HAND/FINGER SUPPORT	ring finger at premolars
COMMENT	finger support usually needs repeated training

Fig 10–52

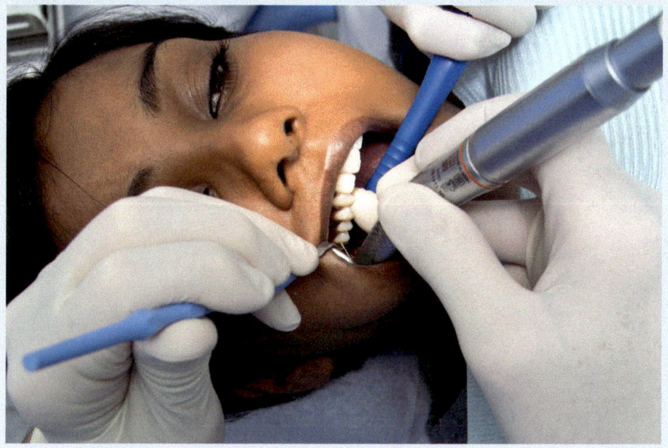

2	
TEETH	17,16
SURFACE	vestibular
HEAD OF PATIENT	back left
BACK OF PATIENT CHAIR	horizontal
VISION	direct
DENTIST POSITION	9
ACTION	parallel to surface crown or polishing
RETRACTION BY ASSISTANT	large suction tube
RETRACTION BY DENTIST	mirror
SMALL ASPIRATION TUBE	retromolar opposite side
INSTRUMENT GRIP	90- to 110-degree pen grip angle, modified until the dentist's right elbow is in slight contact with the body
HAND/FINGER SUPPORT	by the dentist's left hand, which is supported on the patient
COMMENT	See Fig 10–53 for step-by-step explanation, repetition training 30–60 times or more is needed.

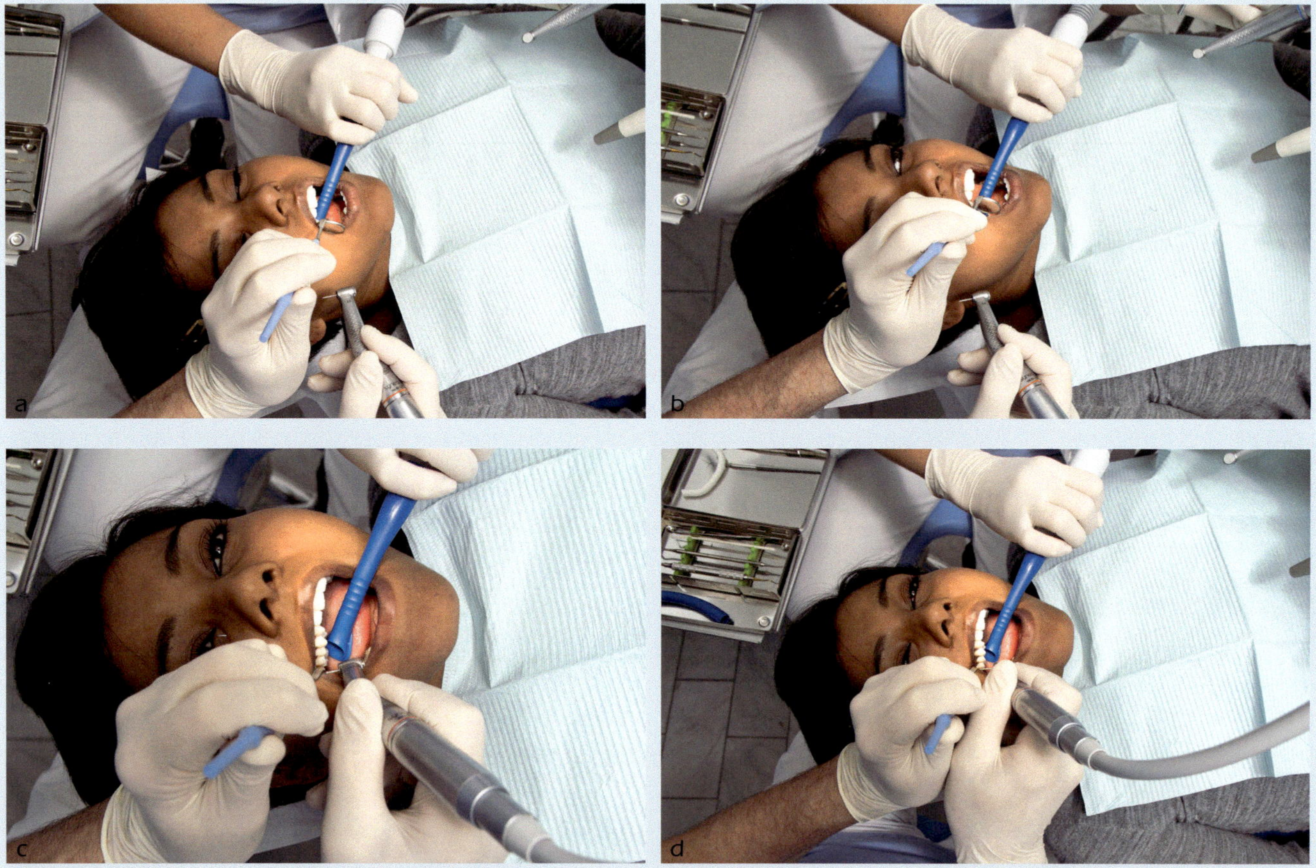

Fig 10–53 *(a) Retraction with the mirror in the left hand. (b) The left hand is supported by the patient's right cheekbone. (c) The diamond and contra-angle is placed correctly for the procedure. The instrument grip is angled in order to keep the dentist's right arm down. (d) Now the dentist's left hand moves to the right in order to provide multiple support for the dentist's right hand, particularly with the ring and small fingers of both hands.*

3	
TEETH	16,17
SURFACE	palatal
HEAD OF PATIENT	back turned right and tilted right
BACK OF PATIENT CHAIR	horizontal
VISION	direct
DENTIST POSITION	12
ACTION	cavity preparation or parallel to surface
RETRACTION BY ASSISTANT	large suction tube
RETRACTION BY DENTIST	ring finger retracts cheek
SMALL ASPIRATION TUBE	right side of retromolar
INSTRUMENT GRIP	110 degree pen grip angle, modified until the dentist's right elbow is in slight contact with the body
HAND/FINGER SUPPORT	ring finger at premolars or the base of the thumb at cheekbone
COMMENT	n/a
Fig 10–54	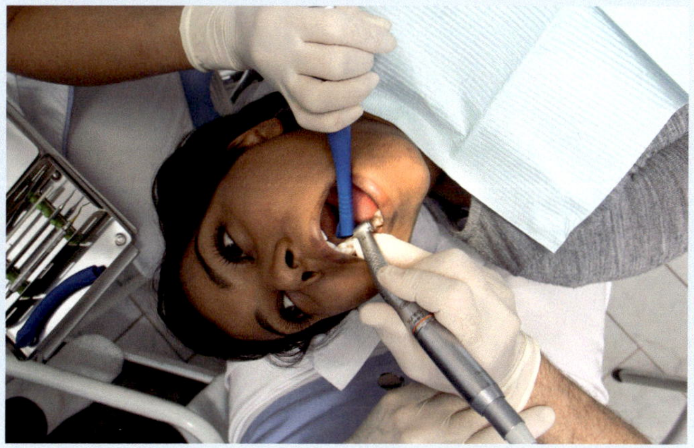

4	
TEETH	17,16
SURFACE	palatal
HEAD OF PATIENT	back slightly right
BACK OF PATIENT CHAIR	horizontal
VISION	mirror kept dry by assistant
DENTIST POSITION	10–11
ACTION	cavity preparation or parallel to the surface
RETRACTION BY ASSISTANT	large suction tube
RETRACTION BY DENTIST	ring finger
SMALL ASPIRATION TUBE	right side of retromolar
INSTRUMENT GRIP	90–110 degree pen grip angle, modified until the dentist's right elbow is in slight contact with the body
HAND/FINGER SUPPORT	ring finger at premolars or base of thumb at patient's cheekbone OR the ring finger is supported by a cotton roll in vestibulum, as shown
COMMENT	n/a
Fig 10–55	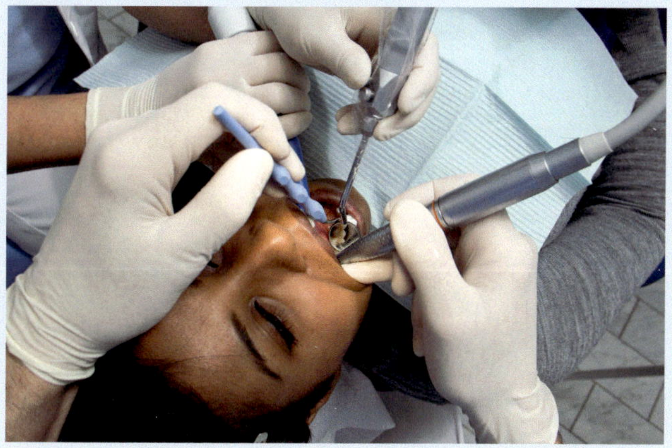

5	
TEETH	17,16
SURFACE	occlusal
HEAD OF PATIENT	as far back as possible – patient may be supported under shoulders and neck by a pillow
BACK OF PATIENT CHAIR	horizontal
VISION	direct
DENTIST POSITION	9
ACTION	initial cavity preparation, finishing composite
RETRACTION BY ASSISTANT	large suction tube
RETRACTION BY DENTIST	mirror
SMALL ASPIRATION TUBE	opposite side retromolar
INSTRUMENT GRIP	90- to 110-degree angled pen grip, modified until the dentist's right elbow is in slight contact with the body
HAND/FINGER SUPPORT	ring finger at premolars, or base of thumb at cheekbone of the patient, or ring finger supported by a cotton roll in vestibulum
COMMENT	Most patients older than 25–30 years cannot move the head enough for direct vision into a cavity
Fig 10–56	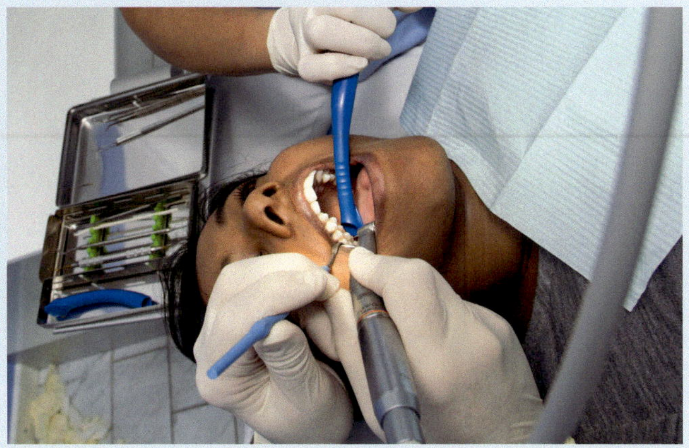

6	
TEETH	17,16
SURFACE	mesial, occlusal, distal
HEAD OF PATIENT	back slightly right
BACK OF PATIENT CHAIR	horizontal
VISION	mirror kept dry by assistant
DENTIST POSITION	11
ACTION	cavity preparation
RETRACTION BY ASSISTANT	large suction tube
RETRACTION BY DENTIST	cotton roll + ringfinger
SMALL ASPIRATION TUBE	opposite side retromolar
INSTRUMENT GRIP	110- to 140-degree pen grip angle (reversed pen grip), modified until the dentist's right elbow is in slight contact with the body
HAND/FINGER SUPPORT	ring finger at premolars, or better a Parotis cotton roll in vestibulum
COMMENT	training needed
Fig 10–57	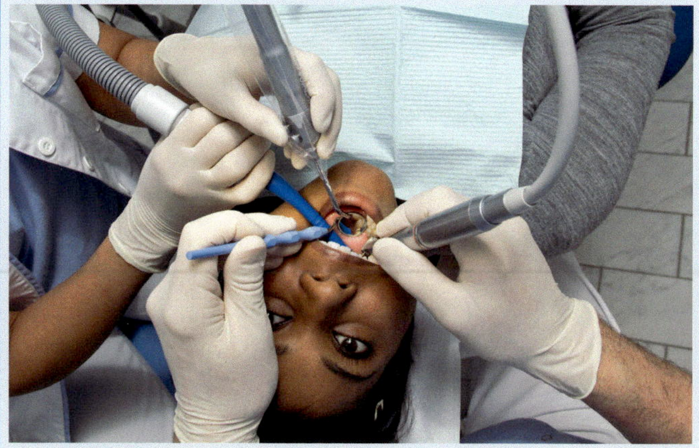

7	
TEETH	15, 14, 13
SURFACE	vestibular
HEAD OF PATIENT	left
BACK OF PATIENT CHAIR	horizontal
VISION	direct
DENTIST POSITION	9
ACTION	cavity preparation
RETRACTION BY ASSISTANT	large aspiration tube for palatal evacuation – palatal retraction in many cases not necessary
RETRACTION BY DENTIST	mirror or left index finger
SMALL ASPIRATION TUBE	left side retromolar
INSTRUMENT GRIP	modified reverse pen grip, angled until the dentist's right elbow is in slight contact with the body
HAND/FINGER SUPPORT	mesial neighboring teeth
COMMENT	training needed – not so easy as it looks
Fig 10–58	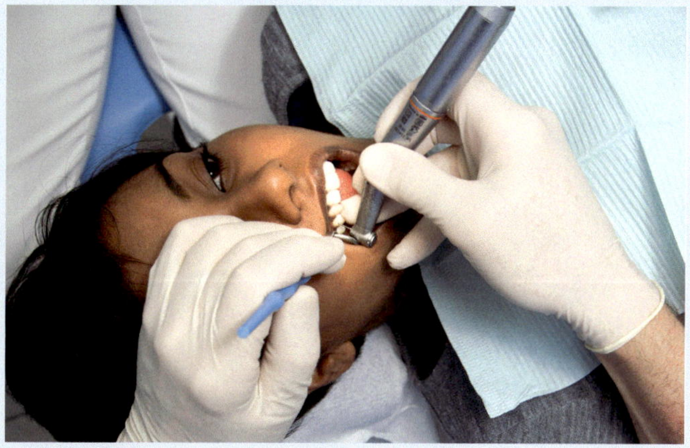

8	
TEETH	15, 14, 13
SURFACE	vestibular
HEAD OF PATIENT	left
BACK OF PATIENT CHAIR	horizontal
VISION	direct
DENTIST POSITION	9
ACTION	parallel to surface
RETRACTION BY ASSISTANT	large aspiration tube for palatal evacuation – in many cases retraction is not necessary
RETRACTION BY DENTIST	mirror or left index finger
SMALL ASPIRATION TUBE	left side retromolar
INSTRUMENT GRIP	modified pen grip, angled until the dentist's right elbow is in slight contact with the body
HAND/FINGER SUPPORT	mesial neighboring teeth
COMMENT	Attention to the biomechanical guided parallel movement of the rotating instrument is required
Fig 10–59	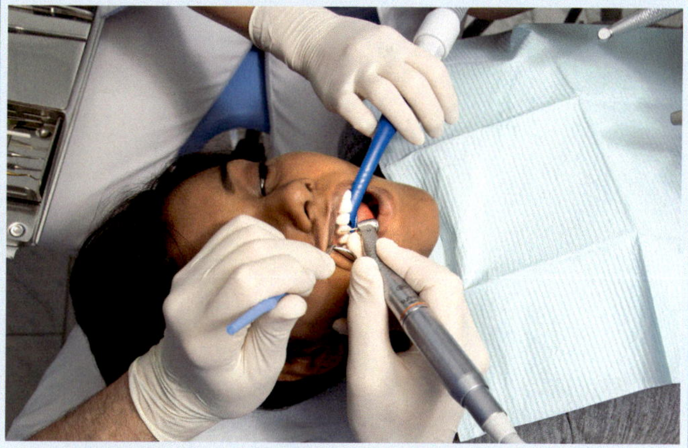

9	
TEETH	15, 14, 13
SURFACE	occlusal/incisal, maybe mesial
HEAD OF PATIENT	left as far back as possible, pillow under neck
BACK OF PATIENT CHAIR	horizontal
VISION	direct
DENTIST POSITION	9
ACTION	cavity preparation, occlusal polishing
RETRACTION BY ASSISTANT	large aspiration tube palatal – in most cases, retraction is not necessary
RETRACTION BY DENTIST	right index finger
SMALL ASPIRATION TUBE	left side retromolar
INSTRUMENT GRIP	modified pen grip angled until the dentist's right elbow is in slight contact with the body
HAND/FINGER SUPPORT	back side of right ring finger and small finger supports on skin over cheekbone of the patient or at adjacent tooth as shown here
COMMENT	If direct vision is not possible in a good work posture, the action is performed with mirror vision (as in case no. 10)
Fig 10–60	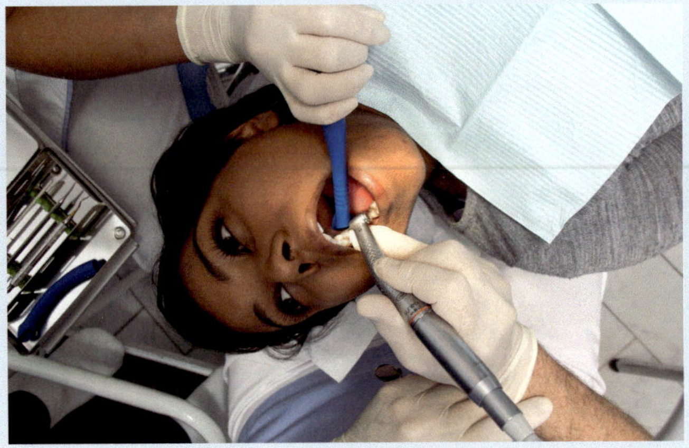

10	
TEETH	15, 14, 13
SURFACE	occlusal/incisal, mesial and distal
HEAD OF PATIENT	middle position
BACK OF PATIENT CHAIR	horizontal
VISION	mirror kept dry by assistant
DENTIST POSITION	11
ACTION	cavity preparation
RETRACTION BY ASSISTANT	aspiration tube palatal for evacuation – in most cases there is no need for retraction
RETRACTION BY DENTIST	right ring finger
SMALL ASPIRATION TUBE	left side retromolar
INSTRUMENT GRIP	modified pen grip angled until the dentist's right elbow is in slight contact with the body
HAND/FINGER SUPPORT	The dentist's hand (the inner part of small finger side of hand) is supported by skin over the patient's right cheekbone – if the mouth is large, support on teeth behind the tooth where the work has to be done
COMMENT	This solution is used when the patient cannot move the head backwards
Fig 10–61	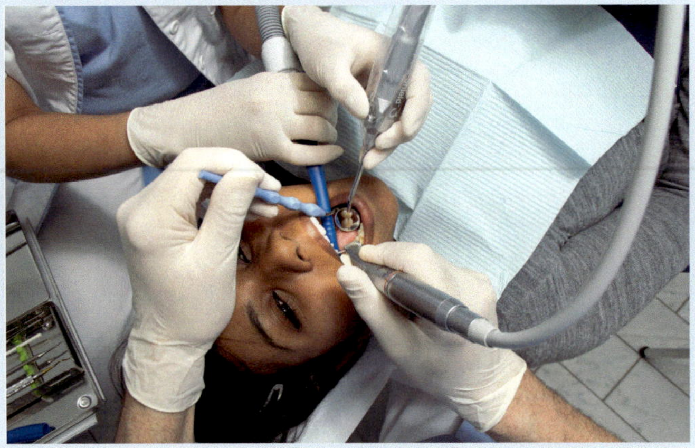

11	
TEETH	15, 14, 13
SURFACE	palatal
HEAD OF PATIENT	middle position
BACK OF PATIENT CHAIR	horizontal
VISION	mirror
DENTIST POSITION	11
ACTION	cavity preparation or parallel to surface
RETRACTION BY ASSISTANT	large aspiration tube
RETRACTION BY DENTIST	not necessary
SMALL ASPIRATION TUBE	opposite side retromolar
INSTRUMENT GRIP	pen grip
HAND/FINGER SUPPORT	vestibular part of occlusal/incisal part of tooth
COMMENT	Direct vision is seldom possible in a good work posture for the dentist
Fig 10–62	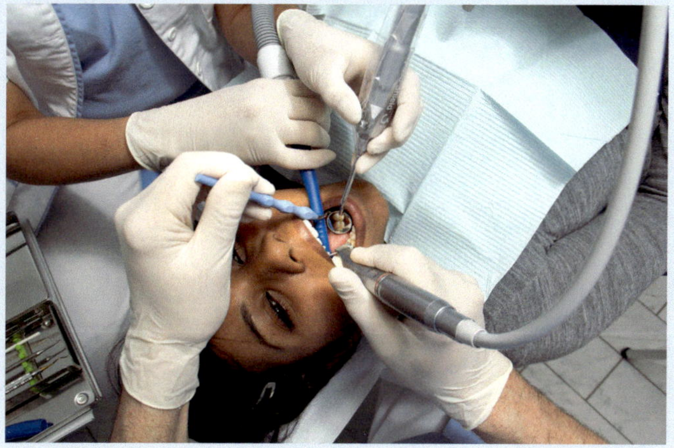

12	
TEETH	12, 11, 21, 22
SURFACE	12, 11 distal 21, 22 mesial
HEAD OF PATIENT	left
BACK OF PATIENT CHAIR	horizontal
VISION	direct
DENTIST POSITION	9 (or 10 or 11 or 12)
ACTION	cavity preparation
RETRACTION BY ASSISTANT	labial or palatal with aspiration tube, and labial retraction may also be done with assistant's left index finger
RETRACTION BY DENTIST	dentist's left index finger or mirror while aspiration tube is placed palatal
SMALL ASPIRATION TUBE	opposite retromolar
INSTRUMENT GRIP	pen grip
HAND/FINGER SUPPORT	neighboring teeth
COMMENT	n/a
Fig 10–63a	Fig 10–63b
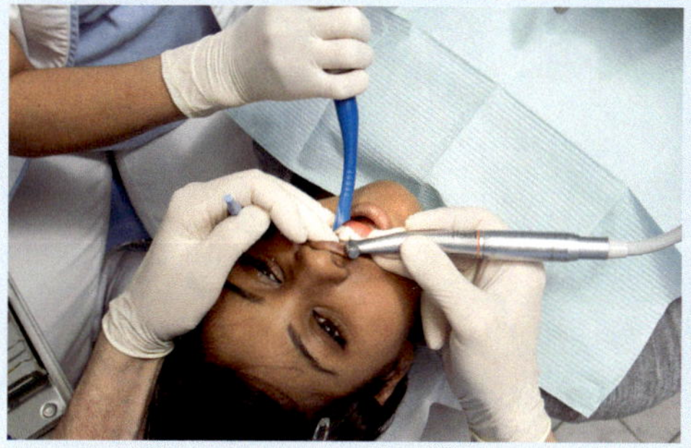	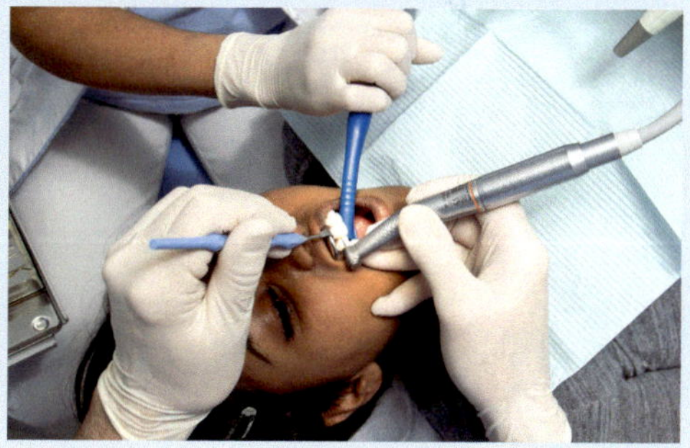

13	
TEETH	12, 11, 21, 22
SURFACE	12, 11, distal – 21, 22, mesial
HEAD OF PATIENT	left
BACK OF PATIENT CHAIR	horizontal
VISION	mirror
DENTIST POSITION	11
ACTION	parallel to surface
RETRACTION BY ASSISTANT	labial with aspiration tube or with assistant's left index finger
RETRACTION BY DENTIST	dentist's left index finger, while aspiration tube is placed palatally to support the assistant's retraction of the lips.
SMALL ASPIRATION TUBE	opposite retromolar
INSTRUMENT GRIP	pen grip
HAND/FINGER SUPPORT	ring finger on neighboring teeth
COMMENT	n/a
Fig 10–64a 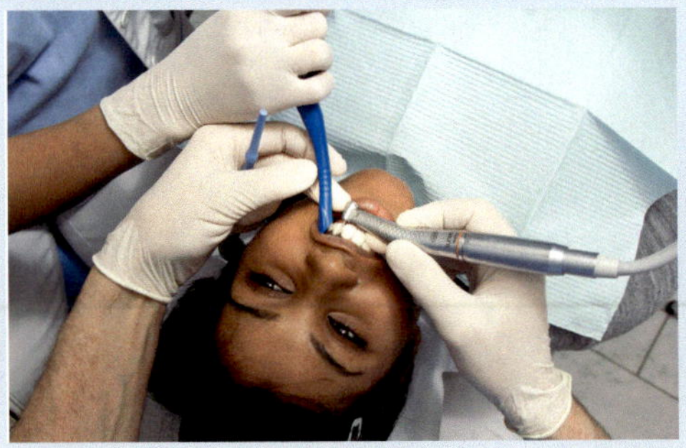	Fig 10–64b 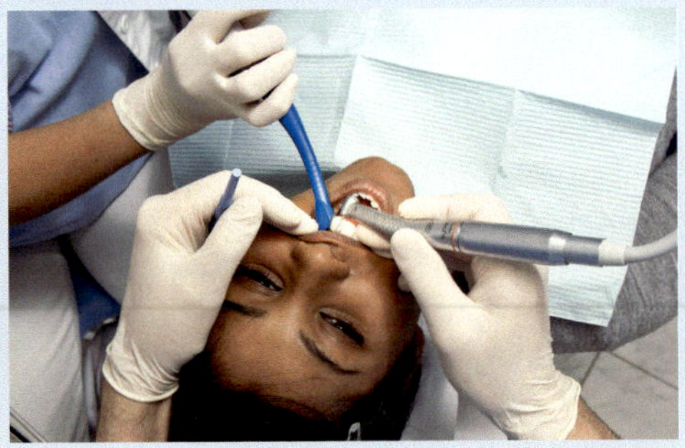

14	
TEETH	12, 11, 21, 22
SURFACE	labial
HEAD OF PATIENT	right
BACK OF PATIENT CHAIR	horizontal
VISION	direct
DENTIST POSITION	9, 10, 11
ACTION	cavity preparation
RETRACTION BY ASSISTANT	labial with aspiration tube or with the assistant's left index finger
RETRACTION BY DENTIST	the dentist's left index finger, while the aspiration tube is placed by the palatal side
SMALL ASPIRATION TUBE	opposite retromolar
INSTRUMENT GRIP	pen grip
HAND/FINGER SUPPORT	ring finger on neighboring teeth
COMMENT	Left index finger may give a extra support to the contra-angle head
Fig 10–65	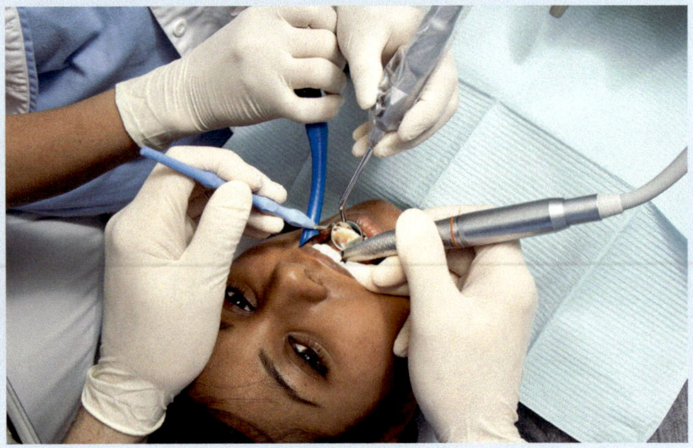

15	
TEETH	12, 11, 21, 22
SURFACE	palatal
HEAD OF PATIENT	middle
BACK OF PATIENT CHAIR	horizontal
VISION	mirror held dry by assistant
DENTIST POSITION	11
ACTION	parallel to surface
RETRACTION BY ASSISTANT	large aspiration tube for evacuation at palatal side, rarely needed for retraction
RETRACTION BY DENTIST	none
SMALL ASPIRATION TUBE	opposite retromolar
INSTRUMENT GRIP	pen grip
HAND/FINGER SUPPORT	ring finger on teeth
COMMENT	n/a
Fig 10–66	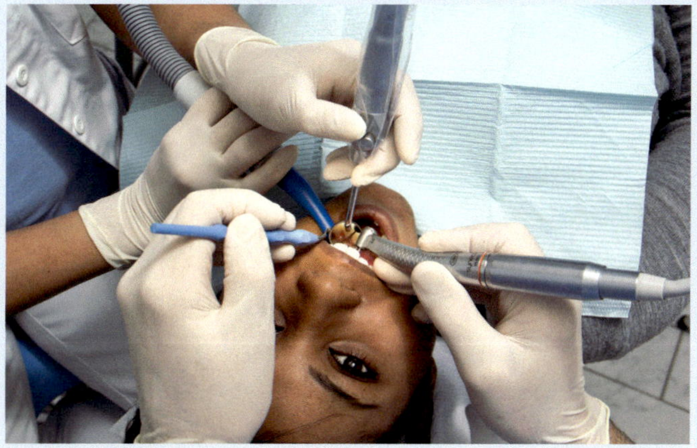

16	
TEETH	23, 24, 25, 26, 27
SURFACE	vestibular
HEAD OF PATIENT	right and tilted right
BACK OF PATIENT CHAIR	horizontal
VISION	direct
DENTIST POSITION	11–12
ACTION	cavity preparation or working parallel to surface
RETRACTION BY ASSISTANT	by large aspiration tube, as the assistant cannot see the teeth – the dentist guides the assistant verbally for correct position of aspiration tube
RETRACTION BY DENTIST	the dentist may give manual support to the aspiration tube with left hand
SMALL ASPIRATION TUBE	retromolar right side
INSTRUMENT GRIP	pen grip
HAND/FINGER SUPPORT	ring finger at teeth in the right side of the mouth
COMMENT	the dentist may support the large aspiration tube
Fig 10–67a	Fig 10–67b
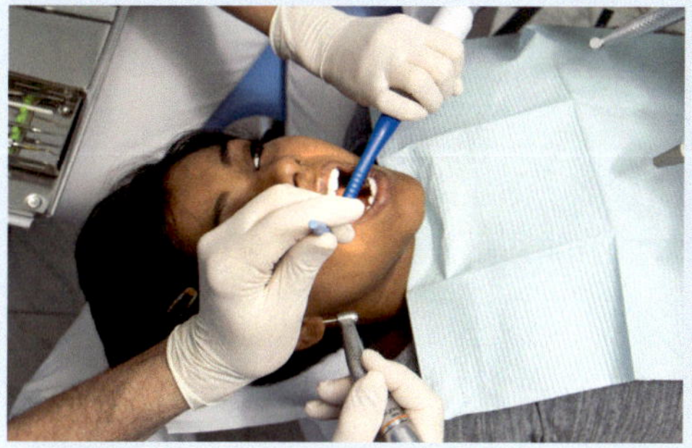	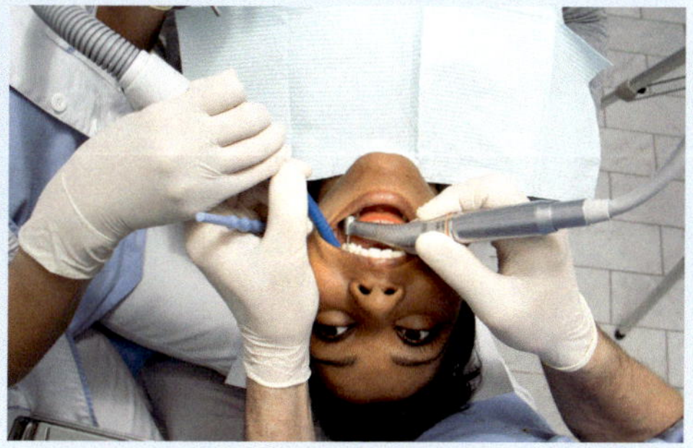

17	
TEETH	23, 24, 25, 26, 27
SURFACE	palatal
HEAD OF PATIENT	left and backwards
BACK OF PATIENT CHAIR	horizontal
VISION	direct
DENTIST POSITION	9
ACTION	cavity preparation or parallel to surface
RETRACTION BY ASSISTANT	left cheek slight retraction with aspiration tube
RETRACTION BY DENTIST	retraction of tongue with mirror (sometimes not necessary)
SMALL ASPIRATION TUBE	left side retromolar
INSTRUMENT GRIP	pen grip
HAND/FINGER SUPPORT	ring finger on teeth, opposite side of mouth
COMMENT	
Fig 10–68	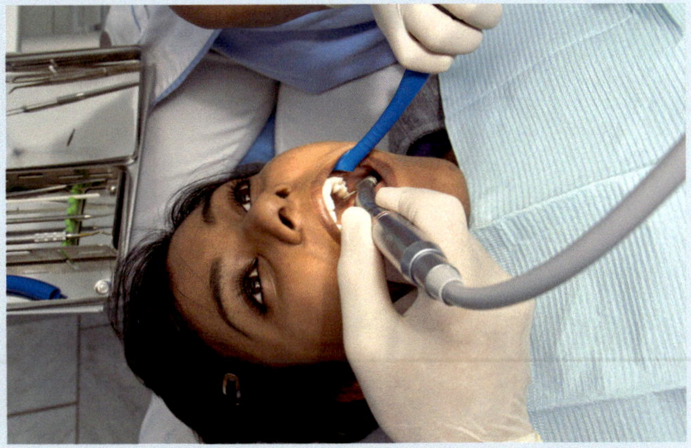

18	
TEETH	23, 24, 25, 26, 27
SURFACE	palatal
HEAD OF PATIENT	middle position
BACK OF PATIENT CHAIR	horizontal
VISION	mirror kept dry by assistant and placed so that the direction of vision is almost horizontal
DENTIST POSITION	11
ACTION	cavity preparation or parallel to surface
RETRACTION BY ASSISTANT	left cheek, slight retraction with aspiration tube
RETRACTION BY DENTIST	none or by mirror while looking in it
SMALL ASPIRATION TUBE	right side retromolar
INSTRUMENT GRIP	pen grip
HAND/FINGER SUPPORT	ring finger on teeth in opposite side of mouth
COMMENT	n/a
Fig 10–69	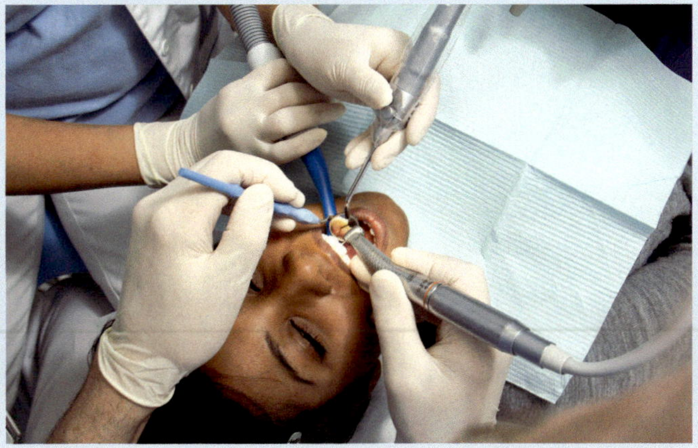

19	
TEETH	23, 24, 25, 26, 27
SURFACE	mesial, occlusal, distal
HEAD OF PATIENT	middle position
BACK OF PATIENT CHAIR	horizontal
VISION	mirror kept dry by assistant
DENTIST POSITION	11
ACTION	cavity preparation or polishing
RETRACTION BY ASSISTANT	cheek and lips with large aspiration tube
RETRACTION BY DENTIST	none
SMALL ASPIRATION TUBE	right side retromolar
INSTRUMENT GRIP	pen grip
HAND/FINGER SUPPORT	teeth of opposite side of mouth
COMMENT	n/a

Fig 10–70

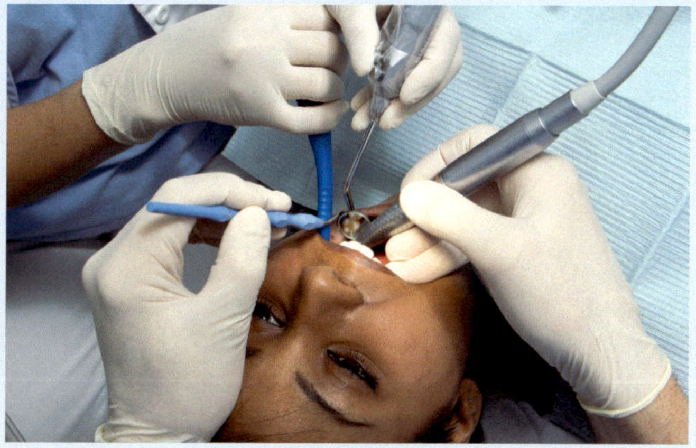

20	
TEETH	23, 24, 25, 26, 27
SURFACE	occlusal, initially mesial
HEAD OF PATIENT	as far back as possible
BACK OF PATIENT CHAIR	horizontal
VISION	direct
DENTIST POSITION	9
ACTION	cavity preparation or polishing
RETRACTION BY ASSISTANT	cheek and lips with large aspiration tube
RETRACTION BY DENTIST	none
SMALL ASPIRATION TUBE	right side retromolar
INSTRUMENT GRIP	pen grip
HAND/FINGER SUPPORT	teeth on opposite side of mouth
COMMENT	n/a

Fig 10–71

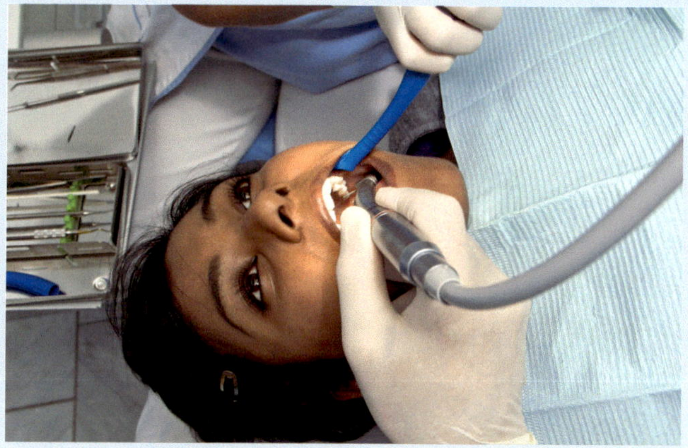

21	
TEETH	47, 46, 45, 44
SURFACE	vestibular
HEAD OF PATIENT	left
BACK OF PATIENT CHAIR	horizontal
VISION	direct
DENTIST POSITION	9
ACTION	cavity preparation or parallel to surface
RETRACTION BY ASSISTANT	tongue with large aspiration tube
RETRACTION BY DENTIST	cheek and lips with mirror or left index finger
SMALL ASPIRATION TUBE	left side retromolar
INSTRUMENT GRIP	modified pen grip angled until the dentist's right elbow slightly touches her/his body
HAND/FINGER SUPPORT	ring finger on front teeth
COMMENT	n/a
Fig 10–72	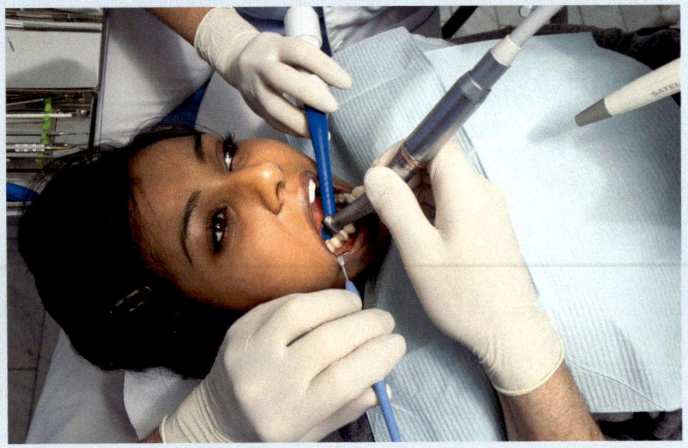

22	
TEETH	47, 46, 45, 44
SURFACE	lingual
HEAD OF PATIENT	turned right and backwards and tilted right
BACK OF PATIENT CHAIR	horizontal
VISION	direct
DENTIST POSITION	12
ACTION	cavity preparation or parallel to surface
RETRACTION BY ASSISTANT	tongue with large aspiration tube
RETRACTION BY DENTIST	If the patient's tongue is strong and active, the dentist helps the assistant to retract the tongue with the left hand
SMALL ASPIRATION TUBE	right side retromolar
INSTRUMENT GRIP	modified pen grip angled until the right elbow of dentist slightly touches her/his body
HAND/FINGER SUPPORT	ring finger on front teeth
COMMENT	n/a
Fig 10–73a	Fig 10–73b
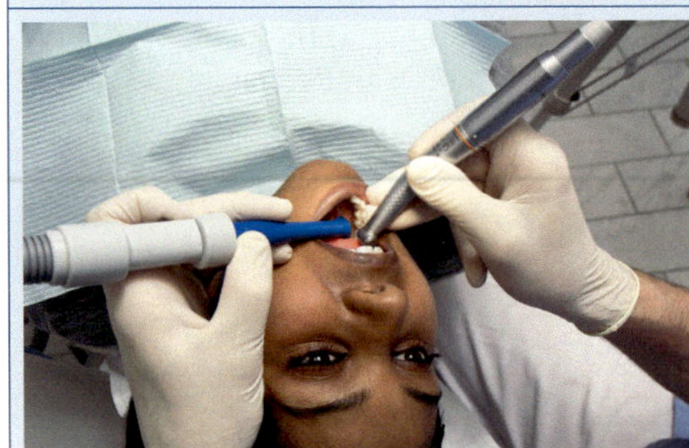	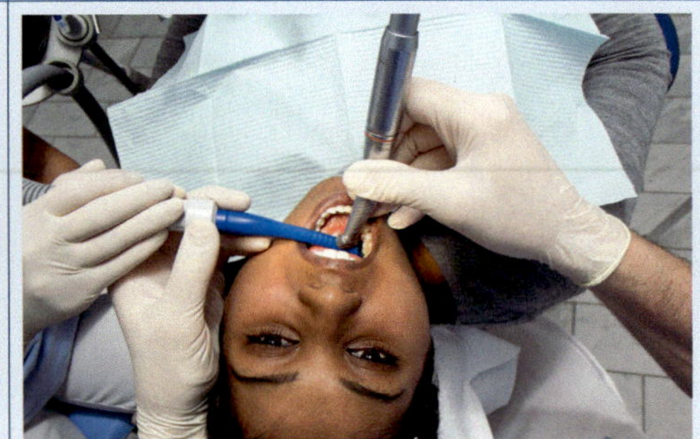

23	
TEETH	47, 46, 45, 44
SURFACE	occlusal, mesial
HEAD OF PATIENT	left,middle and right
BACK OF PATIENT CHAIR	horizontal
VISION	direct
DENTIST POSITION	11
ACTION	cavity preparation
RETRACTION BY ASSISTANT	tongue with large aspiration tube, which may be supported by the dentist's left hand
RETRACTION BY DENTIST	cheek and lip with mirror or left index finger to retract lip (if left hand of dentists is not supporting aspiration tube)
SMALL ASPIRATION TUBE	right side retromolar
INSTRUMENT GRIP	modified pen grip angled until the dentist's right elbow slightly touches the body
HAND/FINGER SUPPORT	back side of ring finger supported extraorally on skin over part of the mandibular jaw
COMMENT	n/a
Fig 10–74	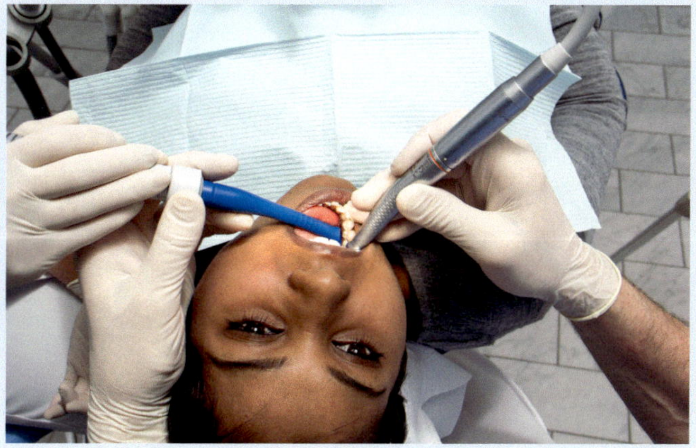

24	
TEETH	47, 46, 45, 44
SURFACE	distal and narrow occlusal cavity
HEAD OF PATIENT	backwards – for last molars, far backwards
BACK OF PATIENT CHAIR	horizontal
VISION	mirror placed behind the tooth/cavity
DENTIST POSITION	11
ACTION	cavity preparation, take care: up is seen as down and down seen as up
RETRACTION BY ASSISTANT	tongue with large aspiration tube
RETRACTION BY DENTIST	right hand ring finger
SMALL ASPIRATION TUBE	left side retromolar
INSTRUMENT GRIP	modified pen grip angled until the dentist's right elbow touches the body
HAND/FINGER SUPPORT	back side of right ring finger is supported extraorally on the skin over part of the mandibular jaw
COMMENT	a small mirror may be used
Fig 10–75	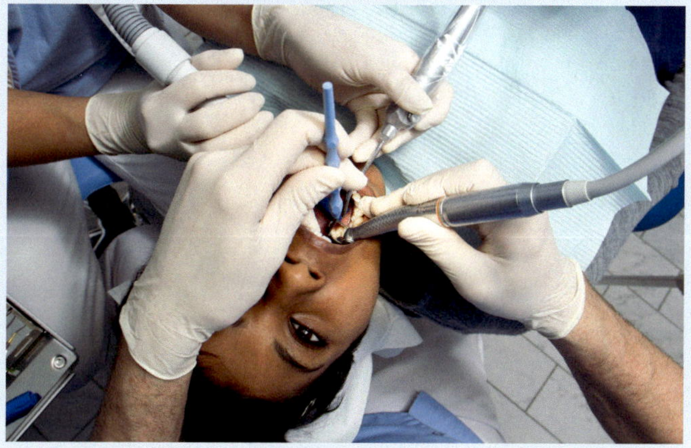

25	
TEETH	45, 44
SURFACE	distal and narrow occlusal cavity
HEAD OF PATIENT	forward and right
BACK OF PATIENT CHAIR	If patient cannot move head forward sufficiently to enable vision into a distal cavity, the patient chair may be adjusted so the backrest is about 30 degrees above horizontal position
VISION	direct
DENTIST POSITION	11
ACTION	cavity preparation
RETRACTION BY ASSISTANT	tongue with large aspiration tube – if the tongue is strong, the dentist may support the assistant while retracting
RETRACTION BY DENTIST	right hand ring finger
SMALL ASPIRATION TUBE	left side retromolar
INSTRUMENT GRIP	modified pen grip angled until the right elbow of dentist touches the body
HAND/FINGER SUPPORT	back side of right ring finger supported extraoral on skin over the mandibular jaw
COMMENT	n/a
Fig 10–76	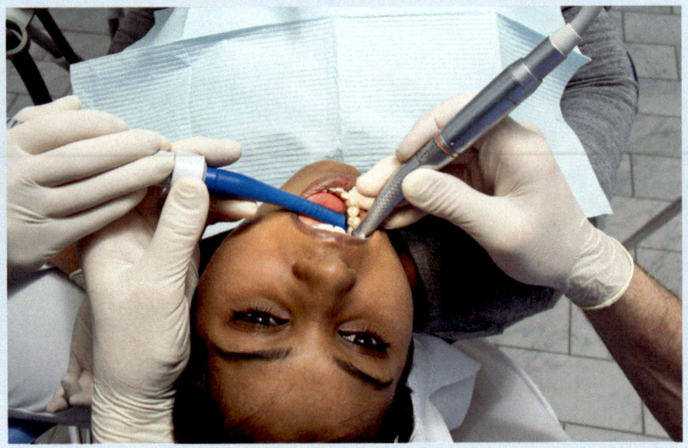

26	
TEETH	43, 42, 41, 31, 32, 33
SURFACE	distal and labial aspects of 43, 42, 41 mesial, and labial 31, 32, 33
HEAD OF PATIENT	left
BACK OF PATIENT CHAIR	horizontal
VISION	direct
DENTIST POSITION	9
ACTION	cavity preparation or parallel to surface
RETRACTION BY ASSISTANT	lip by large aspiration tube or by assistant's left index finger
RETRACTION BY DENTIST	by left hand index finger or thumb, as shown in Fig 10–77b
SMALL ASPIRATION TUBE	left side retromolar
INSTRUMENT GRIP	pen grip
HAND/FINGER SUPPORT	on neighboring teeth
COMMENT	n/a
Fig 10–77a	Fig 10–77b
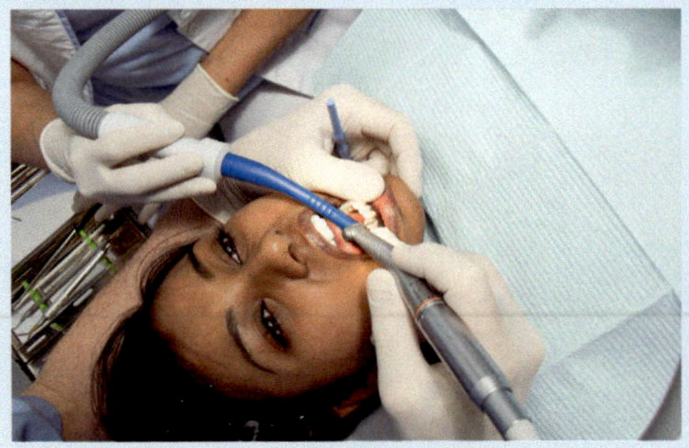	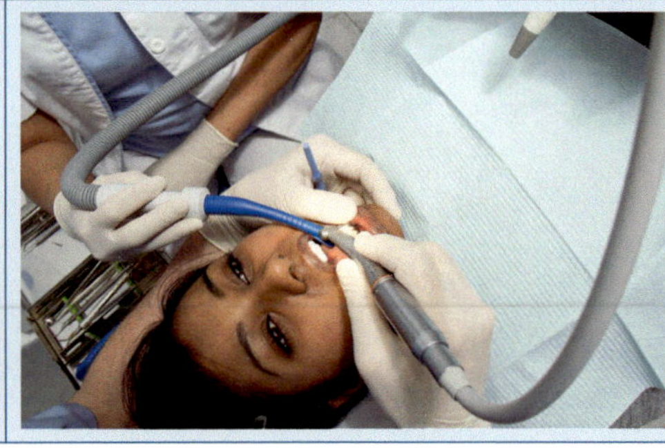

27	
TEETH	43, 42, 41, 31, 32, 33
SURFACE	mesial 43, 42, 41, distal 31, 32, 33
HEAD OF PATIENT	turned more or less right depending on specific position
BACK OF PATIENT CHAIR	horizontal
VISION	direct
DENTIST POSITION	11–12
ACTION	cavity preparation or parallel to surface
RETRACTION BY ASSISTANT	lip by large aspiration tube or with assistant's left index finger
RETRACTION BY DENTIST	by the left hand index finger or by mirror
SMALL ASPIRATION TUBE	left side retromolar
MIRROR	at photo used for light reflection
INSTRUMENT GRIP	pen grip
HAND/FINGER SUPPORT	on neighboring teeth
COMMENT	n/a
Fig 10–78	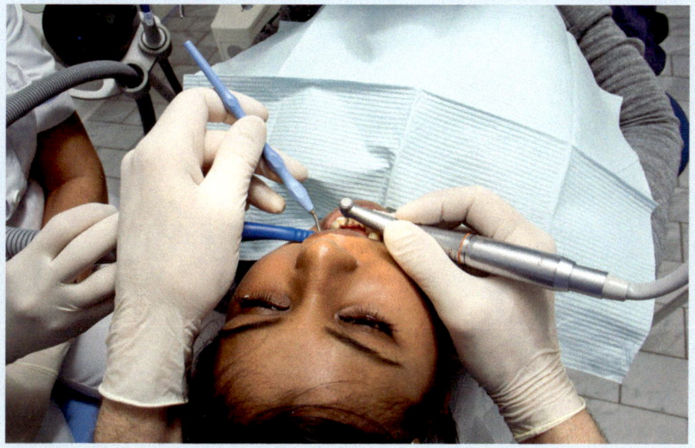

28	
TEETH	43, 42, 41, 31, 32, 33
SURFACE	lingual
HEAD OF PATIENT	forward
BACK OF PATIENT CHAIR	If patient cannot move head sufficiently forward to enable visibility of lingual surface, the patient chair may be adjusted so the backrest is about 30 degrees above the horizontal position
VISION	direct
DENTIST POSITION	11
ACTION	cavity preparation or parallel to surface
RETRACTION BY ASSISTANT	tongue with large aspiration tube and maybe lip, with assistant's left index finger
RETRACTION BY DENTIST	none
SMALL ASPIRATION TUBE	left side retromolar
INSTRUMENT GRIP	pen grip
HAND/FINGER SUPPORT	ring finger on neighboring teeth
COMMENT	n/a
Fig 10–79	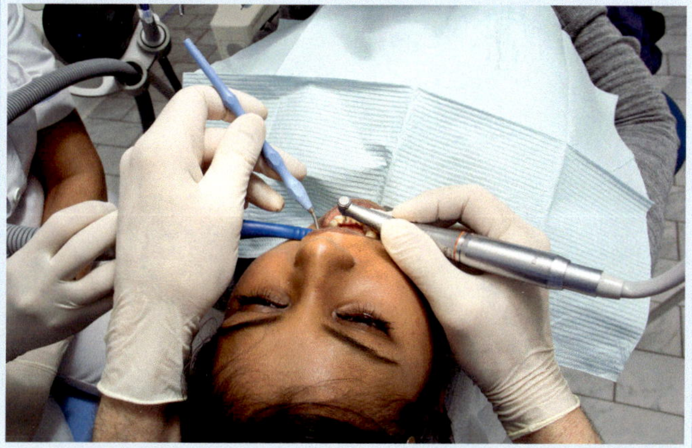

29	
TEETH	43, 42, 41, 31, 32, 33
SURFACE	lingual
HEAD OF PATIENT	slightly right and forward
BACK OF PATIENT CHAIR	if patient cannot move head sufficiently forward to look at lingual surface, the patient chair may be adjusted so the back rest is about 30 degrees above horizontal position
VISION	mirror is kept dry by assistant or for scaling with ultrasonic scaler, looking through mirror with water film on surface
DENTIST POSITION	11
ACTION	cavity preparation (and scaling) – take care: labial direction (up by the lying patient) is seen as downward and lingual direction is seen as up
RETRACTION BY ASSISTANT	tongue by large aspiration tube
RETRACTION BY DENTIST	none
SMALL ASPIRATION TUBE	left side retromolar
INSTRUMENT GRIP	pen grip
HAND/FINGER SUPPORT	ring finger on teeth at right side of mouth, or support of back side of ring finger extraorally on skin of the left mandibular jaw
COMMENT	n/a
Fig 10–80a	Fig 10–80b
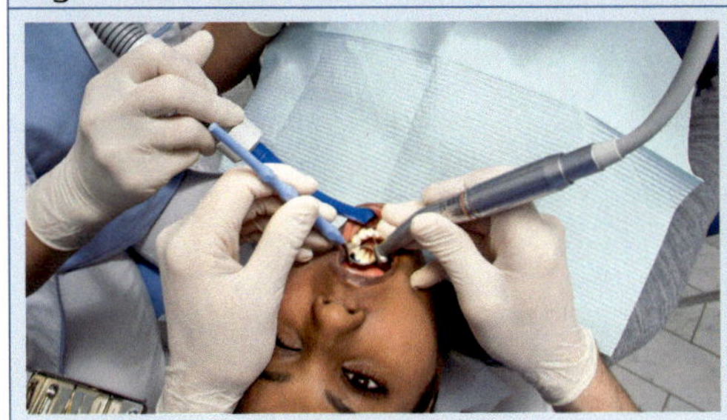	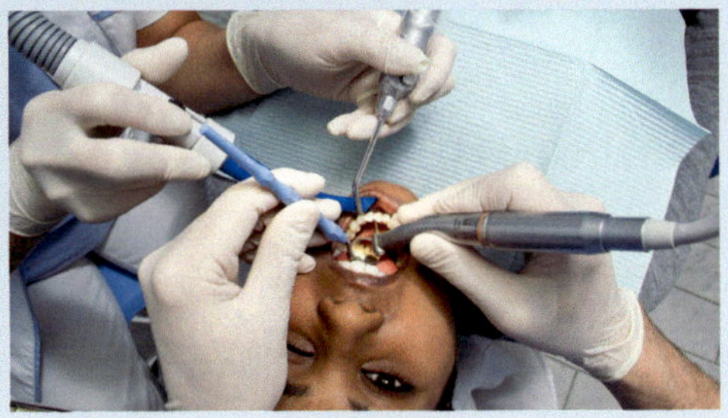

30	
TEETH	34, 35, 36, 37
SURFACE	lingual
HEAD OF PATIENT	left
BACK OF PATIENT CHAIR	horizontal
VISION	direct
DENTIST POSITION	9 to10
ACTION	cavity preparation and parallel to surface
RETRACTION BY ASSISTANT	chin by large aspiration tube
RETRACTION BY DENTIST	tongue with mirror – retraction towards the right requires less force than depressing the tongue
SMALL ASPIRATION TUBE	right side retromolar
INSTRUMENT GRIP	about a 90-degree angled pen grip, so the elbow of the dentist's right arm slightly touches the body
HAND/FINGER SUPPORT	ring finger on teeth at right side of mouth, or support on back side of ring finger extraorally on skin of patient's left mandibular jaw
COMMENT	n/a
Fig 10–81	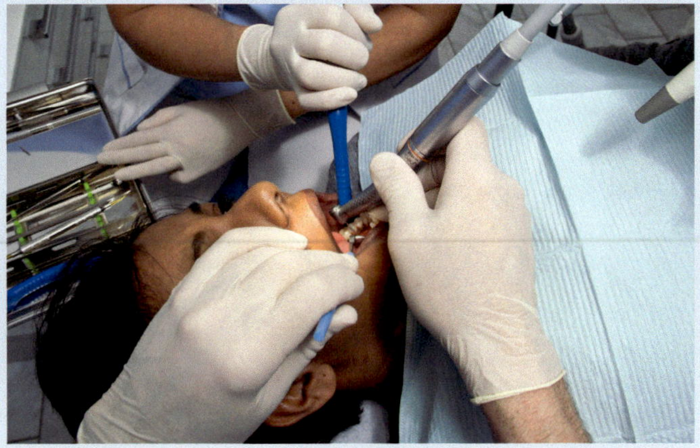

31	
TEETH	34, 35, 36, 37
SURFACE	occlusal, mesial
HEAD OF PATIENT	left/slightly right
BACK OF PATIENT CHAIR	horizontal and backwards as much as possible
VISION	direct
DENTIST POSITION	10 –11
ACTION	cavity preparation
RETRACTION BY ASSISTANT	cheek with large aspiration tube
RETRACTION BY DENTIST	lateral retraction with mirror with reversed side grip
SMALL ASPIRATION TUBE	right side retromolar
INSTRUMENT GRIP	pen grip
HAND/FINGER SUPPORT	ring finger at teeth at right side
COMMENT	n/a
Fig 10–82	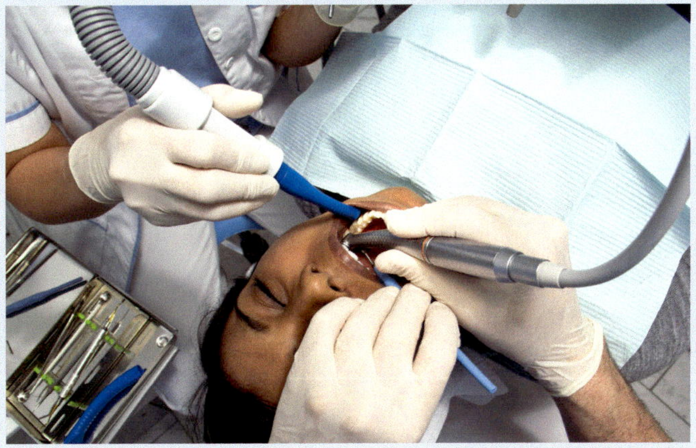

32	
TEETH	34, 35, 36, 37
SURFACE	occlusal, distal
HEAD OF PATIENT	left, right and backwards
BACK OF PATIENT CHAIR	horizontal
VISION	mirror kept dry by assistant
DENTIST POSITION	11
ACTION	cavity preparation – take care: up is seen as down and down is seen as up
RETRACTION BY ASSISTANT	cheek with large aspiration tube
RETRACTION BY DENTIST	mirror with reversed side grip
SMALL ASPIRATION TUBE	right side retromolar
INSTRUMENT GRIP	pen grip
HAND/FINGER SUPPORT	ring finger extraorally in chin region, or ring finger at mandibular front teeth
COMMENT	n/a
Fig 10–83	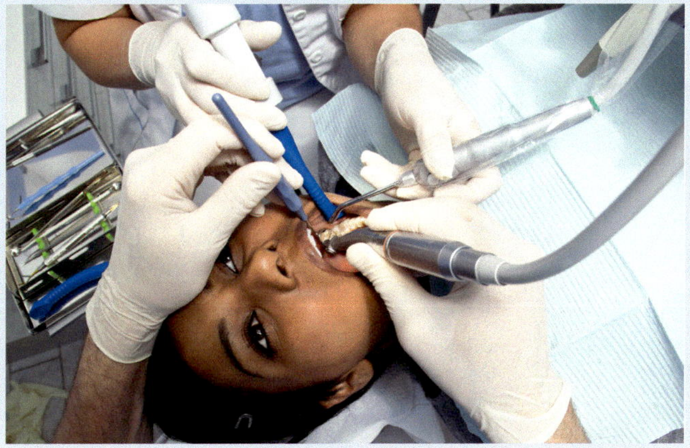

33	
TEETH	34, 35, 36, 37
SURFACE	vestibular
HEAD OF PATIENT	turned and tilted right
BACK OF PATIENT CHAIR	horizontal
VISION	direct
DENTIST POSITION	12
ACTION	cavity preparation or parallel to surface
RETRACTION BY ASSISTANT	cheek with large aspiration tube
RETRACTION BY DENTIST	the dentist may assist assistant to hold the aspiration tube
SMALL ASPIRATION TUBE	right side retromolar
INSTRUMENT GRIP	pen grip
HAND/FINGER SUPPORT	ring finger extraoral in chin region or ring finger at mandibular front teeth
COMMENT	n/a
Fig 10–84	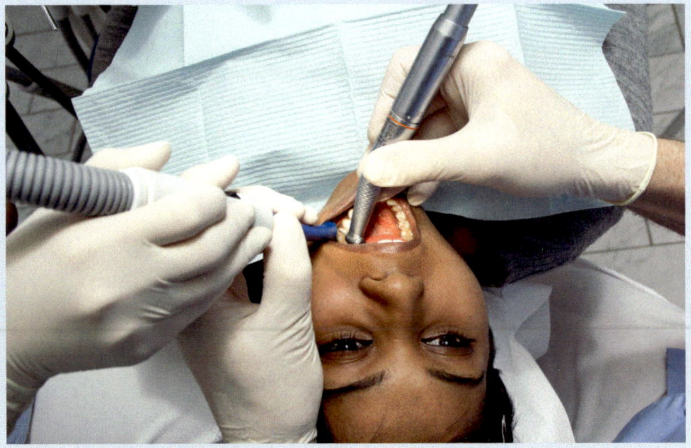

Chapter 11

ORGANIZATION AND DESIGN OF THE TREATMENT ROOM

INTEGRATION OF COMPUTER, SCREENS, KEYBOARDS AND MICE

In the modern, digital dental practice, the computer is essential. But where should it be placed, who uses it and for what purpose?

The dentist must have a screen, mouse and keyboard

This screen runs the practice administration program that is able to show digital radiographs and intraoral photos. The dentist must also have a keyboard and mouse (Figs 11–1 and 11–2).

Here the dentist can study radiographs, registrations and diagrams in order to develop a treatment plan for the patient and input information, which the assistant may not do.

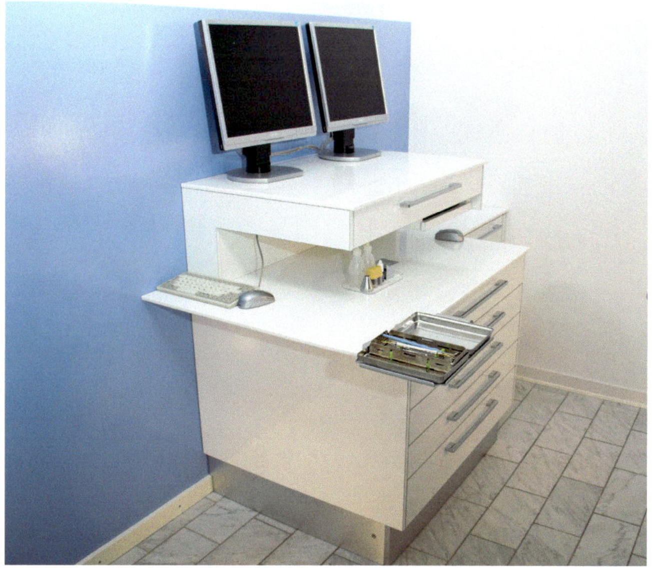

Fig 11–1 Dentist's computer screen, keyboard and mouse on the MEGASPACE.

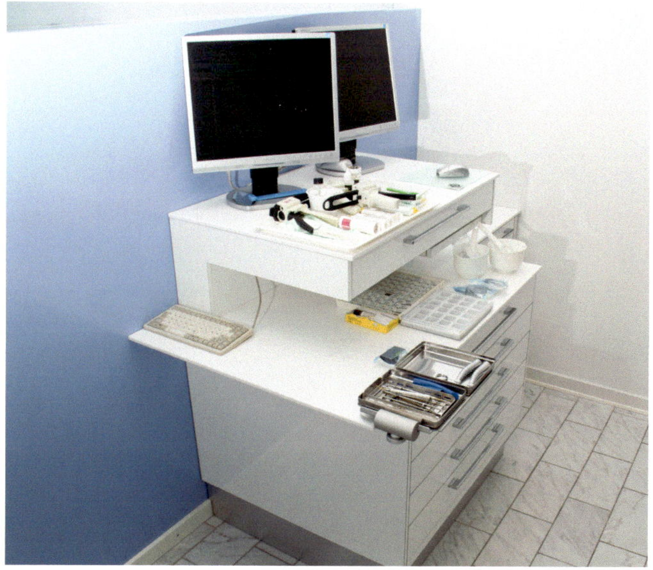

Fig 11–2 The dentist's computer screen is turned towards him/her to avoid reflexes. This is the reason the dentist and assistant cannot share a computer screen.

The assistant must have her own screen, mouse and keyboard

The assistant can fill in registration diagrams for present teeth, fillings, caries, bleeding points, periodontal pockets, biofilm, etc, inputting information of finished treatments and printing off patient invoices (Figs 11–3 and 11–4).

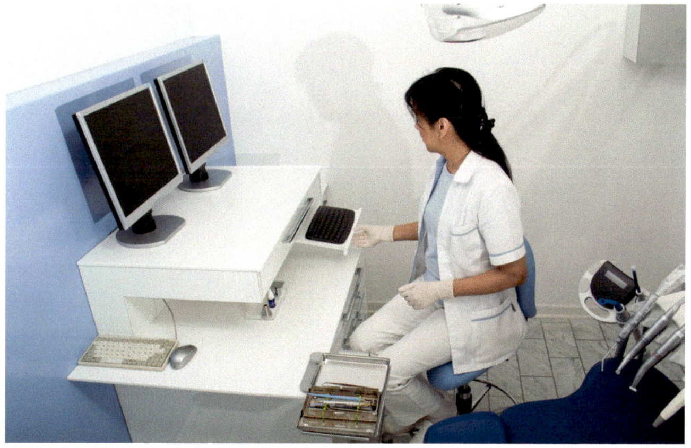

Fig 11–3 The assistant's keyboard has a resting position that does not disturb visibility to the materials on the work table. The assistant pulls her keyboard to the working position.

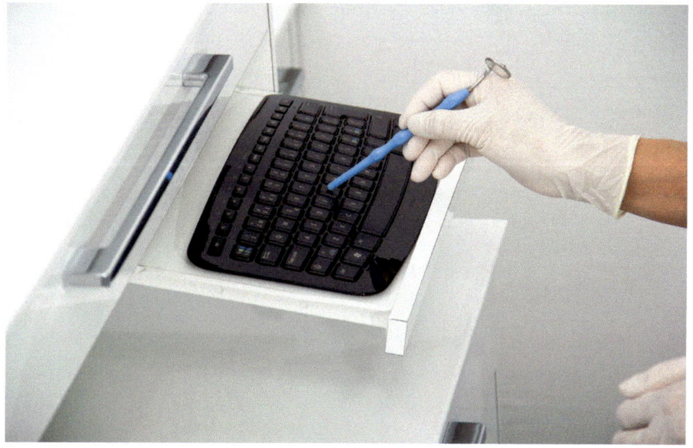

Fig 11–4 The assistant must have her own screen, mouse and keyboard.

The patient must have a screen too

The patient when horizontal should see this computer screen, so a change of position is not necessary (Fig 11–5).

The horizontal position is also necessary in order to use an intraoral camera for photos and video for

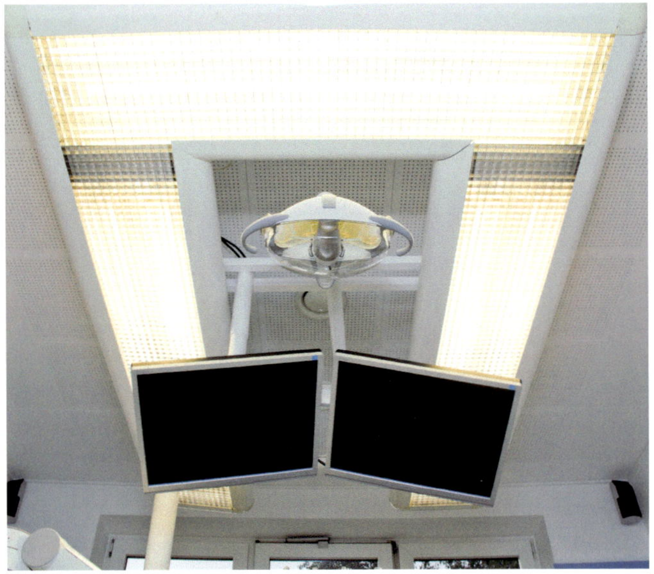

Fig 11–5 The patient's screen.

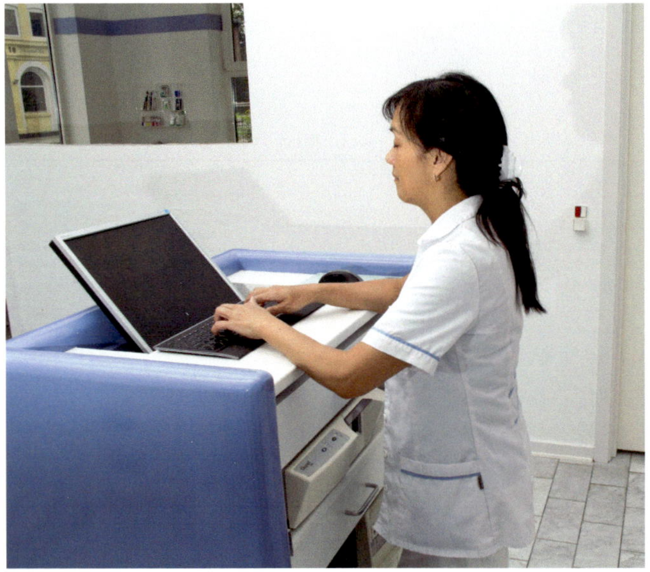

Fig 11–6 Stand up workplace, also used for scanning intraoral radiographic plates.

gathering information from the patient. The patient screen can be suspended in the ceiling, or as seen here, in the armatures for general light.

The patient's screen is used for showing diagrams, radiographs, intraoral photos, and live video using an intraoral camera. The patient's screen is an interactive part of case presentations.

The screen on the left is placed at a neutral position, where it does not disturb the dental unit, unit instrument arms or the arm of the operation lamp. If two screens are mounted, as done so here in the author's treatment room, the right one is used for patient information and the left one for an entertainment program for the patient. As the right hand screen may come into conflict with the operating lamp, it therefore needs a very precise position. It is advised to only use the left screen to show the patient selected radiographs during certain treatment procedures.

One computer can be easily served by two keyboards and two mice, and the use of a splitter can create an unlimited number of computer screens.

Stand up computer workplace

For writing in the patient's record book after the appointment is over, a stand up workplace provides a pleasant variation (Fig 11–6).

The stand up computer workplace is also used to give information to the patient, where both can see the screen in a relaxed fashion.

ONE TREATMENT ROOM, NEXT PATIENT IN CHAIR – NOW!

Fast patient changes

A fast patient change is important if the dentist works in one single workplace. The following procedure may save 5 minutes per patient change, and if, for example, there are 12 patient appointments per day, this equals to a saving of 1 hour per day. If the dentist has more than 12 appointments per day, then even more time is saved.

The assistant does not leave the treatment room alone; the dentist accompanies the patient to the reception area and says goodbye. The dentist goes to the waiting room and asks the next patient to come with him to the treatment room. In between patients, the assistant has prepared the patient chair, the operation lamp and the cuspidor, napkins, etc, and has disinfected the equipment. The dentist asks the patient to sit in the patient chair. In the meantime, the hand instrument table is cleaned up and new hand instruments made ready. The dentist brings the patient to the treatment position and now the dental unit is finally ready too. If the dentist works in only one treatment room, you can have a predisinfection container for the used instruments, so the assistant does not need to leave the treatment room.

Workplaces like MEGASPACE and WORKPLACE 2 make fast patient changes possible without having to leave the treatment room, except for carrying used cassettes to the sterilization area (if no other is available for doing it).

The assistant stays in the treatment room while the dentist says goodbye to the departing patient, and arrives together with the next patient. The patient change may be done in 2 minutes, if trained properly.

THE SUPERTEAM CONCEPT

When patient care, functionality of the patient chair, dental unit, suction, and work station are combined with optimal assistance and best practice working methods, we call it the "superteam concept." The superteam concept is not a new idea, but its principles have been used at excellent dental practices for decades.

Here are the principles for the superteam concept:

- The dentist has permanent chairside assistance, for the transfer of hand instruments, unit instruments and materials to the dentist's hand.
- The dentist can therefore keep undisturbed concentration on the patient.
- The manual skills of the dentist in macro and micro level are highly trained.
- Turbine (air rotor) is replaced by a second micromotor with high-speed contra-angle.
- Two micromotors are used: one is mostly used with the blue contra-angle, and the second with the red 1:5 multiplication contra-angle.
- Unit instruments are placed between assistant and dentist, over the patient and within reach of both.
- Patient chair, stool, workstation, and organization are all as described previously in this book.

The team of one dentist and two assistants work at two identically-equipped treatment rooms. Both assistants have the same competencies and can replace each other.

One assistant works chairside, and the other prepares the other treatment room for the next patient. She guides the patient to the patient chair, and helps them to be seated. Clinical procedures like scaling, polishing and even making fillings (which in some European countries, assistants are now allowed to perform), are not normally performed by the assistant because both treatment rooms are in use for the dentist, and the second assistant will be very busy performing many other tasks.

The two treatment rooms give a large amount of flexibility, a relaxed workflow and a high efficiency. The patient changes are also very quick. Short examinations are easy to make. Patients can have an anesthetic 15 minutes before the treatment begins. Emergencies are much more easy to handle. Delays are easier to cope with. The assistant can take bitewings, apical radiographs, full mouth radiographic status, intraoral photos, BOP index, biofilm registration using disclosing solution, inform and train mouth hygiene, and advise about treatment plans and treatment.

The time gained from using two treatment rooms as described above may be about 20%. The time gain from using four-handed assistance, compared to working with an assistant where the dentist takes "everything" themselves may be around 20%, including a time gain because the patient does not have to rinse themselves during the treatment.

The time gain from using four-handed assistance, compared to solo work, is about 40%. Dentists with highly trained micro skills may have a time gain of 10 to 20%, depending on their start level. All estimates are based on the use of the unit suction holder and workstation as described earlier in this book. All estimates will of course depend on the starting level of function. Recall patients are divided in groups, according to the time needed.

The patient flow will of course depend on the type of dental practice. In a practice with many recall patients and a complete instrument cassette system, the instrument washing machine and autoclave will be in almost continuous use.

Sometimes it is argued that there are advantages to a shared dental practice, eg, sharing a sterilization area. As explained previously, this is not the case. There is no free capacity in a sterilization area for a superteam.

Even in a group practice with two or more dentists, it will be an advantage to have separate sterilization rooms for each superteam. Ideally, the sterilization room could be placed between the two treatment rooms, so the route for the assistants is the shortest possible. When each superteam has their own sterilization room, then the instruments, burs and materials are not mixed with those of other dentists. Having a rational organization of instruments also reduces the time spent in the sterilization room.

One assistant working chairside

If one assistant is working chairside, then the other assistant takes care of reception, makes appointments according to the information on the patient record, takes care of the waiting room service, and looks after the sterilization room. She also refills the workstations, writes the patients' record book notes (perhaps dictated by the dentist) and writes the patient invoice, so the patient can pay in cash or with a credit card after the visit. When needed, she assists the chairside assistant in preparing for unexpected treatments.

The superteam is very efficient and busy, so there is no possibility of time for an assistant to perform supragingival scaling and polishing, as permitted in some countries. Well-trained four-handed work saves much more time. The superteam may be extended with a dental hygienist, if she has her own treatment room. This means having three treatment rooms all together.

The hygienist could, however, cause a capacity problem in the autoclave. The hygienist uses hand instruments packed in sterile plastic bags as they do not take up so much room in the autoclave, to solve this problem.

A flexible team concept

Two superteams work 6 to 7 hours a day and share a practice as described above. The practice is open 10 to 11 hours a day with 2 hours of overlap in the middle of the day. In the overlap time, where there is only one treatment room per dentist, long treatments are scheduled. This concept provides optimal use of the practice resources.

Large practices have large-scale disadvantages, which can be reduced using the decentralized superteam concept. This also allows the teams to develop in different areas with different specialisms and levels of activity, without running into the conflicts often seen.

The advantages of large practices include a collegial and social community, the possibility of specialization, collegial sparring, mutual coaching, flexible working hours and holidays, and common marketing. On the negative side, there are the possibilities of internal rivalry or competition about patients, and differing opinions for future developments in the practice.

The superteam concept may profit from the positive elements, and avoid the negative ones.

AN EXTRAORDINARY DENTAL PRACTICE

Here is a description of an extraordinary dental practice in Japan, as seen in the 1980s.

After leaving one's shoes outside and changing into Japanese slippers, one enters the practice. A good-natured receptionist receives the patients and in a side room, a bookkeeper is working. The new patient is seated and a specially trained assistant examines the patient, registers caries, periodontal status, and takes a full mouth radiograph.

The dentist politely greets the patient and they have a relaxed conversation. The examination just carried out by the assistant is confirmed and a treatment plan is proposed. The ambience is active, kind and relaxed. Now the assistant takes over to explain the details of the treatment plan with illustrations (no photos are available on the practice computer at that time).

For treatments, the dentist performs irreversible actions such as preparations, excavations, endodontic treatment, and crown and bridge preparations. Then so-called "expanded duty dental auxiliaries" take over. They are assistants who have undertaken special training to take on additional responsibilities. They make fillings, take impressions for crowns and bridges and cement them later, and also check for occlusion, etc. They are assisted by chairside assistants, as is the dentist.

Two dental hygienists take care of the periodontal treatment and preventive procedures, and in the event of surgery, the dentist takes over. All treatments are high quality, unhurried, and full concentration and a tremendous sense of productivity are always maintained.

How many were working in the practice:

- 1 dentist
- 1 receptionist
- 1 bookkeeper
- 1 case presentation assistant
- 2 expanded duty assistants
- 2 hygienists
- about 6 or 7 assistants
- 3 lab technicians
- and then we hope the dentist never is sick!

TREATMENT ROOM REDESIGN

Step-by-step improvements of the physical conditions for assistance and four-handed dentistry

If a new dental unit, chair, lamp, assistant and workplace is not an option right now, where is the best place to start, and what is most important – is there a step-by-step solution?

This question is made after almost all training courses. The answer will depend on whether the first priority is to achieve better working postures and/or improvement of assistance and efficiency. If the dentist has problems with working postures caused by tensions in the back, lumbar region, neck, headaches, aching shoulders, and general muscular pains, then a better patient chair and dentist's stool has a high priority.

Patient chair

The patient chair must:

- Have a thin back, be comfortable in a horizontal position, and move in so high a position – up to 90 cm – that the dentist does not need to bend down to achieve a working distance (when necessary) of about 32 cm. The base of the chair must be so small that the foot controller can be placed under the left side of the back of the patient chair.
- Have an adjustable headrest and the back of the chair must not be too long.
- Allow the dentist to (sometimes) work in a 12 o'clock position. A free space of 60 cm behind the headrest of the horizontal patient chair is necessary. (For a more detailed description, see page 147.)

Dentist's stool

The dentist's stool must be constructed for a balanced sitting position. The dentist sits higher in this position, which means that the patient chair must also be adjusted to a higher position. (For a more detailed description, see page 15.)

If the objective is to work in a more relaxed manner, improve concentration, reduce fatigue, and save time (for shorter working hours or improved economical turnover), then the workstation for the assistant and dentist has first priority.

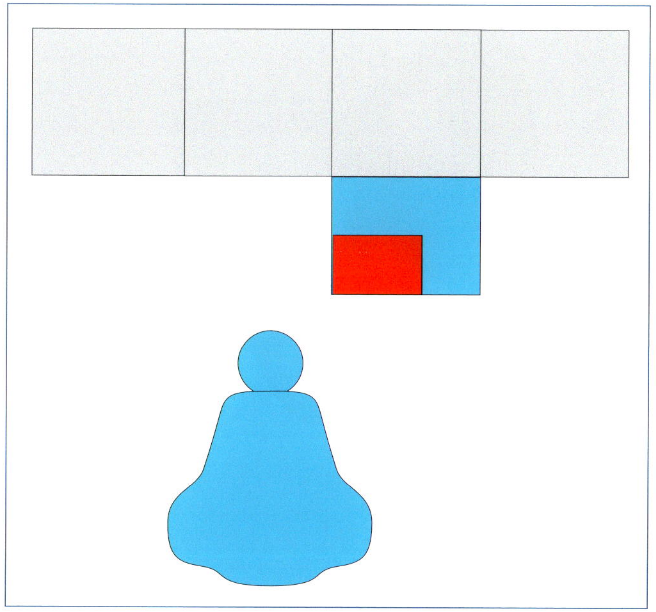

Fig 11–7 Temporary hand instrument table on a drawer.

Using the MEGASPACE workstation, the assistant can prepare for almost all treatments without leaving the patient, and she can assist with hand instrument and material transfers to the dentist.

Temporary hand instrument table and workplate for assistant

A temporary solution may be – if possible in the treatment room – to use a drawer as a support for the hand instrument tray (Fig 11–7). The drawer is fitted with a plate of composite plastic (like Corian, HiMac or similar) and serves as a working table as well (its above-floor height is about 75 to 80 cm).

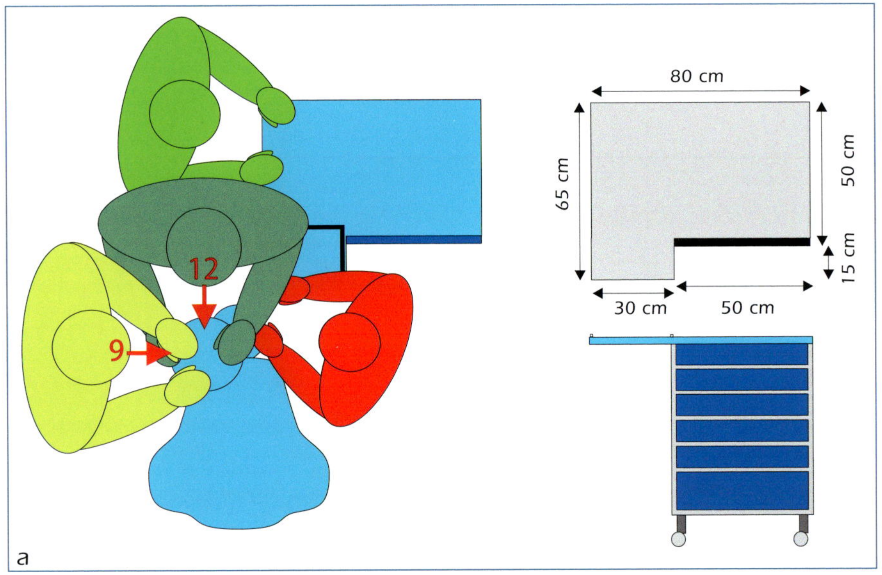

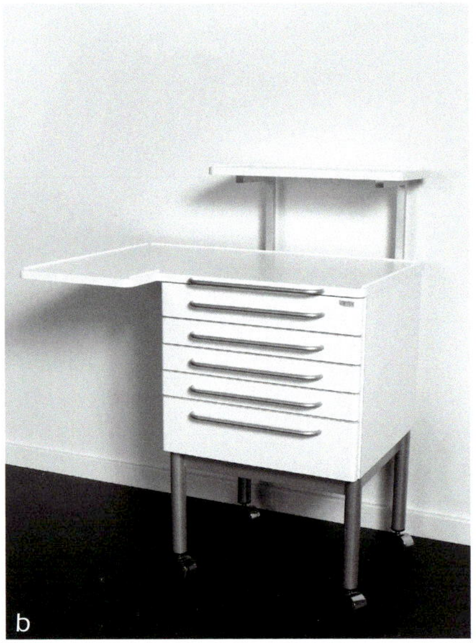

Fig 11–8 (a) Working positions of dentist and assistant. (b) Workplace 3.

Mobile module

Another possibility is to use a mobile element with an extended work plate, serving both dentist and assistant for support of the hand instrument tray and for preparing materials.

- For a start, it may be an existing mobile module fitted by an extended work plate, as in the work place.
- The measurements are indicated on the illustration (Fig 11–8).
- The workplate is used by the assistant.
- The extension closest to the patient is support for the hand instrument tray.
- The extension on the dentist's side is for his use.

New workplace designed for optimal assistance

It is unfortunate to note that most cabinet arrangements in dental practices – the older as well as the newer – do not support the principles of good assistance. Compared to the time-saving advantages (eg, 1 hour a day) of having a workplace such as the MEGASPACE, and replacing existing modules, this will probably have a pay back time of some weeks if this is applied along with slightly shorter patient appointments. The removed modules may be reused at other positions.

If the dentist goes for a better, faster and more precise use of rotating instruments, the confirmed solution is to substitute the turbine with a red 1/5 multiplication contra-angle mounted at the micromotor. Ideally, the dental unit has two micromotors: the most-used with a blue 1/1 contra-angle, and the other mounted with a red contra-angle and substitution turbine.

The dental unit completes the treatment room

The dental unit must be constructed for high-end assistance, with balanced unit instruments placed over the patient, and between the dentist and assistant. The assistant takes over the preparation of unit instruments and can integrate this into instrument transfer. Unit instruments must be able to be placed so high up that they can be placed over the lying patient's body in a horizontal patient chair to a height of 80 cm, and up to 90 cm (for dentists 175 cm in height or more).

When the suction holder is placed 12 cm from the unit instrument closest to the assistant, then the workplace is ready for "dancing hands."

The 3-in-1 syringe, two micromotors and scaler

The dental unit does NOT need to have many instruments:

- a good 3-in-1 syringe, which can dose spray at soft, medium and hard intensities
- two micromotors and an ultrasonic scaler.

No more is needed.

LED composite polymerization lamp

There are now super effective rechargeable LED composite polymerization lamps on the market – cheaper than a unit-mounted polymerization lamp and much more easy to replace. The assistant transfers the polymerization lamp to the dentist's hand or holds it herself while it is used.

Intraoral camera

The intraoral camera is an excellent tool for patient examination. It may be placed on the dental unit, but could also be connected directly to the computer and integrated in the practice's computer-based administration program. In most cases, it is positioned on the upper part of the MEGASPACE or workplace.

Conclusion

Four unit instruments are sufficient, mounted on the assistant's side with a 3-in-1 syringe, two micromotors and a scaler. Sometimes one gets the impression that a very expensive dental unit and patient chair are supposed to lead to better treatments. This is not the case.

Better treatments depend on the skills of both the dentist and assistant, combined with functional optimal equipment and workplace.

TREATMENT ROOM DESIGN

Using the all-in-one workstation MEGASPACE by Skovsgaard, the treatment room design is very simple (Fig 11–9).

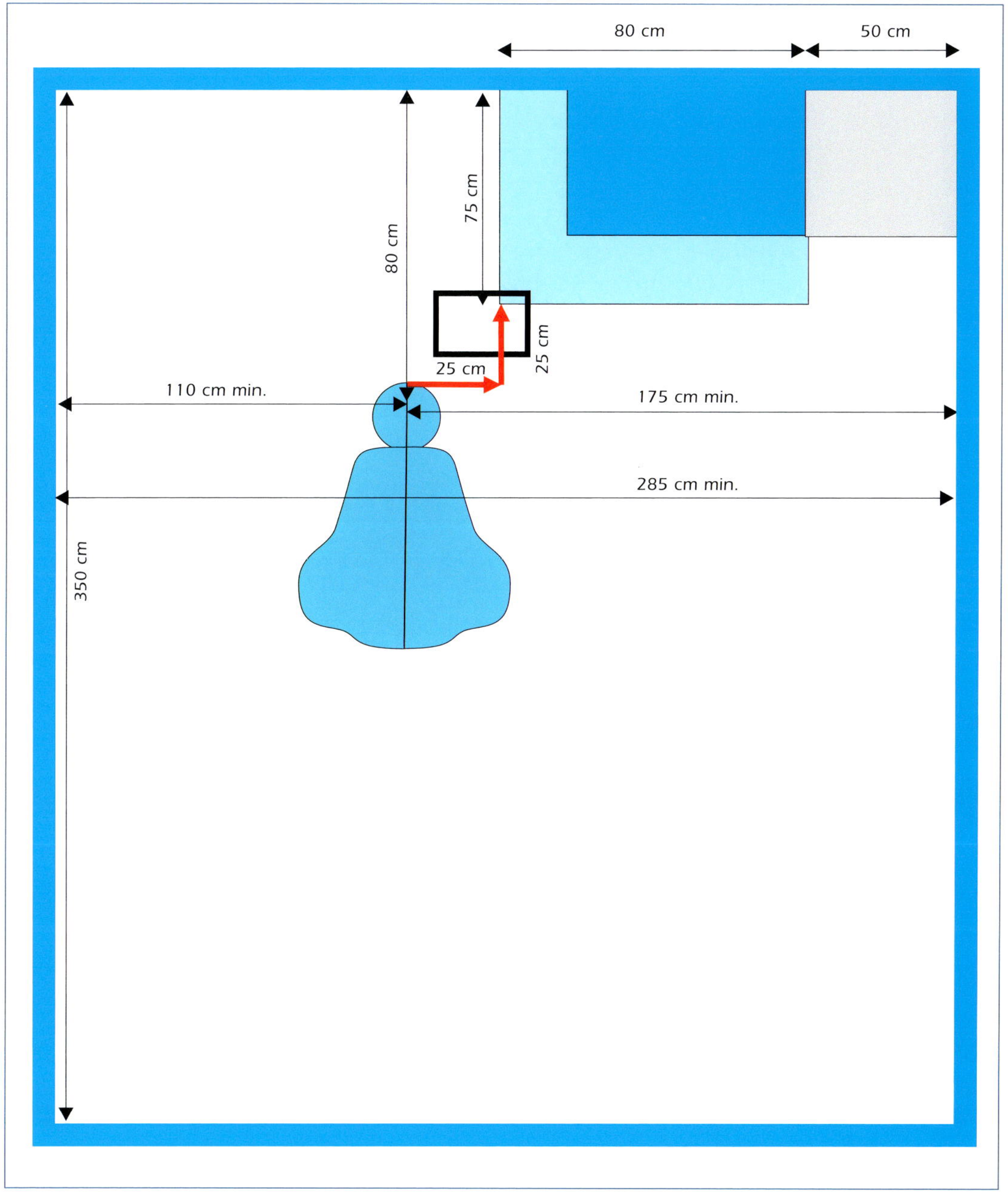

Fig 11–9
Measurements of the treatment room with MEGASPACE.

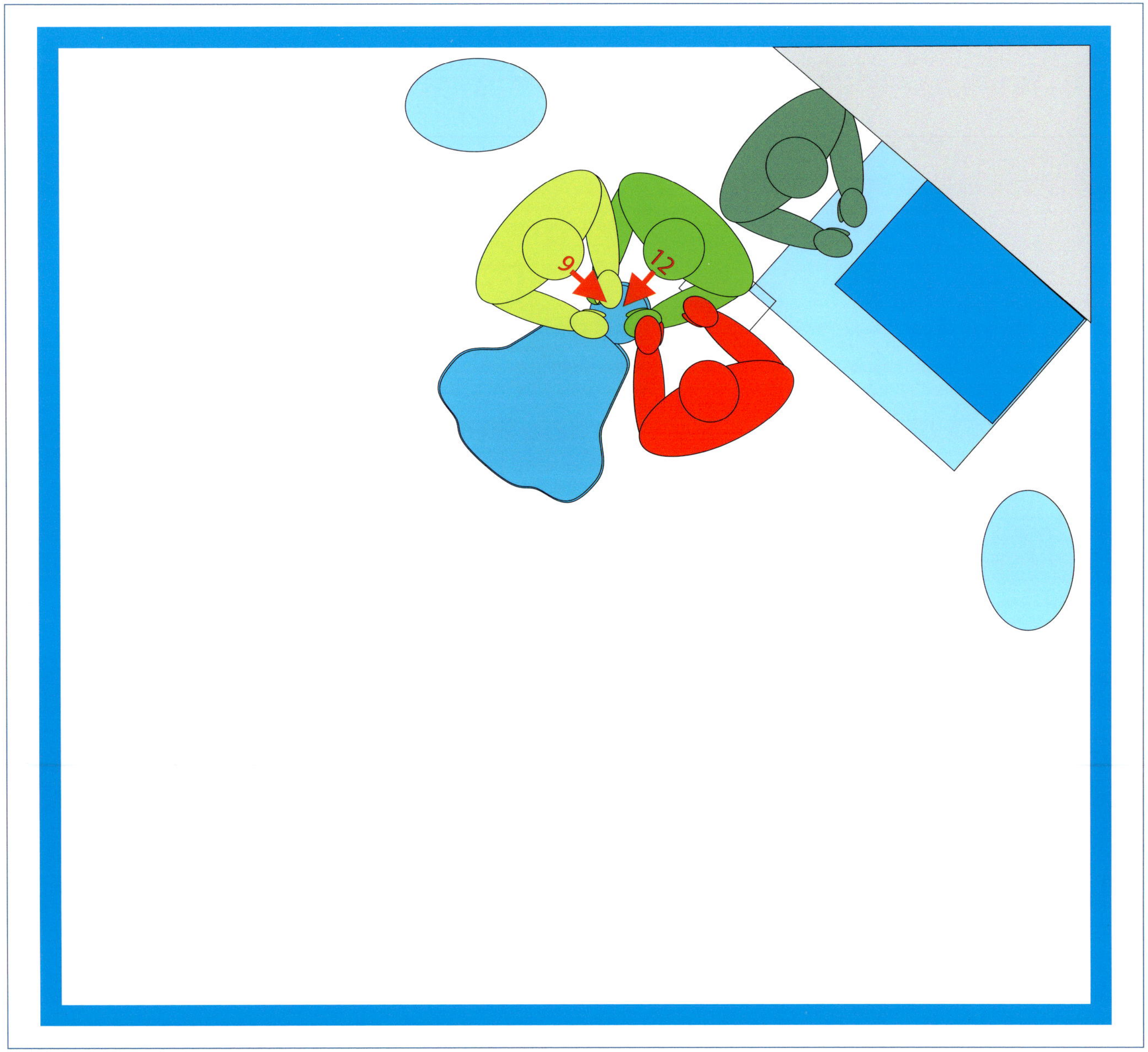

Fig 11–10 Corner arrangement with the MEGASPACE.

MEGASPACE, width 102 cm, depth 76 cm

- The distance from the wall at the assistant's side is 50 cm.
- If using a unit with a parking position at the assistant's side, a 60 cm space to the wall is more convenient.
- The module shown at the assistant's side of the MEGASPACE may be a storage module for hand instrument cassettes, or a wash module and a wall-mounted module for soap, alcogel, serviettes, gloves, cups for water, etc.
- Wash elements and doors may be placed freely, if not disturbing the area around the MEGASPACE.
- Detailed examples can be seen at www.neter-gonomie.com.

Corner designs are tricky to make, because one has to be careful not to reduce the free space around the MEGASPACE, and in most cases are not space saving. Here the space is sufficient (Fig 11–10).

The ideal practice for a dentist has two treatment rooms, with a sterilization room between them. If the reception area is very close to the sterilization room, it is easier for one assistant to take care of both.

LEFT-HANDED DENTIST: TWO SOLUTIONS

1. Working on the right side of the patient chair
2. Working on the left side of the patient chair.

1. Left-handed dentist working on the left side of the patient chair

To do this, the equipment should be arranged so that the dental unit, workplace, positions, use of the dentist's hands and of the assistant is MIRRORED. If all the photos in this book are looked upon as if in a mirror, then mirrored left-handed work is perfectly illustrated.

The dental unit

Say for example the dentist is working on the left side of the patient chair, and the assistant on the right side. The unit must be made in a left-handed version with the suction tube holder on the right side. Few units have this variation (see www.netergonomie.com). The unit base can remain on the patient's left side.

The suction holder can be placed on an arm system, so it can be placed either on the patient's left side for a right-handed dentist, OR on the patient's right side for a left-handed dentist. The unit instruments must be placed so that the syringe is closest to the assistant on the right side, as it is much used by her. The micromotors and other instruments then follow.

MEGASPACE

The workstation must be mirrored too, and the hand instrument table is placed on the assistant's side.

Assistance

The assistant uses her left hand for holding the large suction tube and the right hand for using the 3-in-1 syringe, eg, to dry the mirror when the dentist is working with mirror and spray.

The transfer of hand and unit instruments is made by the right hand. If the assistant is right-handed and is trained to work with a right-handed dentist, it will – for most assistants – be easy to "mirror" the functions of the hands in order to assist a left-handed dentist working on the left side. To assist a left-handed dentist as a right-handed assistant is in fact ideal, because the most "difficult" functions are now done by the assistant's right hand.

The author has had to learn to work left-handed in order to demonstrate and instruct teamwork training for the left-handed dentist. This was surprisingly easy, and both examples indicate that our manual abilities are located in the brain, as well as in the hands.

2. Left-handed dentist working on the right side of the patient chair

Is it possible to work in good working positions as a left-handed dentist working on the patient's right side?

The workplace is the same as for a right-handed dentist, so yes that is possible. Instrument grip, instrument transfer, aspiration and retraction are special and not a mirroring of the work of a right-handed dentist (Figs 11–11 to 11–16).

Workplace for use of both right-handed (working on the right side of the patient) and left-handed dentist (working on the left side of the patient)

This is certainly complex but there is a solution. The dental unit must have a suction holder, which can be placed either on the left side for right-handed dentists, or on the right side for left-handed dentists working on the left side. The workplace must have a special design (see www.netergonomie.com)

A MEGASPACE in left/right version

The construction is symmetrical with a tabletop extension at both sides and an adaptor for the hand instrument table on both sides.

The MEGASPACE is mounted with sturdy wheels, allowing the whole MEGASPACE module to roll sideways for a left-to-right slide of the patient chair. A rail in the floor, to ensure the wheels stay on track, guides the back wheels. The movement to the sides is 180 cm.

- When the right-handed dentist is working, the MEGASPACE is placed on the left side of the patient chair.
- When the left-handed dentist is working, the MEGASPACE is placed on the right side of the patient chair (see www.netergonomie.com).

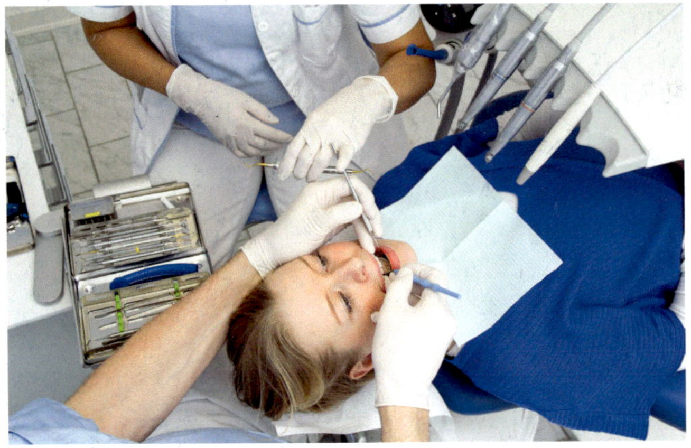

Fig 11–11 The hand instrument transfer.

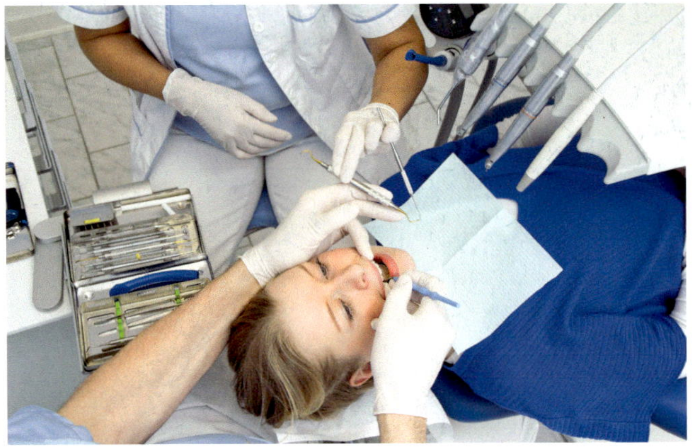

Fig 11–12 A special hand instrument transfer to a left-handed dentist working on the right side of the patient chair.

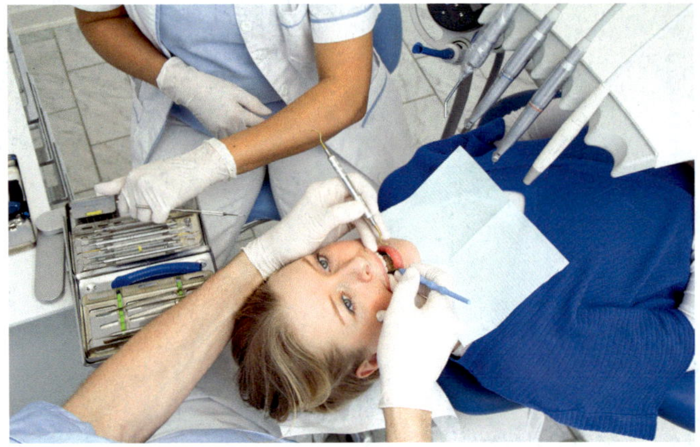

Fig 11–13 Used instrument replaced on tray.

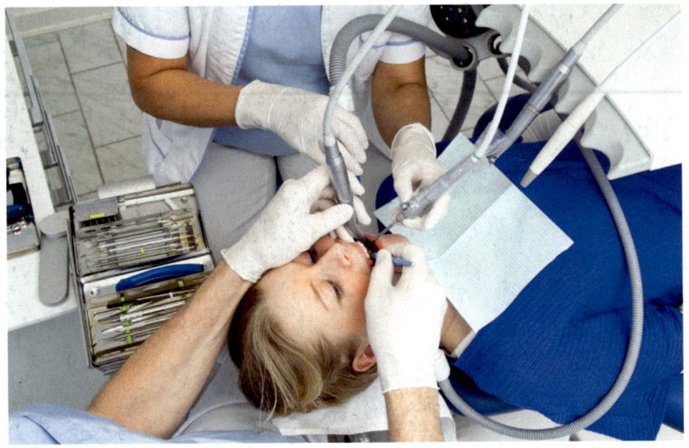

Fig 11–14 Working with a mirror, dried by the assistant.

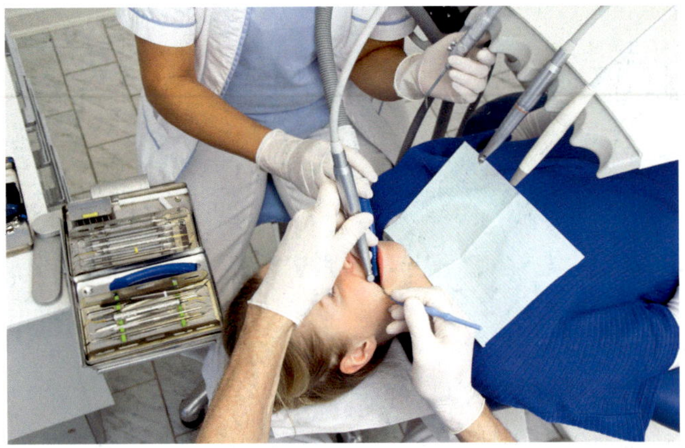

Fig 11–15 Working in the maxillary right region.

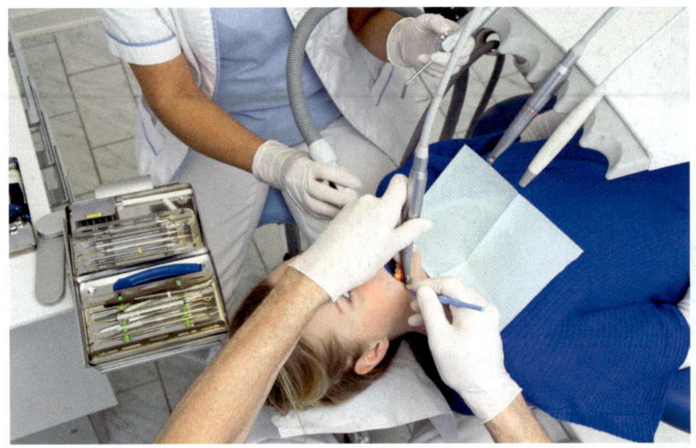

Fig 11–16 Working in the mandibular right region.

CONCLUSIONS

STRAIGHT TALKING

Dancing Hands presents knowledge, skills and solutions that a dental team can take into practice after a few days.

The author has learned that expressions, case stories, descriptions, and presentations in some countries have to be both colorful and very direct. This is particularly true when communicating the shortcomings of some traditional habits. In this section, the reader will find such straight and direct descriptions.

However, if the reader comes from a country and culture where such direct language is considered as impolite and disrespectful, then please see this chapter as an exotic example of how communication may differ in other cultures.

MENTAL BLOCKS FOR FINE WORK POSTURES, ASSISTANT, PRECISION VISION AND PRECISION WORK

Dentists are very often unaware of certain knowledge and skills of practical work. This can be revealed in specific questions like – what is your instrument grip or instrument support when working at *x* tooth at *y* surface. So, this is said with a humoristic touch – dentists often do not know what they are doing! This may be a starting point, and an eye opener for acquiring new knowledge.

There is often no teaching in universities of manual skills, and dentists most often have not attended post-graduate courses on this subject. Neither have the dental teachers in universities. Most dentists think that training in manual skills is not necessary. This expression can be compared to a musician or a dancer who trains repeatedly and intensively before a performance. If you do not know what you do not know and which skills you do not have, then you have no reason or motivation for acquiring the knowledge and skills. Dentists are adapting to unfortunately constructed dental equipment and workplaces. This should be changed. Dentists should be very conscious about best working methods and buy dental equipment that is adapted to these methods.

One cannot blame the dental industry – to sell what dentists are buying. But one can blame the dentist – without seeking prior knowledge and acquiring skills – to buy equipment obstructive to fine working positions, fine assistance, and time and energy saving working methods.

Dentists unaware about insufficient assistance

Dentists have often not learned how to train the manual skills of both the assistant and themselves. They are often unaware about bad working postures, the reason for them, and do not know and do not have the skills to prevent them. If they had the skills, surely one would not see so many dentists adopting bad working postures?

Dentists are often unaware that work postures are a result of: vision; retraction; their own position and instrument/finger/hand/arm position; and of assistance and of the dental unit; patient chair; suction system and hand instrument position; and workstation.

Some dentists believe it is possible to work in a good posture, in just one "clock position." And others believe that the horizontal patient can see unit instruments placed centrally over the patient. Dentists often believe that patients cannot be treated in a horizontal position, although millions of patients have been treated in this way for about 50 years. Perhaps they forget to politely ask the patients for permission to move their chair down?

There are dentists who believe the patient relates to the equipment, when the truth is that the patient relates to the dentist (with her/his face 30 cm from the patient) and to the assistant.

Many dentists think that a change of habits is difficult, whereas hundreds of post-graduate hands-on courses show that they can be learned in just 1 or 2 days.

Dentists in a few countries believe that the assistant must sit higher than the dentist to be able to look into the patient's mouth. The fact is that if patient moves their head to the right to improve vision for the dentist, the assistant in all cases cannot see anything in the left side of the mouth, and the dentist must therefore guide the assistant to the correct suction position. The assistant should instead sit facing the patient, which also improves the assistant's access to the unit instruments over the patient.

This is strange!

The patient chair and the dental unit stand in the treatment room, without close relation to the work tables and storage areas. The dentist believes that the unit instruments are all that is necessary to be able to work.

However, it is the unified whole that is important:

- The skills of dentist and assistant are most important.
- These skills interact with unit instruments, suction systems, hand instrument tables and workstations.

A lack or insufficiency of one or more of these elements obstructs the work. In fact it is the workstation that is used more than the unit instruments, and is therefore very important. Many dentists believe that their work cannot be performed in fine postures. This opinion is confirmed by the bad postures in colleges. The fact is that almost all procedures can be performed in good work postures, if the dentist and assistant have the necessary knowledge and skills.

SOME EXAMPLES OF MISUNDERSTANDINGS

Patient's acceptance of centrally placed equipment

The patient sees the unit instruments placed in a central position (over the patient and between dentist and assistant, to be used by both). The horizontal patient cannot see the unit instruments (the patient does not have eyes like snails). But the patient might see balanced instrument support.

Centrally placed unit instruments support full assistance and working methods, where the dentist can be calm and concentrate on the task. The patient will experience a calm, relaxed and focused dentist, while avoiding the need for looking away and back, perhaps more than 200 times just during a composite molar filling.

Patients do not accept treatment in a horizontal position

The patient's acceptance is completely dependent on the dentist's motivation of the patient, a stepwise change of the patient chair, and if necessary, rinsing with aspiration tube and spray from the 3-in-1 syringe.

Every year, many millions of patients in many countries are treated in a horizontal position with centrally placed unit instruments, with a good standard of assistance, and relaxed, undisturbed concentration from the dentist.

"Save time and energy, concentrate" – this fine principle cannot be performed with a unit at the right side of the patient. A dental unit on the right side disturbs the concentration of the dentist (and the assistant cannot reach the unit instruments).

Working alone with assistant, or 50% assistance from a full-time assistant

Many dentists work alone, but with an assistant sitting beside them.

The assistant does not transfer unit instruments or hand instruments to the dentist. So what is she doing then? She is holding an aspiration tube, while finding and preparing instruments and materials in a kitchen-like cabinetry.

This is SOLO dentistry with an assistant. The assistant is present but the dentist takes the hand instruments and unit instruments her/himself.

Horizontal forearms

Very often you see illustrations showing the dentist and assistant in working positions with horizontal forearms.

This is a good positioning, but unfortunately no one can work like this. The reason is that the eye-to-tooth distance is too long by far for precision vision, so when starting to work, down to an eye-to-tooth distance sufficiently close to achieve precision vision (this is about 30 to 35 cm). So the result is a very poor working posture.

The solution is to sit upright in a good posture and move the horizontal patient up until the eye-to-

tooth distance is sufficiently close enough to achieve precision vision. This implies that the forearms are inclined upwards. They should be less inclined if the dentist is below average height, and more inclined for taller dentists. (More precisely: it should be less if the eye-to-elbow distance is below average, more if eye-to-elbow distance is long.) Performing precision work with an eye-to-tooth distance of 45 to 50 or even 60 cm is not recommended.

Turbines

With turbines, the speed cannot be adapted to the task performed. The speed regulation can be compared to driving a car through a city in 6th gear, and regulating the speed by switching off the motor.

High-speed contra-angles are superior to the turbines. When under load, it runs faster and the torque is much higher. The speed can also be regulated according to task, tooth substance, tactility, skill of the dentist, access to tooth, visual access, etc. The precision and the tactile feedback are much better.

A recommendation: do as tens of thousands of dentists have done. Quit the turbine and replace it with a second micromotor fitted with a 1:5 multiplication contra-angle.

Fixed clock position of the dentist

A dentist working in a fixed 9 o'clock position will not be able to look at some surfaces and into some cavities without severely twisting the body, neck and head.

Reasons for a fixed 9 o'clock position

The cabinetry may be placed so close to the chair that the dentist cannot sit in an 11–12 o'clock position. A dentist working in a fixed 11–12 o'clock position will not be able to look at some surfaces and into some cavities without severely twisting the body, neck and head.

Reasons for a fixed 11 to 12 o'clock position:

The dental unit is placed on the right side of the patient. If the patient chair base is so big that the foot controller cannot be placed under the chair, but has to be placed at the right side of the patient chair base, it makes it impossible to work in a 9 o'clock position.

Equipment obstructions for fine work postures and for assistance

The patient chair cannot be positioned horizontally and does not move sufficiently upwards (horizontal back positioned 80 cm above floor, and for dentists taller than 175 to 180 cm, placed 90 cm above the floor).

A centrally placed unit must be able to be positioned above the horizontal patient, with the unit instruments about 30 cm above the horizontal patient chair. Many units are constructed so they cannot be placed over a horizontal lying patient, even with balanced unit instruments. The balanced arm of the unit is too short and placed too low.

The base of the patient chair (with the chair positioned horizontally) is too large, leaving no place for the foot controller under the chair. If the foot controller is placed to the right side of the chair base, then working in a 9 to 10 o'clock position is very bad for the dentist.

Unit instruments at right side of patient

Lost concentration on the working area

Maintaining concentration on the working area in the patient's mouth is not possible if the dental unit is placed on the patient's right side. The dentist is repeatedly interrupted by having to look away from the patient's mouth to pick up and replace unit instruments every time when turning away from the patient.

This also changes the direction of vision, causing the convergence of eyes and accommodation to another distance, and the most tiring, adaptation to a different intensity of light.

If the dentist also takes the hand instruments himself, the number of interruptions and changes of vision fields may exceed several hundred to many hundred per hour. It is easy to imagine how tiring this is.

Poor unit instrument grip for the dentist in 9 to 10 o'clock position

To place a dental unit on the right side is like placing the gear lever of a car in the back seat. Uninterrupted concentration on the working field is just not possible.

Having the unit instruments placed on the right side of the patient hinders assistance. The assistant cannot prepare the unit instruments or pass them to the dentist's hand, so that she/he can maintain undisturbed concentration.

Disadvantages of unit instruments at the patient's right side

The dentist has to prepare and take the unit instruments by himself. The patient experiences the dentist's head filling out most of the visual field, repeatedly looking away and losing concentration in order to pick up and replace unit instruments.

As unit instruments are unbalanced, the dentist has to carry the weight of the unit instrument and hose in hand. This is interacting with the precise movements of the dentist's hand.

The seated patient sees the unit instruments right in front while waiting to be reclined.

Solutions to these obstructions

Centrally placed and balanced unit instruments over the horizontal patient enable the dentist to take the unit instruments in all positions, and the assistant can reach them, prepare them and transfer them to the dentist's hand.

Suction holder

The suction holder is placed behind the assistant. The assistant cannot pick up the suction or 3-in-1 syringe without twisting or turning herself. If the 3-in-1 syringe is also placed by the suction holder, it is inconvenient for the assistant.

One solution is that the assistant uses the 3-in-1 syringe beside the unit instrument, which also is used by the dentist. The syringe is placed at the assistant's side of the unit instruments. The suction holder is fixed in a position with the tip of the large suction tube about, 12 cm from the tip of the 3-in-1 syringe. This implies a "parking position" for the unit at the assistant's side.

Another solution is that the suction holder is separated from the unit instrument, but is adjusted so the large suction tube is placed exactly as described above. This positioning of the 3-in-1 syringe and large suction tube enables an important assistant's technique: simultaneous pick up of the large suction tube with the right hand and 3-in-1 syringe with the left hand. This is used for rinsing the patient's mouth, and for drying the dentist's mirror.

Unit instruments

If too many unit instruments are placed in a central position, they can be difficult to access. Four unit instruments are enough, considering that the assistant prepares unit instruments with contra-angles, burs and diamonds, so the dentist does not need to do so.

- A 3-in-1 syringe at the assistant's side of the unit instruments is easy to use by both assistant and dentist.
- Two micromotors, one for general use with blue contra-angles and one with a red high-speed contra-angle replacing the turbine, are also used with an ultrasonic scaler.
- An airscaler may also be mounted as a fifth instrument, used for patients with sensitive root surfaces.

Other instruments such as polymerization lamps, intraoral camera, endo motor, etc, are used with cordless rechargeable battery power. New versions of these instruments are very effective, and repair or replacement is easier and cheaper.

Hand instrument table

The hand instrument table is placed so that the assistant cannot prepare, take and transfer hand instruments to the dentist.

A solution for this could be that the hand instrument tray is placed between the assistant and dentist at the upper left side of the patient's head. Here the assistant can pick up unit instruments by the left hand and transfer them to the dentist's hand close to the patient's mouth.

The dentist can also pick up a hand instrument with the left–right hand method. Each method can be learned and trained in about 20 minutes. Meanwhile, the hand instrument table is mounted at, and is a part of, the workstation – not of the dental unit.

Cabinetry

A high-level workstation is as important as a dental unit, suction system and patient chair. Insufficient kitchen-like cabinetry is a problem.

Most of the cabinetry the author has seen in dental practices and at exhibitions do not support assistance, and rather obstruct certain aspects of it. They look like kitchen cabinets with some special inserts in the drawers, with no hand instrument tray and insufficient or lacking work surface for the seated assistant. Also, there is often no storage area within reach of the patient. "The most important drawer" is also missing.

This is in contrast to a workstation that is a deeply integrated part of the working methods and organization of materials and instruments.

The working methods presented in Dancing Hands is the central part of the manual competence of dentist and assistant. Therefore it is suggested that every dentist and assistant learns to use them.

A FINAL WORD...

Very many dentists are unaware of the knowledge, methods and skills presented in this book.

Dancing Hands presents knowledge and skills to all practicing dentists, to all hygienists and assistants, and to clinical teachers and students in universities. Work postures depend on the visibility in the working field, combined with retraction, the possible use of mirror, manual flexibility and support, instrument grip, dentist and patient position, assistance and of the dental equipment. It is necessary to integrate all these elements, knowledge, and well-trained skills.

Working methods that save time and energy will depend on an undisturbed concentration on a task, which to a high degree will depend on assistance, and dental equipment that supports good assistance. A highly developed workstation integrated into the organization of materials and instruments will reduce the time the assistant uses for treatment preparation, and enable her to focus on providing treatment assistance.

Training skills is essential and can be done in a few hours! A perfect organization of materials and instruments saves much time and energy for both assistant and dentist.

If working DUO/SOLO, sometimes with and sometimes without assistance, the workstation and organization of instruments and materials take even higher priority for the time spent working SOLO.

The mental processes for sensomotoric precision work can for many dentists be simplified for relaxed and timesaving precision work. Selection of the best tools – like a high-speed, red contra-angle – is very important. When training the skills for movement, simplification is essential.

The author finds working as a dentist a highly privileged and relaxing career. For a large part of your working hours you can sit and be relaxed with your patients in good working postures, and enjoy your hands performing precise and fast movements during the manual parts of dentistry. If working with an assistant – you are also enjoying the pleasure of perfect coordinated teamwork.

With kind regards,
And good luck to you.
Herluf Skovsgaard

INDEX

T